眼科学聚焦

Ophthalmology

INfocus

注意

医学是一个不断进步的领域。由于新的研究与临床经验不断扩展着我们的知识，我们在遵守标准的安全预防措施的同时，也有必要在治疗和用药方面做出适当的变动。建议读者对每一用药都要学其生产厂家所提供的最新产品信息，以确定药物的推荐剂量、服用方法、持续时间及相关禁忌证。根据自己的经验和患者的病情，决定每一位病人的服药剂量和最佳治疗方法，是经治医师的责任。不论是出版商还是著者，对于由于本出版物引起的任何个人或财产的损伤或损失，均不承担任何责任。

出版者

眼科学聚焦

Ophthalmology

IN *focus*

原　著　Jack J Kanski
　　　　Brad Bowling

译　者　崔　浩　张丽琼

北京大学医学出版社
Peking University Medical Press

Ophthalmology, 1st edition
Jack J Kanski , Brad Bowling
ISBN-13: 978-0-443-10030-7
ISBN-10: 0-443-10030-6

978-981-259-563-8
981-259-563-5

Elsevier (Singapore) Pte Ltd.
3 Killiney Road, #08-01 Winsland House I, Singapore 239519
Tel: (65) 6349-0200, Fax: (65) 6733-1817
First Published 2006
2006 年初版

北京市版权局著作权合同登记号：图字：01-2006-1818

YANKEXUE JUJIAO

图书在版编目（CIP）数据

眼科学聚焦 /（英）坎斯基（Kanski, J.J.），（英）
鲍林（Bowling, B.）著；崔浩，张丽琼译. —北京：北
京大学医学出版社，2006.9
书名原文：Ophthalmology in focus
ISBN 7-81071-987-4

I.眼… II.①坎… ②鲍… ③崔… ④张…
III.眼科学 IV. R77

中国版本图书馆 CIP 数据核字（2006）第 107574 号

眼科学聚焦

译　　者：崔浩　张丽琼
出版发行：北京大学医学出版社 (电话：010-82802230)
地　　址：(100083) 北京市海淀区学院路 38 号　北京大学医学部院内
网　　址：http://www.pumpress.com.cn
E-mail：booksale@bjmu.edu.cn
印　　刷：莱芜市圣龙印务有限责任公司
经　　销：新华书店
责任编辑：赵　曼　　责任校对：程　明　　责任印制：郭桂兰
开　　本：880mm × 1100mm　1/32　印张：8.5　字数：272 千字
版　　次：2006 年 12 月第 1 版　2006 年 12 月第 1 次印刷
书　　号：ISBN 7-81071-987-4 /R・987
定　　价：59.90 元

译者前言

《眼科学聚焦》是一本论述眼科学基本理论、基本概念和基本知识的专著。其主要特点是：

1. 图文并茂。彩图丰富、精美而翔实。令读者一目了然，印象深刻。

2. 重点突出。抓住了眼科学的基本内容、主要内容和重点内容。

3. 文字叙述少而精。删繁就简，阐述简洁明了。

这是一本既适合自学，也适合教学；既适合专业教育，也适合科普教育的应用范围广泛，多方咸宜的好书。

在本书的翻译过程中，得到了北京大学医学出版社的大力支持和指导，在此一并致谢。

由于译者水平有限，错误之处难以避免，敬请专家、同仁、读者批评指正。

崔浩　张丽琼

2006 年 6 月

目录

Contents

睑缘炎

定义 眼睑缘常见的慢性炎症。

分类 分成前部和后部两型，前部型由葡萄球菌感染或皮脂溢出造成，而混合型较为典型。

病因学 诱发因素

- *葡萄球菌感染*：患者睫毛根部慢性感染——患者普遍伴有湿疹
- *皮脂溢出*：通常伴随脂溢性皮炎——包含眼睑腺产生过量脂质被细菌分解为有刺激性的脂肪酸
- *后部的*：后部睑缘的睑板腺功能障碍——患者通常伴有酒渣鼻

临床特征 *症状*：通常晨起严重，包括眼睑异物感、烧灼感、充血和眼睑粘着和结痂。

体征：

- *葡萄球菌感染*：睫毛根部的鳞屑（图 1）
- *脂溢性*：脂质碎屑附着在睫毛周围，导致它们前部粘连（图 2）
- *后部的*：泡沫状泪膜（图3）和睑板腺口的堵塞（图4）

所有类型常见症状为睑缘充血（图 5），结膜充血和泪膜不稳定。

并发症 角膜上皮病变，角膜瘢痕和边缘性角膜炎（见图102）；复发性细菌性结膜炎，睑板腺囊肿（见图7）和睑腺炎（见图10）。睫毛脱落和乱睫（倒睫，图6）。

治疗

- 睑缘卫生：用婴儿洗发剂的稀溶液清洗。
- 泪液替代品（丙甲纤维素，卡波姆等）。
- 抗生素油膏（夫西地酸钠、氯霉素等）涂抹睑缘。
- 全身应用抗生素。

1 Blepharitis

Definition

Very common chronic inflammation of the eyelid margins.

Classification

Divided into anterior and posterior forms: the former may be staphylococcal or seborrhoeic; a mixed picture is typical, however.

Aetiology

Causative factors:

- *Staphylococcal*: chronic infection of the bases of the lashes - common in patients with eczema
- *Seborrhoeic*: usually associated with seborrhoeic dermatitis - involves excess lipid production by eyelid glands, converted to fatty acids by bacteria
- *Posterior*: dysfunction of the meibomian glands of the posterior lid margins - common in patients with acne rosacea.

Clinical features

Symptoms: usually worse in the morning, include grittiness, burning and redness, stickiness and crusting of the lids.

Signs

- *Staphylococcal*: dandruff-like scaling, mainly around the eyelash bases (Fig. 1)
- *Seborrhoeic*: greasy debris around the lashes causing them to adhere to one another (Fig. 2)
- *Posterior*: frothy tear film (Fig. 3) and plugging of the meibomian gland orifices (Fig. 4)

All types usually manifest hyperaemia of the lid margins (Fig. 5) and conjunctiva, and tear film instability.

Complications

Corneal epitheliopathy, scarring, and marginal keratitis (see Fig. 102); recurrent bacterial conjunctivitis, chalazia (see Fig. 7) and styes (see Fig.10). Loss of lashes (madarosis) and misdirection (trichiasis; Fig. 6).

Management

- Lid margin hygiene using a weak solution of baby shampoo
- Tear substitutes (e.g. hypromellose, carbomers)
- Antibiotic ointment (e.g. fusidic acid, chloramphenicol) rubbed into the lid margins
- Systemic tetracycline.

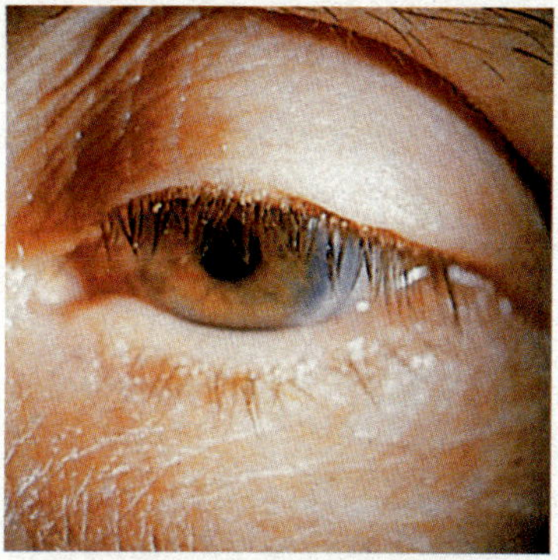

图 1 葡萄球菌性前部睑缘炎，皮屑在眼睑基部周围
Scales around eyelash bases in staphylococcal anterior blepharitis

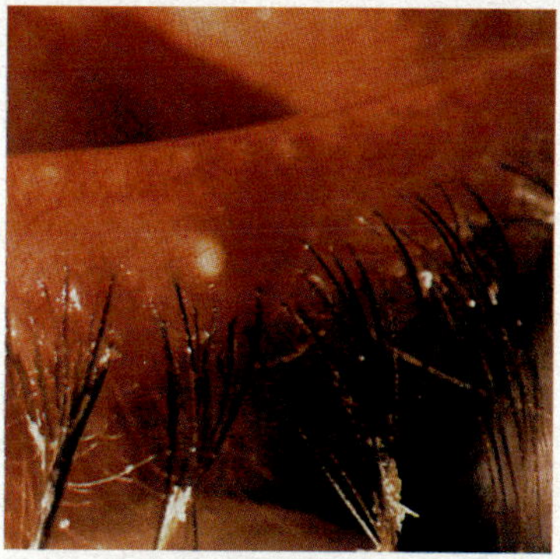

图 2 皮脂溢出性后部睑缘炎，睫毛上的油腻附着物
Greasy adherent lashes, in seborrhoeic posterior blepharitis

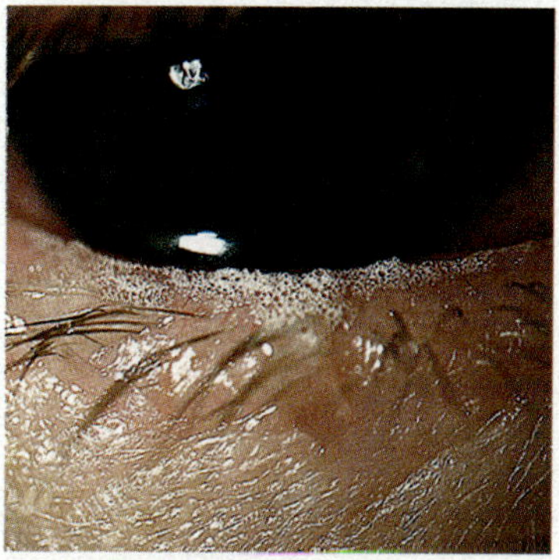

图 3 泡沫状泪膜
Foam in the tear film

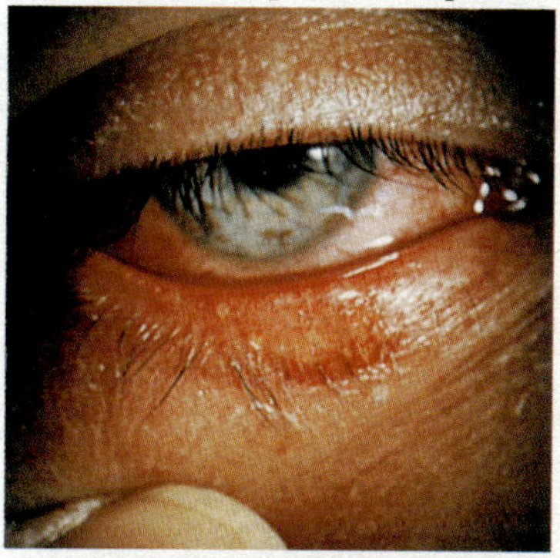

图 4 后部睑缘炎腺体出口阻塞
Blocked meibomian gland orifices in posterior blepharitis

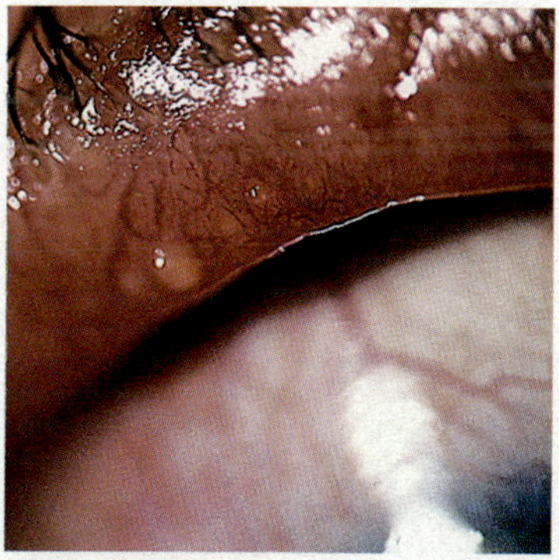

图 5 睑缘充血
Hyperaemia of lid margin

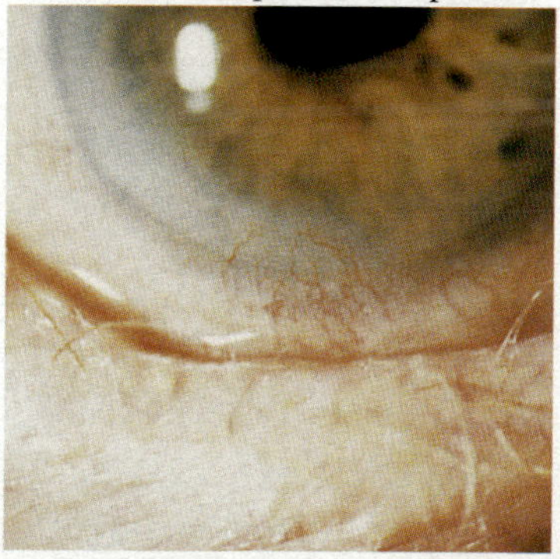

图 6 长期前部睑缘炎导致睫毛乱生
Eyelash misdirection in long-standing anterior blepharitis

2 非新生肿物性眼睑结节（睑腺病）

睑板腺囊肿（霰粒肿）

定义 睑板腺异常，以肉芽肿性炎症为主。

临床特征 患者多半有后部睑缘炎，病程进行缓慢，通常为睑板内的单个、无痛性隆起（图 7），可以继发于睑板腺的急性感染（见下），可继发结膜肉芽肿（图 8）。

治疗 小的囊肿可自行消退，大的囊肿则需行手术切开和刮除术。

内睑腺炎（急性霰粒肿）

定义 睑板腺的急性细菌感染。

临床特征 睑板内的炎性肿块，它可伴发眶隔前部蜂窝织炎（图9）。

治疗 局部涂抹抗生素软膏和全身应用抗生素（青霉素等）治疗眶隔前部蜂窝织炎。热敷能促进内容物排出。对于大的脓肿和继发的慢性病变需手术切开和刮涂术。

外睑腺炎（麦粒肿）

定义 睑缘的小脓肿。

临床特征 位于睑缘前部的急性、疼痛的炎性肿块，通常脓头可穿破皮肤（图 10）。

治疗 切开排脓和热敷。局部应用抗生素软膏。大的病灶需切开排脓。

Zeis 腺和 Moll 腺囊肿

临床特征 Zeis腺囊肿是小的、白色的、慢性的、无痛的、不透明的位于睑缘的结节（图11）。Moll腺囊肿相似，但是半透明的。

治疗 切除。

传染性软疣

临床特征 单个或多个、小的、苍白的、蜡样的脐形小疣（图12），它们能引起继发性、慢性同侧结膜滤泡病（见图 55），在 AIDS 患者，病毒导致的损伤普遍且更严重。

治疗 挤出法和烧灼法。

Non-neoplastic eyelid nodules

Meibomian cyst (chalazion)

Definition A lesion consisting of lipogranulomatous inflammation centred on a dysfunctional meibomian gland.

Clinical features Extremely common, particularly in patients with posterior blepharitis. A chronic, usually solitary, painless, firm swelling in the tarsal plate (Fig. 7); can follow an acute meibomian gland infection (see below). May be associated with a secondary conjunctival granuloma (Fig. 8).

Management Spontaneous resolution may occur, although usually only if the lesion is small. Surgical incision and curettage is often required.

Internal hordeolum (acute chalazion)

Definition An acute bacterial meibomian gland infection.

Clinical features An inflamed swelling within the tarsal plate which may be associated with (mild) preseptal cellulitis (Fig. 9).

Management Topical antibiotic ointment and systemic antibiotics (e.g. flucloxacillin) for preseptal cellulitis. Hot bathing may promote discharge. Incision and curettage may be required for a large abscess, or for a secondary chronic lesion.

External hordeolum (stye)

Definition A small abscess of an eyelash follicle.

Clinical features An acute, painful inflamed swelling on the anterior lid margin, usually pointing through the skin (Fig. 10).

Management Removal of the associated lash, and hot bathing. Topical antibiotic ointment. Large lesions may require incision.

Cysts of Zeis and Moll

Clinical features A cyst of Zeis is a small, whitish, chronic, painless, opaque nodule on the lid margin (Fig. 11). A cyst of Moll is similar but translucent.

Management Simple excision.

Molluscum contagiosum

Clinical features Single or multiple, small, pale, waxy umbilicated nodules (Fig. 12), which may cause a secondary chronic ipsilateral follicular conjunctivitis (see Fig. 55). These virally transmitted lesions are common and more severe, in AIDS patients.

Management Expression or cautery.

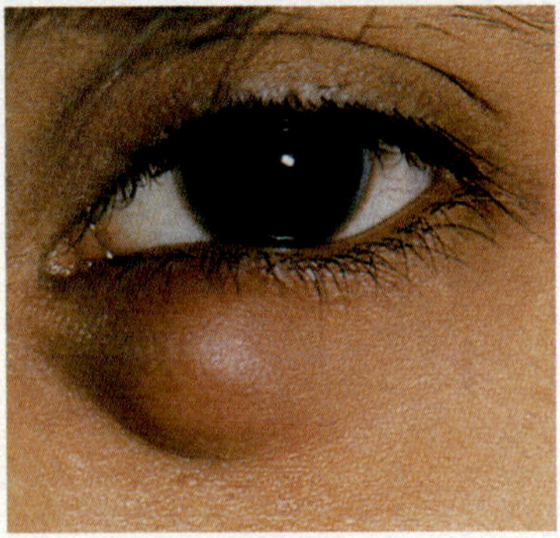

图 7　大睑板腺囊肿
Large meibomian cyst

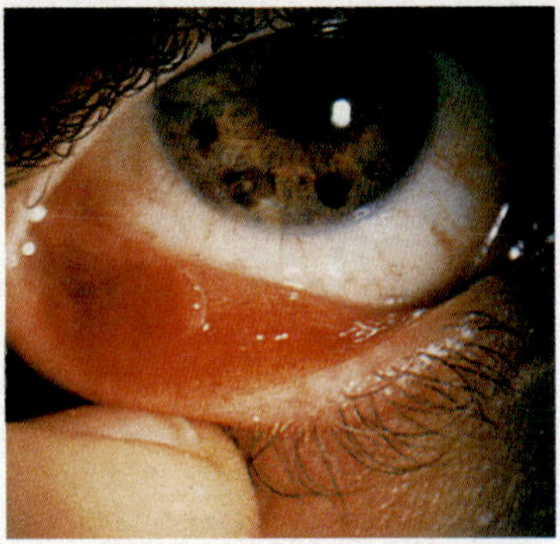

图 8　继发结膜肉芽肿性睑板腺囊肿
Conjunctival granuloma secondary to meibomian cyst

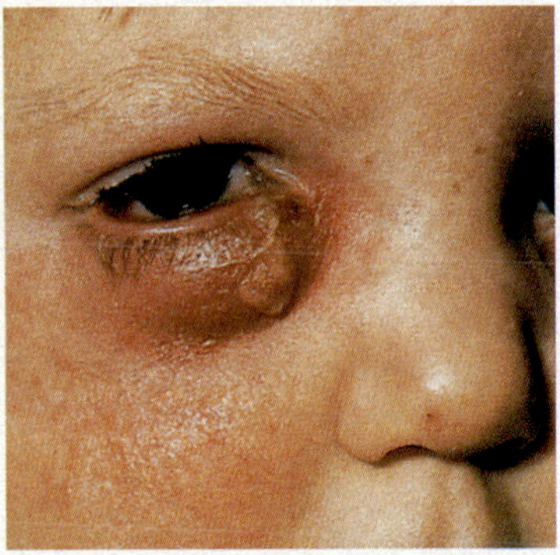

图 9　内睑腺伴发眶隔前部蜂窝织炎
Internal hordeolum with preseptal cellulitis

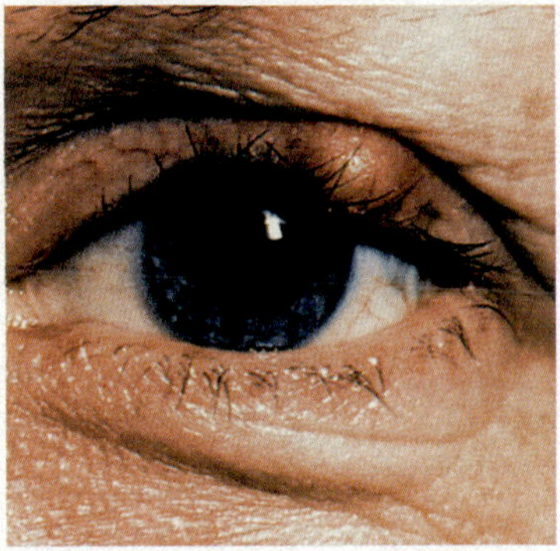

图 10　外睑腺炎
External hordeolum (stye)

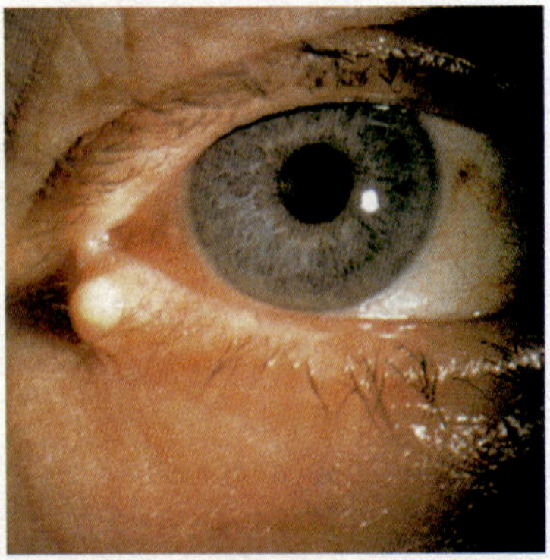

图 11　Zeis 腺囊肿
Cyst of Zeis

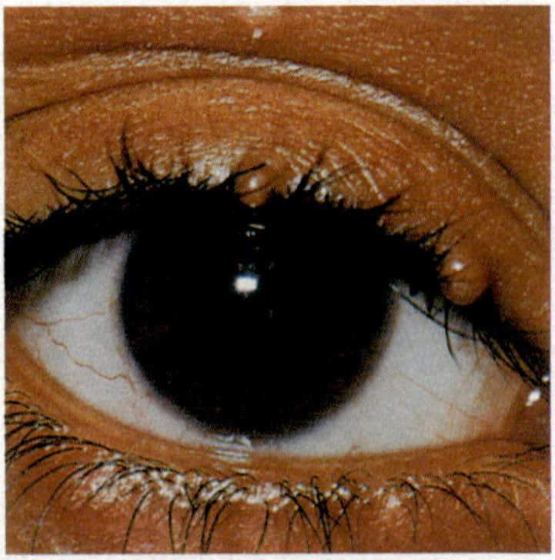

图 12　传染性软疣的损害
Lesions of molluscum contagiosum

鳞状细胞乳头状瘤（病毒瘤）

临床特征 为眼睑最常见的良性肿瘤，分宽基底的(无蒂的)或有蒂的（图 13）。

治疗 切除、烧灼或激光光凝术。

基底细胞乳头状瘤（皮脂溢出性角化病）

临床特征 为老年人常见的肿瘤，是缓慢扩大的褐色的呈脂样的病变，表面脆（图 14）。

治疗 切除或刮除术。

角化棘皮瘤

临床特征 是少见的、生长迅速的硬性粉红色结节。中央下凹充满角化物质（图15），可能被误认为恶性肿瘤。在病变消退前几个月，病变是处于静止的。

黑色素痣

皮内痣 隆起病变，有的色素多，有的色素少。当位于睑缘时可突出于睫毛（图 16），无恶变趋势。

交界痣 一般是平的，境界清楚，呈一致褐色。之所以称交界痣是因为痣细胞位于表皮和真皮交界处，有低度恶变趋势。

复合痣 一般是隆起的，呈均匀的黄褐色或褐色。由皮内痣和交界痣成分结合在一起，有低度恶变趋势。

毛细血管瘤（草莓痣）

临床特征 婴儿出现的不规则红色病变，可导致机械性上睑下垂和弱视（图 17）。

治疗 如需要可局部注射类固醇，但许多逐渐自发消退。

丛状神经纤维瘤

典型存在的多发性神经纤维瘤，睑缘形成特有的“S”型或上睑下垂（图 18）。

3 Benign tumours of the eyelids

Squamous cell papilloma (viral wart)

Clinical features The most common benign tumour of the eyelid which may be broad-based (sessile) or pedunculated (Fig. 13).

Management Simple excision, cautery or laser ablation.

Basal cell papilloma (seborrhoeic keratosis)

Clinical features This common tumour, usually found in the elderly, is a slowly-enlarging brownish papillary lesion with a greasy, friable surface (Fig. 14).

Management Simple excision or curettage.

Keratoacanthoma

Clinical features An uncommon, fast-growing, firm, pinkish nodule that develops a keratin-filled crater (Fig. 15) and may be mistaken for a malignancy. Remains static for several months before involution.

Melanocytic naevus

Intradermal naevus An elevated lesion with variable pigmentation. When located on the lid margin may be associated with protruding lashes (Fig. 16). No malignant potential.

Junctional naevus A flat, well circumscribed lesion with a uniform brown colour, so-called because the naevus cells are located at the junction of the dermis and epidermis. Low malignant potential.

Compound naevus Usually elevated, with a homogeneous tan to brown colour. Consists of both intradermal and junctional components, the latter conferring a low malignant potential.

Capillary haemangioma (strawberry naevus)

Clinical features An irregular red lesion in an infant which may cause a mechanical ptosis and amblyopia (Fig. 17).

Management Local steroids if necessary, but frequently undergoes gradual spontaneous involution.

Plexiform neurofibroma

Typically occurs in neurofibromatosis-1, characteristically giving rise to an S-shaped lid margin and ptosis (Fig. 18).

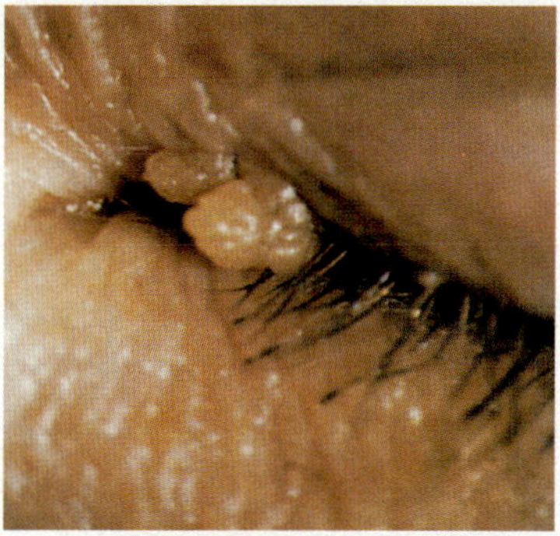

图 13 鳞状细胞乳头状瘤（病毒瘤）
Squamous cell papilloma (viral wart)

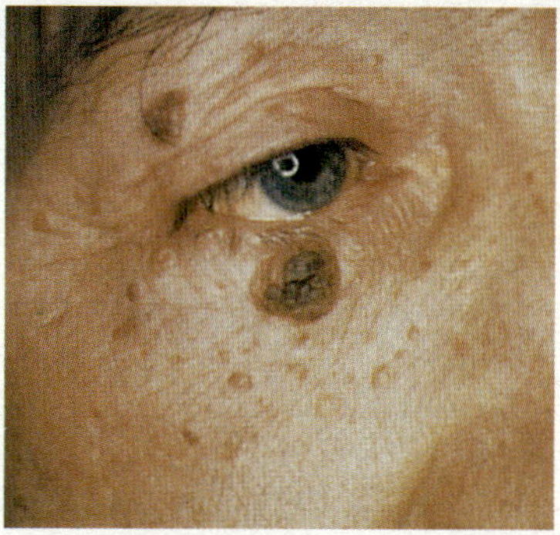

图 14 基底细胞乳头状瘤（脂溢性角化病）
Basal cell papilloma (seborrhoeic keratosis)

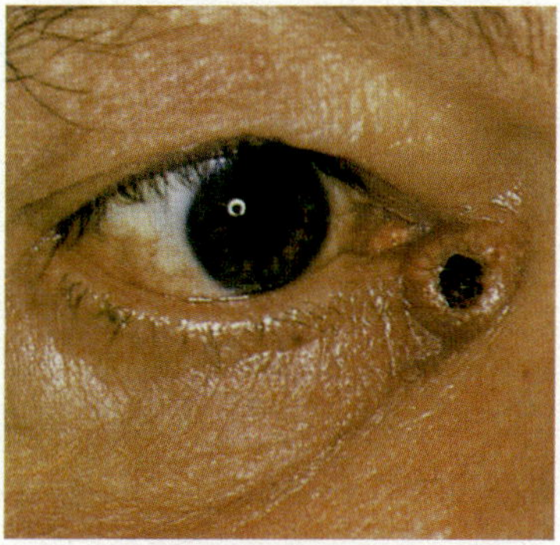

图 15 角化棘皮瘤
Keratoacanthoma

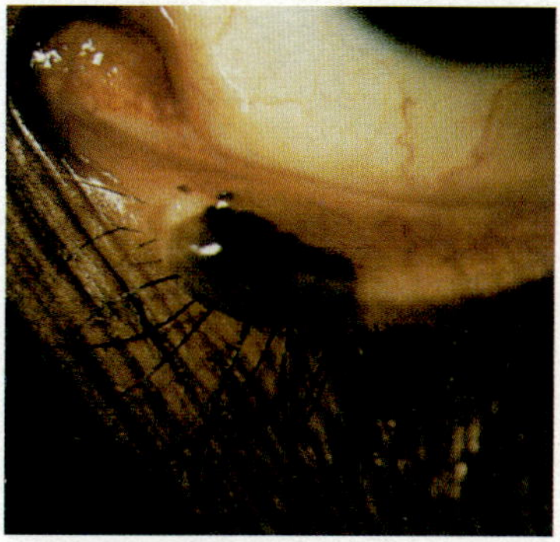

图 16 皮内痣
Intradermal naevus

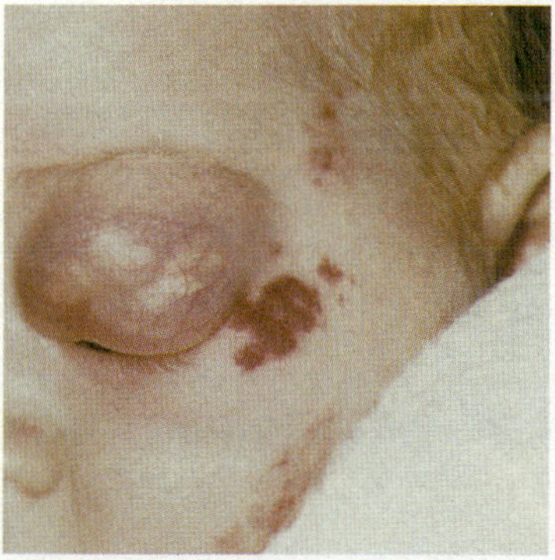

图 17 毛细血管瘤（草莓痣）
Capillary haemangioma (strawberry naevus)

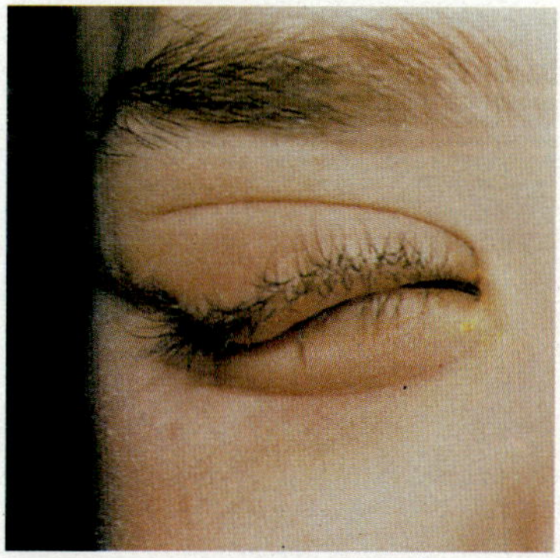

图 18 丛状神经纤维瘤
Plexiform neurofibroma

光化性（日光性）角化病

临床特征 虽然本病罕见，但为浅肤色人眼睑最常见的癌前病变，它是由于过度的日光照射造成的，呈现永久性的鳞状性皮肤改变（图 19），需做病理检查。

基底细胞癌

临床特征 基底细胞癌（BCC）为眼睑最常见恶性肿瘤，局部侵袭，罕有转移。大约 50% 好发于下眼睑，30% 发于内眦。

结节溃疡型 表现为侵蚀性溃疡，常有金箔样过度角化边缘和中心溃疡（图 20），溃疡逐渐扩大超过 1 ~ 2 年。单纯结节型的外观并无特异性（图 21）。

硬化型 表现为浅色硬结，边缘不清，表面的睫毛脱落（图 22），表现像慢性睑缘炎。

鳞状细胞癌

临床特征 鳞状细胞癌（SCC）比基底细胞癌少见，它生长迅速并可转移，可以自发，亦可起自癌前病变，如光化性角化病（看上面）。

结节型 SCC 起自过度角化的结节或斑，以后形成硬皮。

溃疡型 SCC 类似侵蚀性溃疡（图 23）。

皮脂腺癌

临床特征 罕见，侵袭性很强的肿瘤，常起源于睑板腺或Zeis腺，为睑缘上或睑板内的坚韧结节（图24），常被误诊为霰粒肿（见图 7）。

治疗
- 手术切除，大范围切除是治疗眼睑恶性肿瘤的首选。
- 放射治疗。

Premalignant and malignant tumours of the eyelids

Actinic (solar) keratosis

Clinical features

Although rare, this is the most common premalignant lid condition and is strongly associated with excessive sun exposure in light-skinned individuals. It usually presents as a persistent scaly plaque (Fig. 19), which must be biopsied.

Basal cell carcinoma

Clinical features

Basal cell carcinoma (BCC), the most common eyelid malignancy, is locally invasive but does not metastasize. About 50% involve the lower lid, 30% the medial canthal area.

Nodulo-ulcerative A 'rodent ulcer', with rolled hyperkeratotic edges and central granulation (Fig. 20), gradually enlarging over 1-2 years. A purely nodular appearance is common (Fig. 21).

Sclerosing A flat indurated plaque with poorly demarcated margins, often with loss of overlying lashes (Fig. 22) that may simulate chronic blepharitis.

Squamous cell carcinoma

Clinical features

Squamous cell carcinoma (SCC) is much less common than BCC. It grows more quickly and may metastasize. It may arise de novo or from a premalignant condition such as actinic keratosis (see above).

Nodular SCC Starts as a hyperkeratotic nodule or plaque which later develops crusting fissures.

Ulcerative SCC Resembles a rodent ulcer (Fig. 23).

Sebaceous gland carcinoma

Clinical features

This is a rare but very aggressive tumour, which may originate in a meibomian or Zeis gland as a firm nodule either on the lid margin or within the tarsal plate (Fig. 24), when it may be mistaken for a chalazion (see Fig. 7).

Management

- Surgical excision with a wide clearance margin is the treatment of choice for most lid malignancies
- Radiotherapy in selected cases.

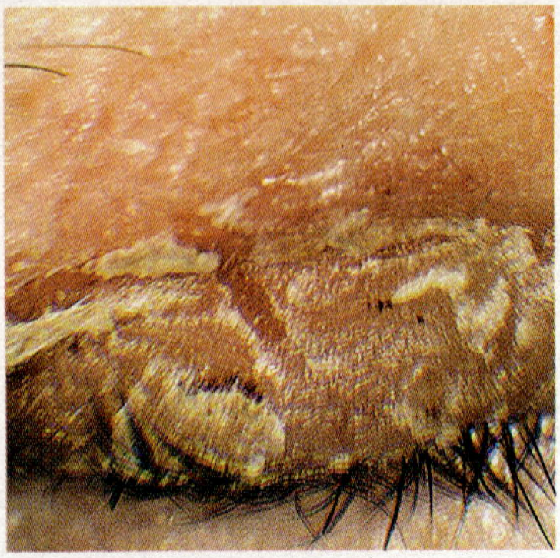
图 19　光化性角化病
Actinic keratosis

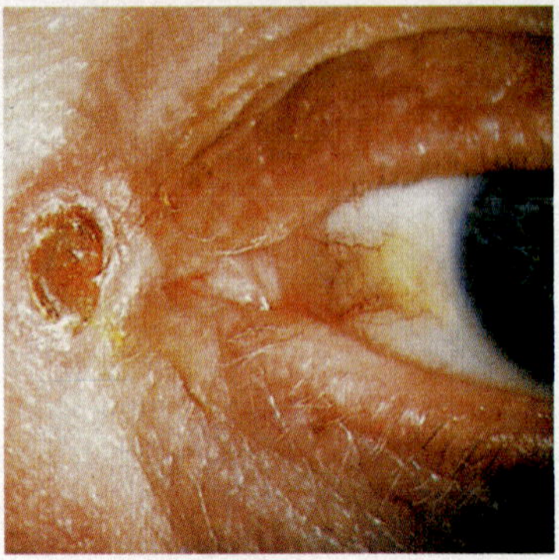
图 20　侵蚀性溃疡
Rodent ulcer

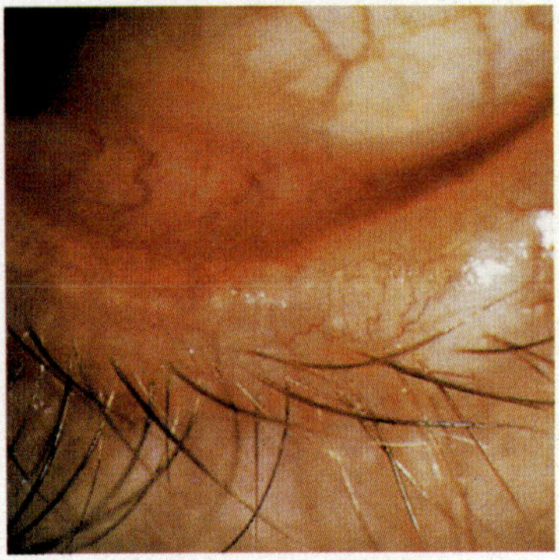
图 21　结节型基底细胞癌
Nodular basal cell carcinoma

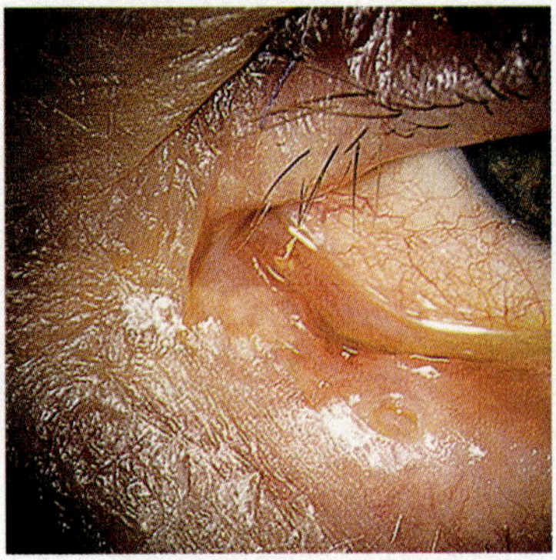
图 22　硬化型基底细胞癌
Sclerosing basal cell carcinoma

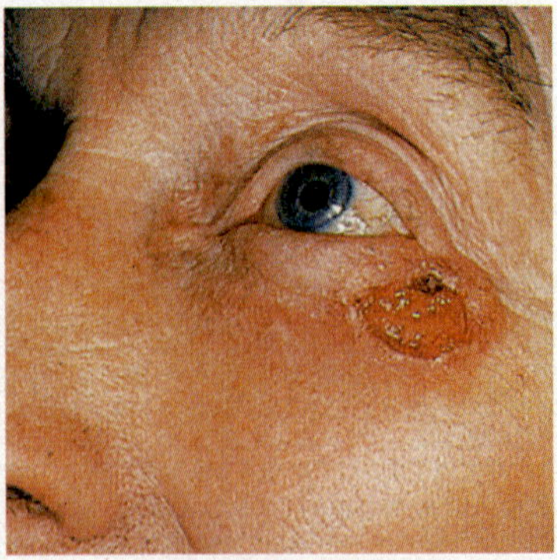
图 23　溃疡型鳞状细胞癌
Ulcerative squamous cell carcinoma

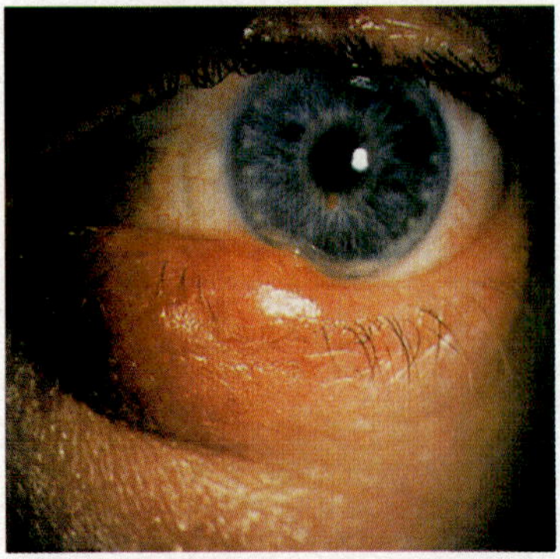
图 24　皮脂腺癌
Sebaceous gland carcinoma

上睑下垂 5

定义 上眼睑低于正常的位置。

分类

神经性

- *第三脑神经（眼球运动）麻痹*（图25）：必须排除“手术”原因（动脉瘤、肿瘤等）压迫神经。
- *Horner 综合征*（图 26）：交感神经传导途径的先天或后天异常。
- *Marcus Gunn（颌-瞬目）综合征*：先天性的，罕见。

腱膜性

- *退化性*：年龄相关性提上睑肌腱松弛（图 27）。
- *手术后*：手术使腱膜伸长。

机械性

- *眼睑重量过重*：水肿、肿瘤（见图17、18），多余皮肤。
- *瘢痕*：上眼睑皮肤或结膜的瘢痕使活动度减少。

肌源性

- *单纯先天性*：单侧或双侧（图 28）。
- *睑裂狭小综合征*：罕见，先天双侧上睑下垂，伴随眼睑和颜面异常（图 29）。
- *后天性*：重症肌无力，眼肌病，强直性肌营养不良（图 30）。

特征

- *第三脑神经麻痹*：瞳孔受累高度怀疑是“手术”病因，再生神经纤维发生“迷路”，导致眼球运动时出现上睑下垂或眼睑退缩。
- *Horner 综合征*：患侧瞳孔缩小，先天性伴异色症，患侧半面无汗。

治疗

- 病因治疗（重症肌无力等）。
- 手术治疗包括提上睑肌或腱膜加固和额肌（额）悬吊。

5 Ptosis

Definition

The upper eyelid rests at a lower position than normal.

Classification

Neurogenic

- *Third (oculomotor) nerve palsy* (Fig. 25): must exclude 'surgical' cause (e.g. aneurysm, tumour) compressing nerve
- *Horner's syndrome* (Fig. 26): congenital or acquired dysfunction of the sympathetic autonomic pathway
- *Marcus Gunn ('jaw-winking') syndrome*: congenital, uncommon.

Aponeurotic

- *Involutional*: age-related laxity of the levator aponeurosis (Fig. 27)
- *Postoperative*: stretching of the aponeurosis during surgery.

Mechanical

- *Excessive lid weight*: oedema, tumours (see Figs 17, 18), redundant skin
- *Cicatricial*: reduced mobility from scarring of the upper lid skin or conjunctiva.

Myogenic

- *Simple congenital*: unilateral or bilateral (Fig. 28)
- *Blepharophimosis syndrome*: rare, congenital bilateral ptosis, associated with other eyelid and facial abnormalities (Fig. 29)
- *Acquired*: myasthenia gravis, ocular myopathy, myotonic dystrophy (Fig. 30).

Salient points

- *Third nerve palsy*: pupillary involvement carries high index of suspicion for 'surgical' aetiology. Misdirection of regenerating nerve fibres may occur, resulting in ptosis or lid retraction on eye movement
- *Horner's syndrome*: ipsilateral miosis, heterochromia if congenital, sweating decreased on affected side dependent on location of lesion.

Management

- Address any treatable cause (e.g. myasthenia gravis)
- Surgical options include levator or aponeurosis strengthening and frontalis (brow) suspension.

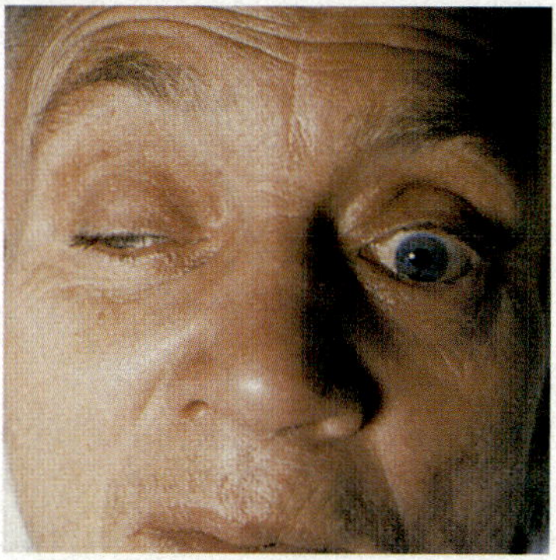

图 25 右侧第三脑神经麻痹
Right third nerve palsy

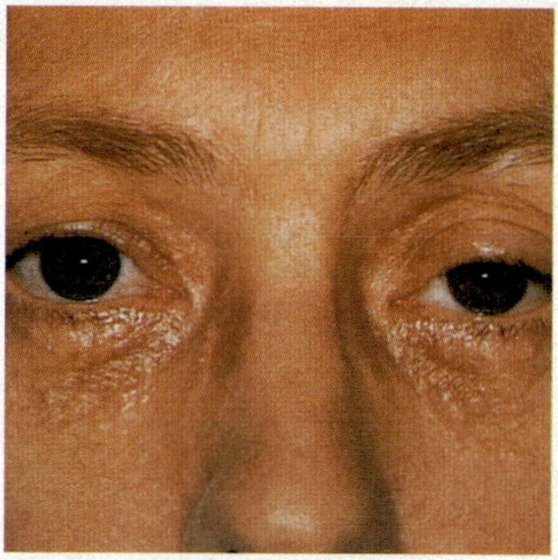

图 26 左侧 Horner 综合征
Left Horner's syndrome

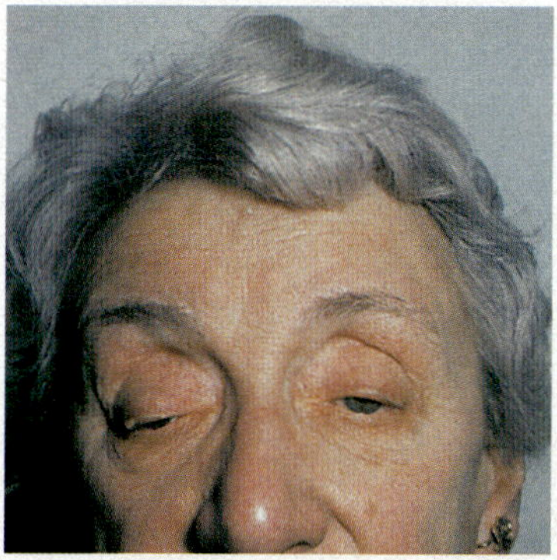

图 27 严重的双侧退化性上睑下垂
Severe bilateral involutional ptosis

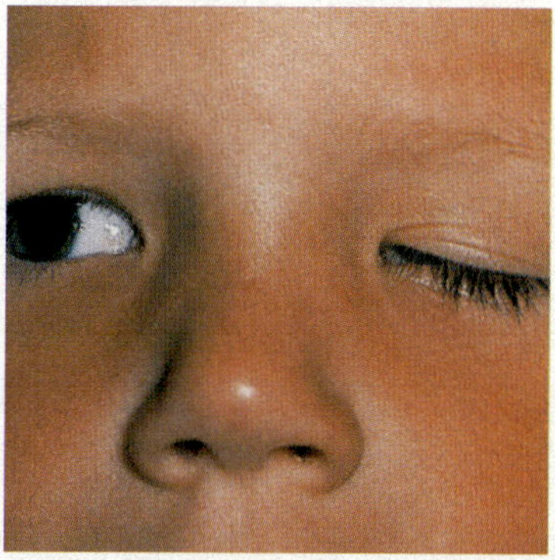

图 28 严重的左侧先天性上睑下垂
Severe left congenital ptosis

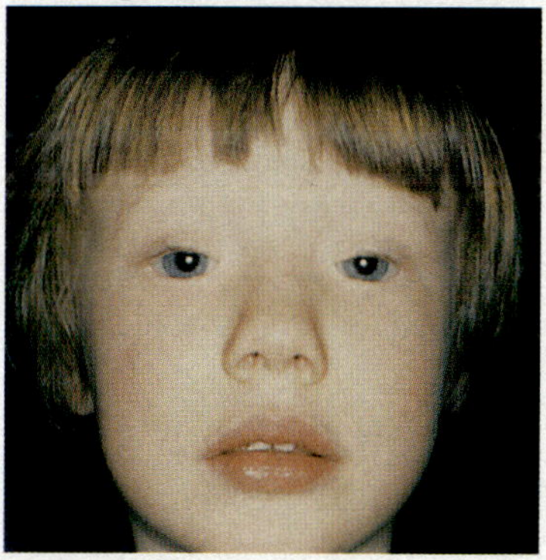

图 29 睑裂狭小综合征
Blepharophimosis syndrome

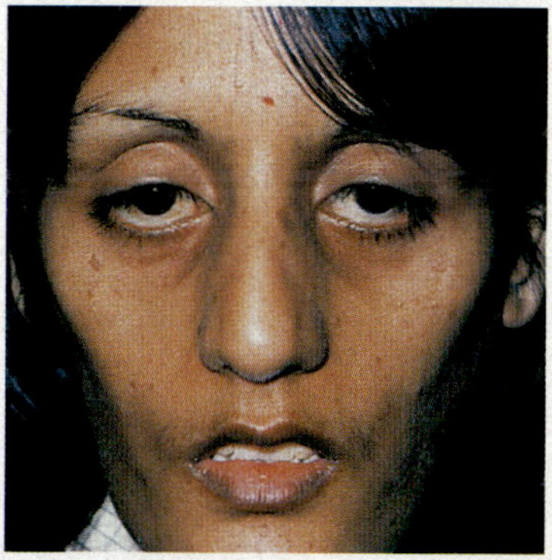

图 30 强直性肌营养不良性双侧上睑下垂
Bilateral ptosis in myotonic dystrophy

6 睑内翻、睑外翻和倒睫

睑内翻

定义 眼睑向内翻转，严重和长期时可形成角膜瘢痕（图31）。

分类

- *退化性*：最常见的原因，是下睑老年性退化的结果。
- *瘢痕性*：主要是上睑结膜的瘢痕所致，比如瘢痕期沙眼（图 32）。
- *痉挛性*：下眼睑痉挛性内翻，由于眼部受刺激或自发性睑痉挛导致眼轮匝肌痉挛而产生，这种痉挛性内翻是暂时的。
- *先天性*：罕见，只累及下眼睑。原因是皮肤和眼轮匝肌肥大。

治疗 手术矫正。

睑外翻

定义 眼睑向外翻转，只累及下眼睑，严重和长期的睑外翻会导致结膜角化（图 33）。

分类

- *退化性*：这是最常见类型，老年性组织松弛。
- *瘢痕性*：烧伤或手术（肿瘤切除等）导致瘢痕形成（图 34）。
- *机械性*：眼睑过重（大肿瘤等）。
- *麻痹性*：面神经麻痹，伴不完全瞬目和眼睑闭合（图 35）。
- *先天性*：睑裂狭小综合征的一部分（见图 29）。

治疗 手术矫正。

倒睫

定义 睫毛不正常向内生长，经常继发于急性或慢性眼睑炎（睑缘炎、沙眼等）。

主要造成角膜刺激，有时出现角膜瘢痕化（图36）。应与双行睫相鉴别，双行睫的额外睫毛（常是先天性）从睑板腺排泄口伸出。

治疗 包括：单纯拔除睫毛、电解法、冷冻疗法和激光光凝术。

Entropion, ectropion and trichiasis

6

Entropion

Definition

An inward-turning of the eyelid. If severe or prolonged may cause corneal scarring (Fig. 31).

Classification

- *Involutional*: most common form; results from age-related changes in the lower lid
- *Cicatricial*: most frequently secondary to scarring of the upper palpebral conjunctiva, as in chronic trachoma (Fig. 32)
- *Spastic*: lower lid; caused by spasm of the orbicularis muscle due to ocular irritation or essential blepharospasm. Frequently temporary
- *Congenital*: very rare; only involves the lower lid. Caused by hypertrophy of skin and orbicularis.

Management

Surgical correction.

Ectropion

Definition

An outward-turning eyelid, virtually exclusively involving the lower lid. If severe and prolonged may cause conjunctival keratinization (Fig. 33).

Classification

- *Involutional*: the most common form; age-related tissue laxity
- *Cicatricial*: scarring resulting from burns or surgery (e.g. tumour resection; Fig. 34)
- *Mechanical*: excess lid weight (e.g. large tumour)
- *Paralytic*: facial nerve palsy; associated with incomplete blinking and lid closure (Fig. 35)
- *Congenital*: may be part of the blepharophimosis syndrome (see Fig. 29).

Management

Surgical correction.

Trichiasis

Definition

Inward misdirection of lashes, often secondary to acute or chronic lid inflammation (e.g. blepharitis, trachoma). Typically causes corneal irritation and sometimes scarring (Fig. 36). Should be differentiated from distichiasis, in which extra lashes (usually congenital) arise from meibomian gland orifices.

Management

Options include simple epilation, electrolysis, cryotherapy and laser ablation.

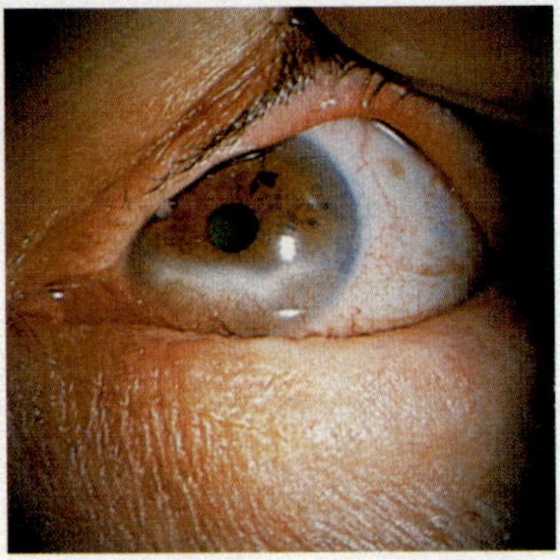

图 31　下睑内翻和角膜瘢痕形成
Entropion of lower eyelid and corneal scarring

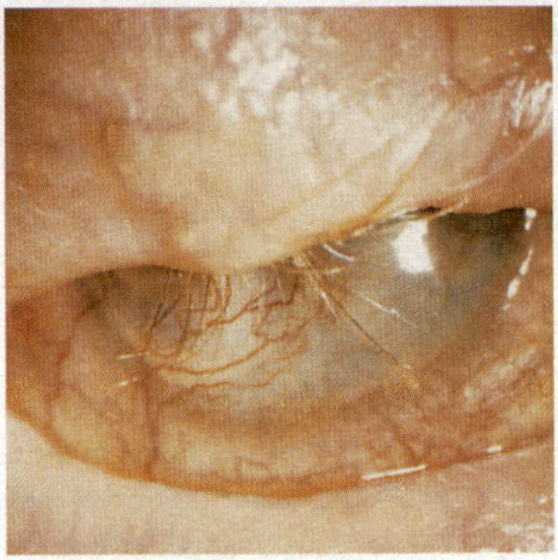

图 32　瘢痕性睑内翻
Cicatricial entropion

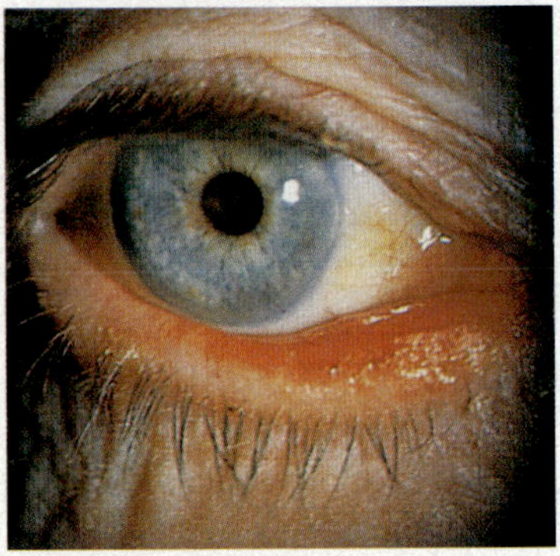

图 33　睑外翻和结膜角化
Ectropion and conjunctival keratinization

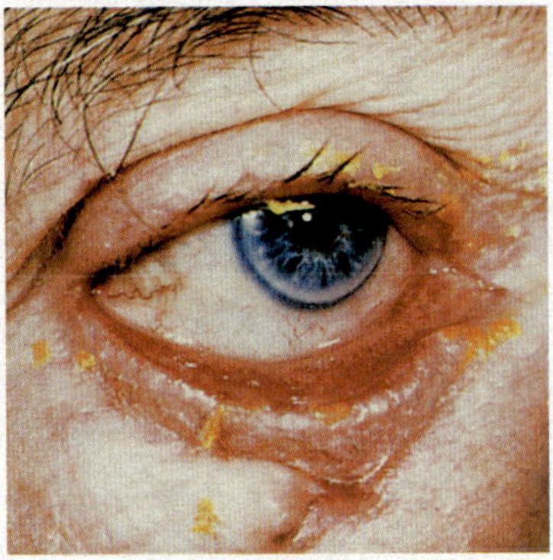

图 34　瘢痕性睑外翻
Cicatricial ectropion

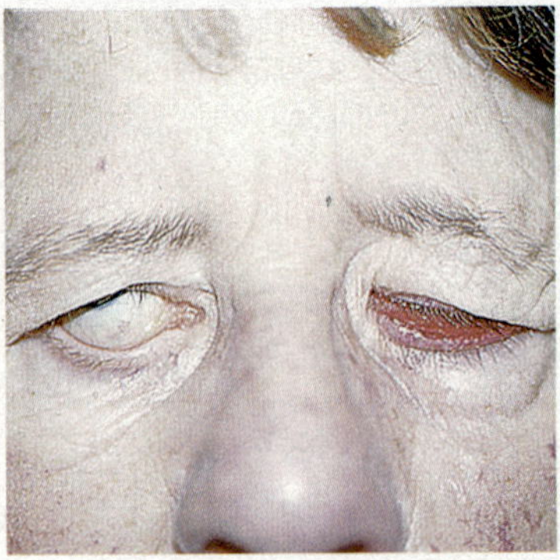

图 35　麻痹性睑外翻伴眼睑缺失
Paralytic ectropian with poor lid closure

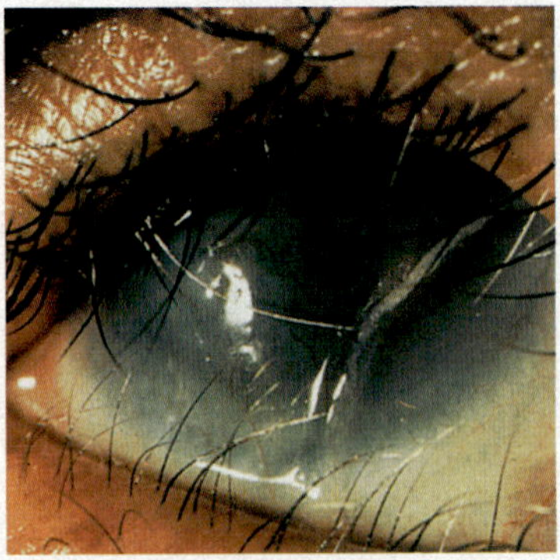

图 36　沙眼导致倒睫
Trichiasis in trachoma

甲状腺眼病

病因学

针对双侧甲状腺和眶组织的自身抗体引起的炎症，眼外肌受累。

临床特征

临床过程包含严重的充血期，通常持续2～3年，随后进入静止期，其后遗症是限制眼球运动为主要特征。

症状

- 充血
- 刺激
- 疼痛
- 眼球呈凝视外观
- 复视

体征

- 眼睑肿胀。
- 结膜充血和水肿（图 37）。
- 突眼：双侧或单侧（图38）。严重时会妨碍眼睑闭合，导致暴露性角膜炎。
- 初期眼睑退缩（图 39），引起眼球突出。
- 眼睑迟落（von Graefe's 征）。
- 早期的炎症和晚期的纤维化导致了眼球突出。下直肌和内直肌常受累。
- 脉络膜褶（图 40）。
- 眶组织肿胀，尤其是眼外肌的肿胀压迫视神经，使之缺血，导致的视神经病变造成视力下降。应做的检查包括色觉、视力和视野。可能有相对性传入性瞳孔阻滞和眼睑水肿。

治疗

- 结膜和角膜受累可滴人工泪液和局部应用类固醇。
- 视神经侵犯常全身应用类固醇。
- 手术治疗：眼球突出（眼眶减压术），复视（肌肉手术矫正）和眼睑回缩。
- 严重充血可用放射治疗。

7 Thyroid eye disease

Aetiology

Autoantibodies to both thyroid and orbital tissue cause inflammation; the extraocular muscles are particularly affected.

Clinical features

The clinical course involves an 'active' congestive stage, usually lasting 2-3 years, followed by a 'quiescent' stage in which residual restriction of ocular movements may be the chief feature.

Symptoms

- Redness
- Irritation
- Aching
- Wide-eyed 'staring' appearance
- Double vision
- Decreased vision in severe cases.

Signs

- Fullness of the eyelids
- Conjunctival hyperaemia and chemosis (Fig. 37)
- Proptosis (exophthalmos): may be unilateral or bilateral (Fig. 38). If severe, may prevent adequate lid closure with resultant exposure keratopathy
- Lid retraction in primary position (Fig. 39), which compounds the cosmetic effect of proptosis
- Lid lag in downgaze (von Graefe's sign)
- Ophthalmoplegia due to inflammation early in the disease and subsequently to fibrosis. The inferior and medial recti are most frequently affected
- Choroidal folds (Fig. 40)
- Optic neuropathy is a sight-threatening complication caused by compression of the optic nerve or its blood supply by swollen orbital tissue, particularly extraocular muscles. Useful tests include colour vision, visual acuity and visual fields. There may be a relative afferent pupillary defect and optic disc oedema.

Management

- Tear substitutes and topical steroids for conjunctival and corneal involvement
- Systemic steroids are usually reserved for optic neuropathy
- Surgery for proptosis (orbital decompression), diplopia (muscle surgery) and eyelid retraction
- Radiotherapy may be appropriate for the congestive phase, if severe.

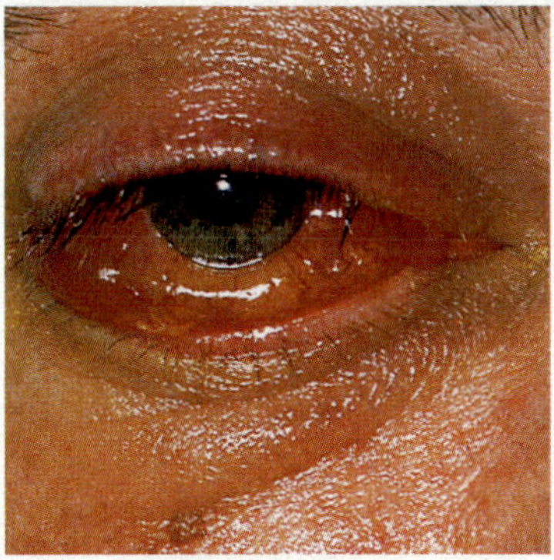

图 37 结膜充血和水肿
Conjunctival hyperaemia and chemosis

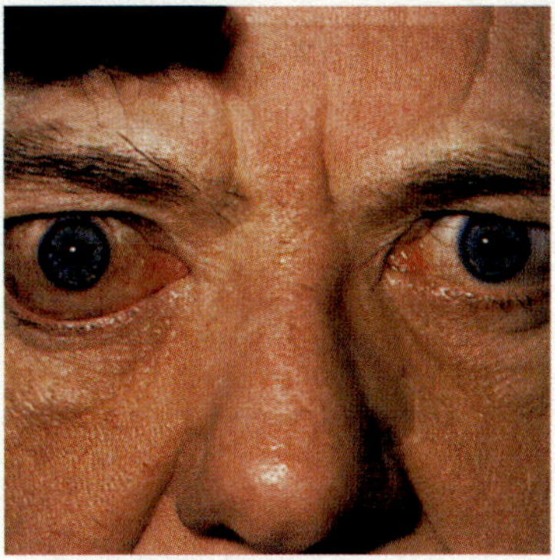

图 38 右侧眼球突出
Right proptosis

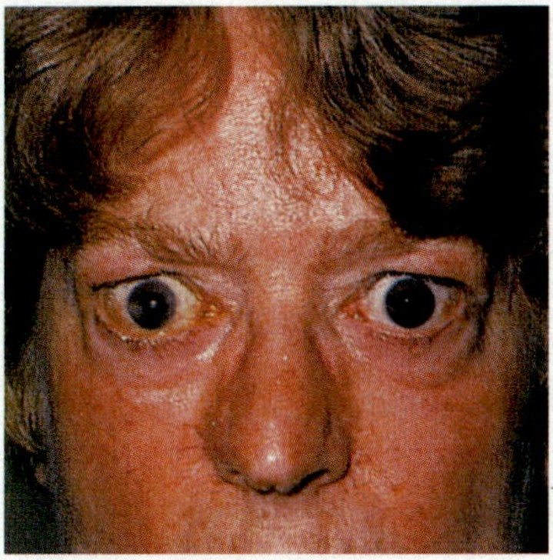

图 39 双侧眼睑退缩
Bilateral lid retraction

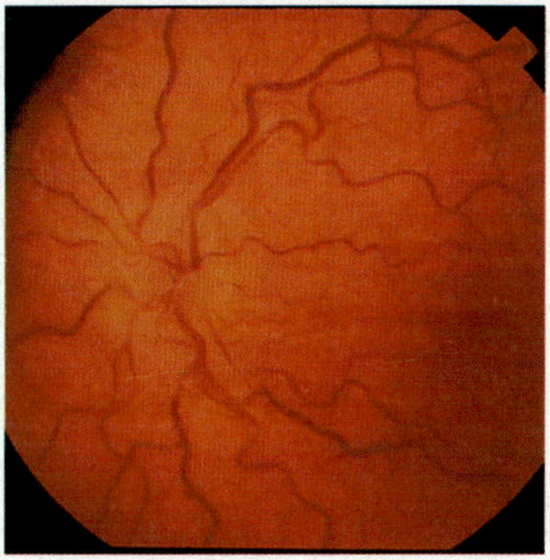

图 40 脉络膜褶
Choroidal folds

眼眶肿瘤

毛细血管瘤

临床特征 婴儿期在眼眶前部出现隆起（图 41），哭闹时肿物增大。可能会出现眼睑皮肤损害，也就是“草莓痣”（见图 17）。

治疗 类固醇肿瘤内注射或全身应用是有效的，但肿瘤经常自行消退。

海绵状血管瘤

临床特征 成人最常见的眶内肿瘤。青年发病，眼球无痛性、进展性轴向突出。

治疗 手术切除。

眶静脉曲张

临床特征 扩张的眶静脉。可出现在任何年龄。

- 间歇性无搏动性眼球突出。
- 眼睑或结膜出现明显病变（图 42）。
- 急性眶内出血和血栓形成（罕见）。

治疗 需手术切除。

横纹肌肉瘤

临床特征 这是罕见、但恶性度高的肿瘤，发病年龄在 7 岁左右，进展性眼球突出，可扪及肿物（图 43）。

治疗 活检后，放射治疗和化学治疗。

神经源肿瘤

视神经胶质瘤 多发病于儿童，进展缓慢。进展性眼球突出和视力丧失，视盘水肿或萎缩（见图 238）。20% ~ 50% 的患者伴有多发性神经纤维瘤。

视神经鞘脑膜瘤 多发于中年女性，眼球突出，且视力慢性进展性丧失（图44）。视盘往往出现视睫状神经旁路血管（图 45）。

治疗 观察、手术和放射治疗。

皮样囊肿

临床特征 可发生于各种年龄，眼球突出和 / 或可扪及肿物（图 46），临床表现取决于位置和大小。

治疗 原则是完全切除。

Orbital tumours

Capillary haemangioma

Clinical features Presents in infancy with an anterior orbital swelling (Fig. 41), which may increase in size when crying. A similar eyelid skin lesion, a 'strawberry naevus' (see Fig. 17), may also be present.

Management Steroids injected into the lesion or given systemically are effective but the tumour often involutes spontaneously.

Cavernous haemangioma

Clinical features The most common benign orbital tumour in adults. Presents in young adults with painless axial proptosis of gradual onset.

Management Surgical excision.

Orbital varices

Clinical features Dilated orbital veins. Presentation is at any age with:

- Intermittent unilateral non-pulsatile proptosis
- Visible lesions in the eyelids or conjunctiva (Fig. 42)
- Acute orbital haemorrhage or thrombosis (less common).

Management Surgical excision may be required.

Rhabdomyosarcoma

Clinical features This very rare but aggressive tumour typically presents at about the age of 7 years with progressive proptosis and a palpable mass may be present (Fig. 43).

Management Incisional biopsy followed by radiotherapy and chemotherapy.

Neural tumours

Optic nerve glioma Presents in childhood with slowly progressive proptosis and visual loss. The optic disc may be swollen or pale (see Fig. 238). 25-50% of patients have neurofibromatosis-1.

Optic nerve sheath meningioma Typically affects middle-aged females and causes slowly progressive visual loss followed later by proptosis (Fig. 44). The optic disc frequently shows opticociliary shunt vessels (Fig. 45).

Management Options include observation, surgery and radiotherapy.

Dermoid cyst

Clinical features Variable age at presentation, with proptosis and/or a palpable mass (Fig. 46) depending on site and size.

Management Excision, which must be complete.

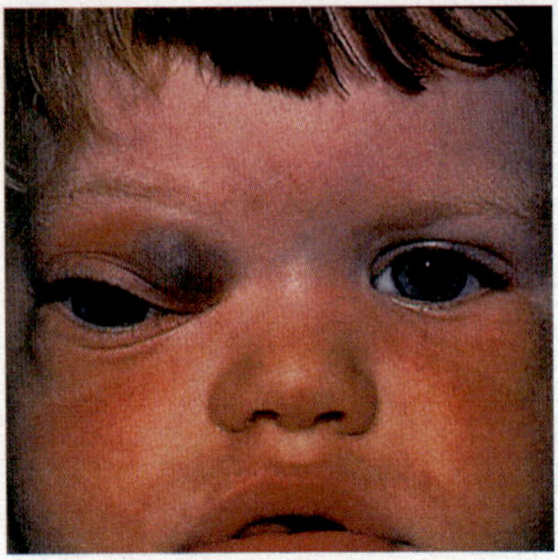

图 41　毛细血管瘤
Capillary haemangioma

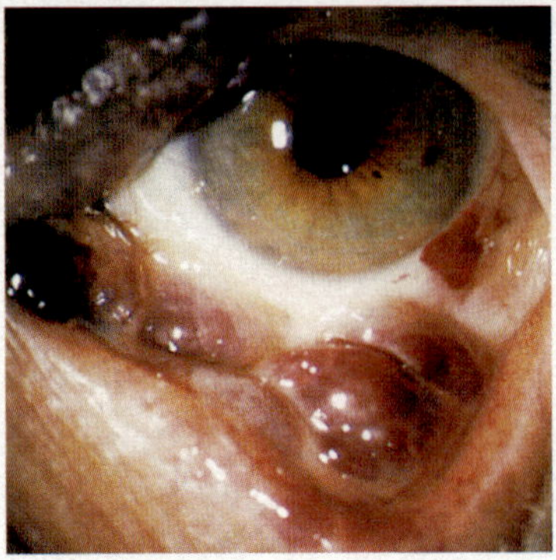

图 42　眶静脉曲张
Orbital varices

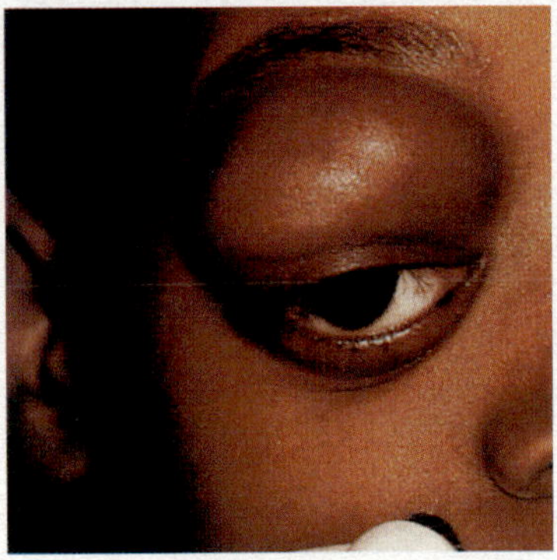

图 43　横纹肌肉瘤
Rhabdomyosarcoma

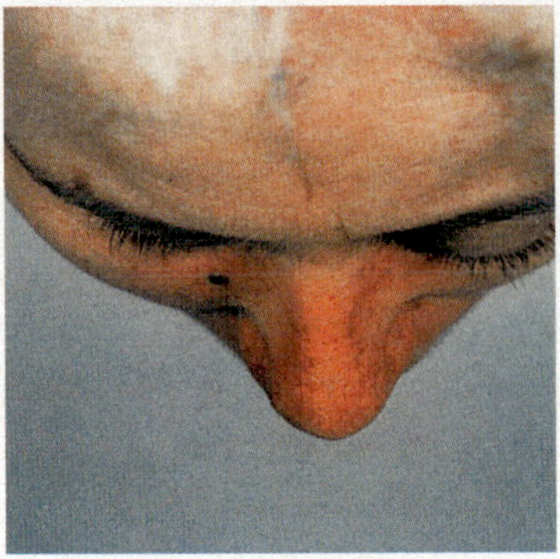

图 44　视神经鞘脑膜瘤导致左侧眼球突出
Left proptosis due to optic nerve sheath meningioma

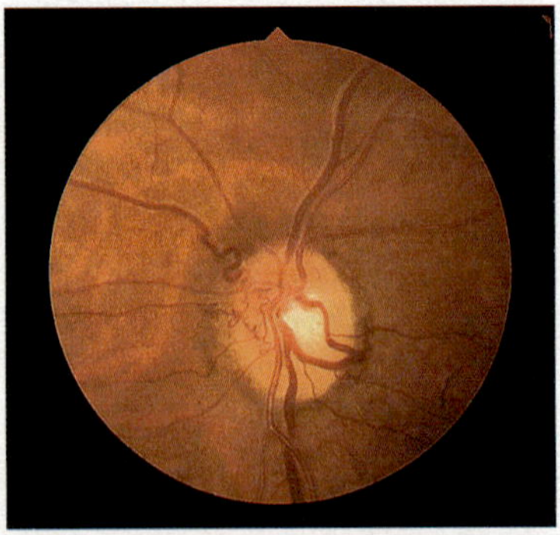

图 45　视睫状神经旁路血管
Opticociliary shunt vessels

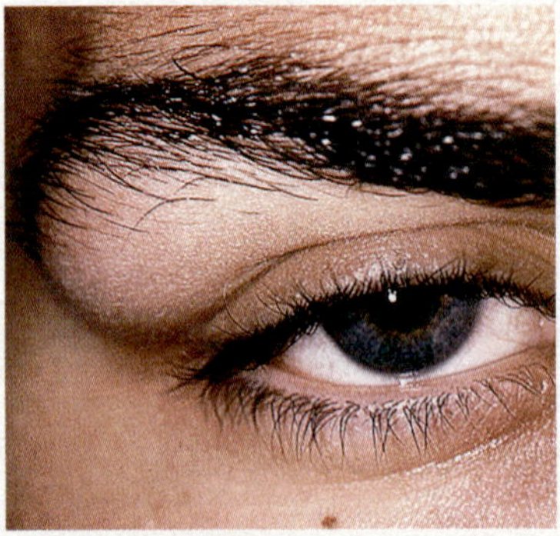

图 46　皮样囊肿
Dermoid cyst

眼眶蜂窝织炎

定义 可危及生命的眼眶软组织急性细菌感染。

病因学
- 继发于鼻窦炎（常见于儿童）。
- 周围结构炎症蔓延（例如泪囊炎）。
- 其次为外伤和手术。

临床特征 *症状* 急性眼睑红肿、疼痛和不适。
体征 视力减退、眼睑红肿（图47）、结膜水肿、眼球突出、眼肌麻痹和视盘水肿。

合并症 颅内感染，海绵窦血栓形成，骨膜下脓肿和失明。

治疗
- 静脉注射抗生素。
- 眶 CT，排除脓肿形成。
- 脓肿引流术或窦道清除术。

特发性眼眶炎症（炎性假瘤）

定义 眶内软组织特发性炎症。

临床特征 亚急性起病的单侧疼痛、眼睑水肿、结膜水肿、眼球突出（图 48）、视力减退和眼肌麻痹。

治疗 全身应用类固醇，放射治疗或免疫抑制剂。

颈动脉海绵窦瘘

定义 颈动脉与海绵窦直接或间接交通，常起自外伤性或自发性颈动脉破裂。

临床特征 头疼，结膜水肿（图49），巩膜外层血管充血（图50），搏动性眼球突出伴随震颤，可闻及杂音，眼肌麻痹，眼压升高和视网膜血管充血、出血（图 51）。

治疗 可放射性介入治疗。

眶底骨折

临床特征 眼眶周围水肿和瘀斑，眼球内陷(图52)，垂直复视，眶下神经知觉丧失和皮下气肿。

治疗 重症必须手术。

9 Miscellaneous orbital disease

Orbital cellulitis

Definition A potentially life-threatening acute bacterial infection of the soft tissues of the orbit.

Aetiology
- Secondary to sinusitis (usually in children)
- Spread from infected adjacent structures (e.g. dacryocystitis)
- Following trauma and surgery.

Clinical features *Symptoms* Acute lid swelling and redness, pain and malaise.

Signs Reduced visual acuity, lid oedema and erythema (Fig. 47), chemosis, proptosis, painful ophthalmoplegia and optic disc swelling.

Complications Intracranial infection, cavernous sinus thrombosis, subperiosteal abscess, and blindness.

Management
- Intravenous antibiotics
- Orbital CT, principally to rule out an abscess
- Surgery for abscess drainage or sinus washout.

Idiopathic orbital inflammation (pseudotumour)

Definition Idiopathic inflammation of the soft tissues of the orbit.

Clinical features Subacute onset of unilateral pain, lid oedema, chemosis, proptosis (Fig. 48), decreased vision and ophthalmoplegia.

Management Systemic steroids, radiotherapy or cytotoxic agents.

Carotid-cavernous fistula

Definition Indirect or direct arterial communication with the cavernous sinus. Usually due to trauma or spontaneous arterial rupture.

Clinical features Headache, chemosis (Fig. 49), dilated episcleral vessels (Fig. 50), pulsatile proptosis with associated thrill and bruit, ophthalmoplegia, raised intraocular pressure and retinal vascular congestion and haemorrhages (Fig. 51).

Management Radiological intervention if appropriate.

Blow-out fracture of orbital floor

Clinical features Periorbital oedema and ecchymosis, enophthalmos (Fig. 52), vertical diplopia, infraorbital nerve anaesthesia and subcutaneous emphysema.

Management Surgery may be necessary in severe cases.

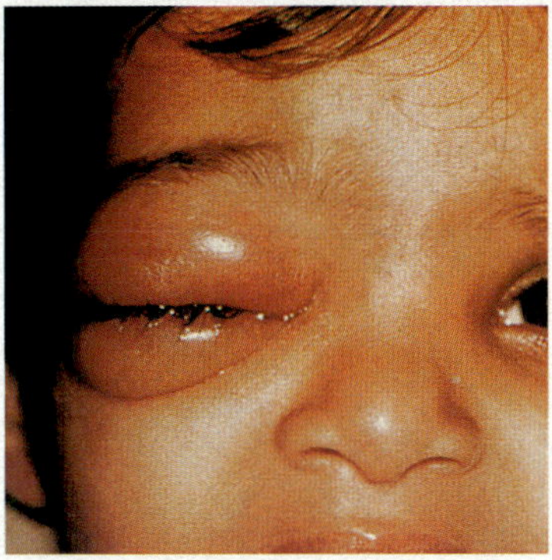

图 47 眼眶蜂窝织炎
Orbital cellulitis

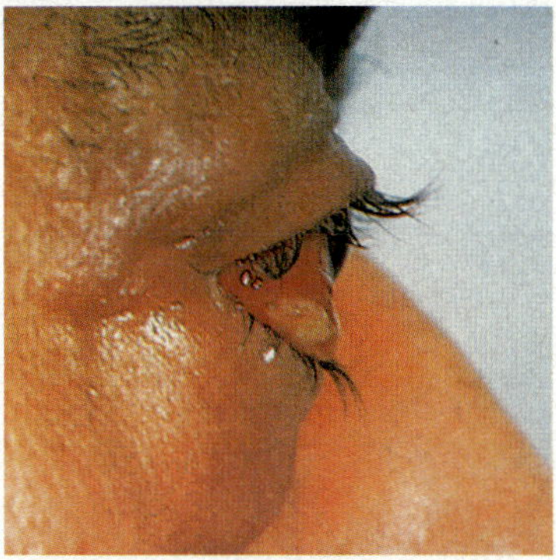

图 48 眼眶假性肿瘤
Orbital pseudotumour

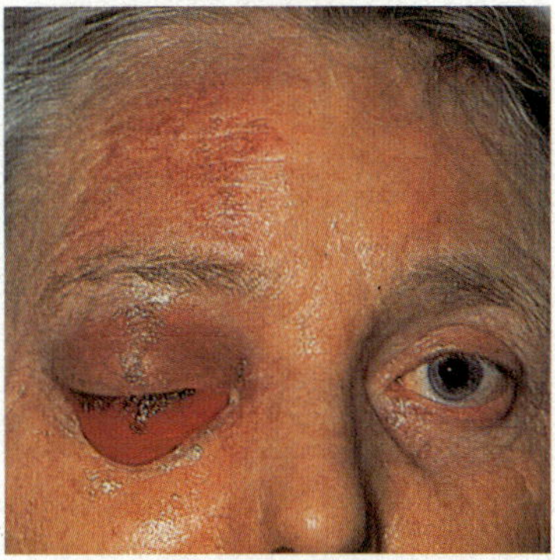

图 49 直接颈内动脉海绵窦瘘引起的严重结膜水肿
Severe chemosis due to direct carotid-cavernous fistula

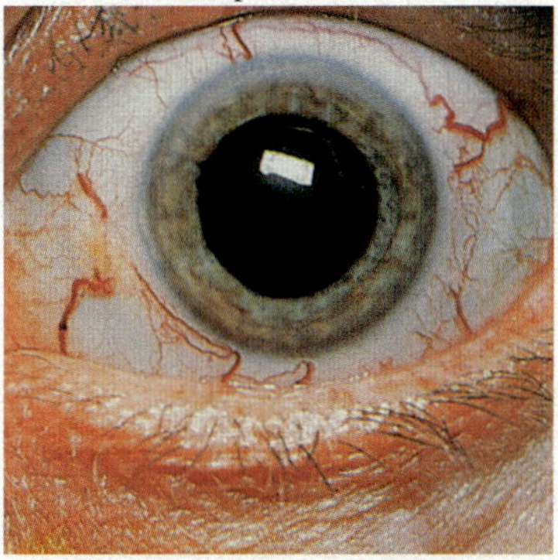

图 50 间接颈内动脉海绵窦瘘引起的巩膜外血管扩张
Dilated episcleral vessels due to indirect carotid-cavernous fistula

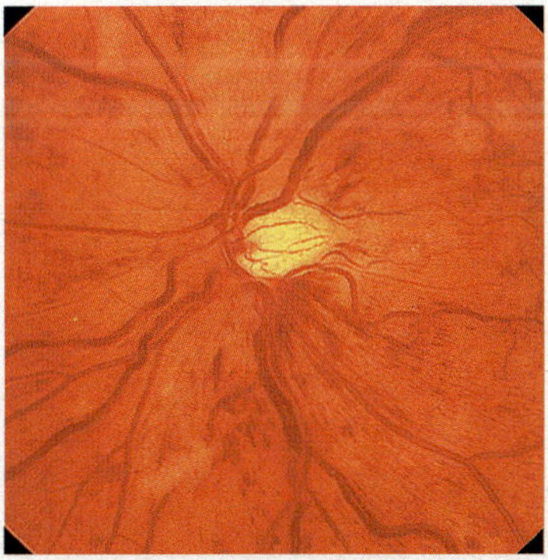

图 51 颈内动脉海绵窦瘘的视网膜出血和静脉扩张
Retinal haemorrhages and dilated veins in carotid-cavernous fistula

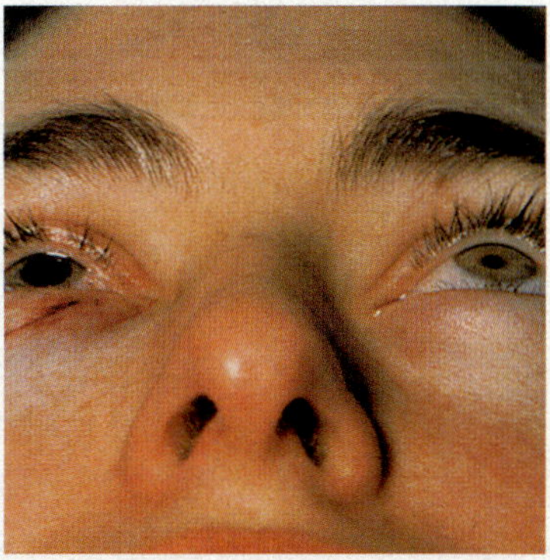

图 52 眶底骨折引起的右侧眼球内陷
Right enophthalmos due to orbital floor blow-out fracture

急性结膜炎

急性变态反应性结膜炎

急性发病，两眼瘙痒，眼睑水肿和结膜水肿 (图 53)。春夏季常见于儿童，由花草引起，几小时内即可发生。

季节过敏性（枯草热）结膜炎

临床特征 在花粉季节持续瘙痒、结膜充血和大量浆液性分泌物。

治疗 抗过敏药物和抗组胺类药物能使症状得到一定缓解。

细菌性结膜炎

临床特征 两眼亚急性发病，但经常不对称、发红、异物感和粘性分泌物。检查可见结膜充血(图 54)和乳头轻度增生。视力，角膜和瞳孔正常。

治疗 局部抗生素应用（如氯霉素, 夫西地酸, 庆大霉素）约 1 星期。

腺病毒结膜炎

临床特征 常双眼急性发作，异物感，发红和水样分泌物。检查可见结膜滤泡（图55)，耳前淋巴结肿大，眼睑水肿，结膜水肿和结膜下出血（图56)。浅层点状角膜炎可逐渐形成永久性深层浸润(图 57)，传染性强。

治疗 局部润滑，角膜炎严重可使用类固醇。

新生儿结膜炎

定义 结膜炎症发病于新生儿出生第 1 个月。

病因学 症状出现时间可以帮助诊断。

- *衣原体属*：最常见（图 58）；发病于出生 1 ~ 3 周。
- *淋球菌*：出生第 1 周。
- *单纯疱疹*：出生 1 ~ 2 周。
- *单纯细菌性结膜炎*：出生 1 周内。

治疗

- 确保角膜未受累。
- 个体化研究和治疗（包含母体感染)。

Acute conjunctivitis

Acute allergic conjunctivitis

Acute onset of bilateral itching, lid oedema and chemosis (Fig. 53), often in children after playing on grass in spring or summer. Settles spontaneously within a few hours.

Seasonal allergic (hay fever) conjunctivitis

Clinical features Persistent itching, conjunctival hyperaemia and excess mucus production during the hay fever season.

Management Topical mast cell stabilizers and antihistamines usually provide adequate symptomatic relief.

Bacterial conjunctivitis

Clinical features Subacute onset of bilateral, but frequently asymmetrical, redness, grittiness and a sticky discharge. Examination shows conjunctival hyperaemia (Fig. 54) and mild papillary changes. Visual acuity, corneas and pupils are normal.

Management Topical antibiotics (e.g. chloramphenicol, fusidic acid, gentamicin) for about a week.

Adenoviral conjunctivitis

Clinical features Acute onset of frequently bilateral grittiness and redness and a watery discharge. Examination shows a follicular conjunctival reaction (Fig. 55), preauricular lymphadenopathy, lid oedema, chemosis and subconjunctival haemorrhages (Fig. 56). A punctate epithelial keratitis may progress to persistent deeper infiltrates (Fig. 57). The condition is highly contagious.

Management Topical lubricants; steroids may be considered for severe keratitis.

Neonatal conjunctivitis

Definition A conjunctival inflammation occurring within the first month of life.

Aetiology The timing of presentation may aid diagnosis.

- *Chlamydia*: the most common (Fig. 58); presents at 1-3 weeks
- *Gonococcus*: during first week
- *Herpes simplex*: 1-2 weeks
- *Simple bacterial conjunctivitis*: end of first week onwards.

Management

- Ensure cornea is uninvoled
- Investigate and treat individual conditions as appropriate (including maternal infection).

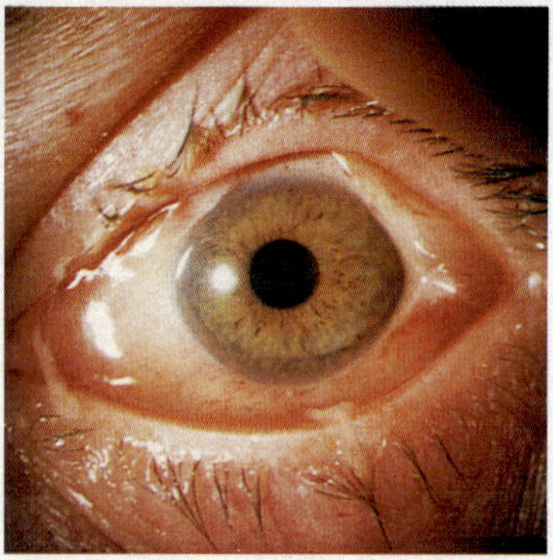

图 53　急性变态反应性结膜炎
Acute allergic conjunctivitis

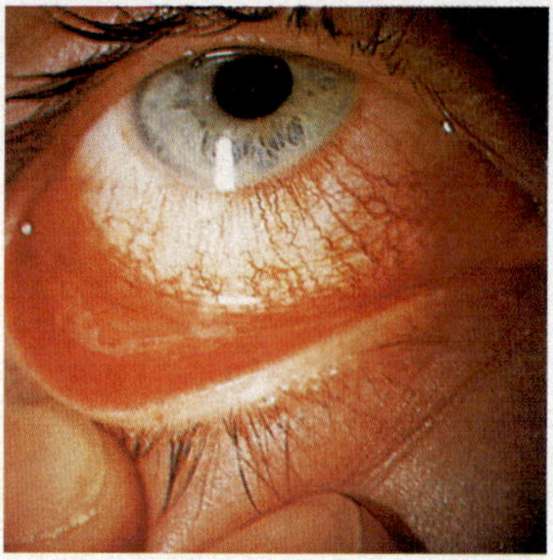

图 54　细菌性结膜炎
Bacterial conjunctivitis

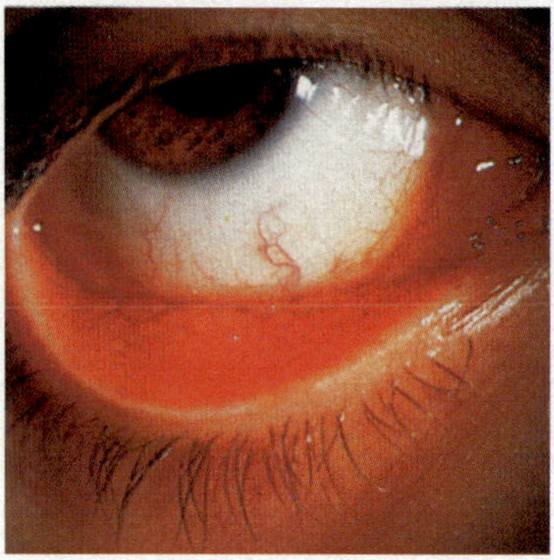

图 55　腺病毒感染的结膜滤泡
Follicular conjunctivitis in adenoviral infection

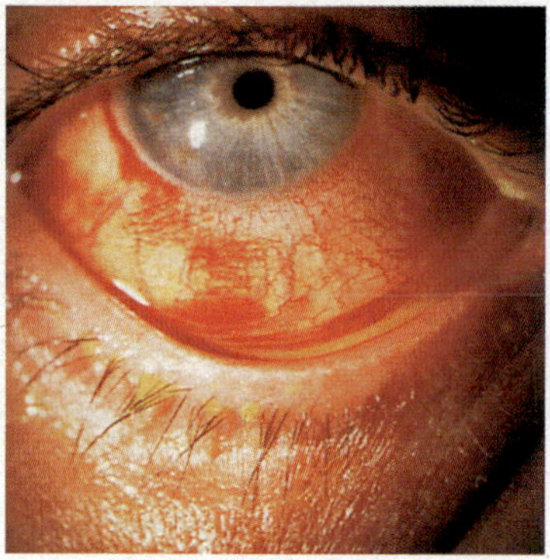

图 56　严重腺病毒性结膜炎的结膜下出血
Subconjunctival haemorrhages in severe adenoviral conjunctivitis

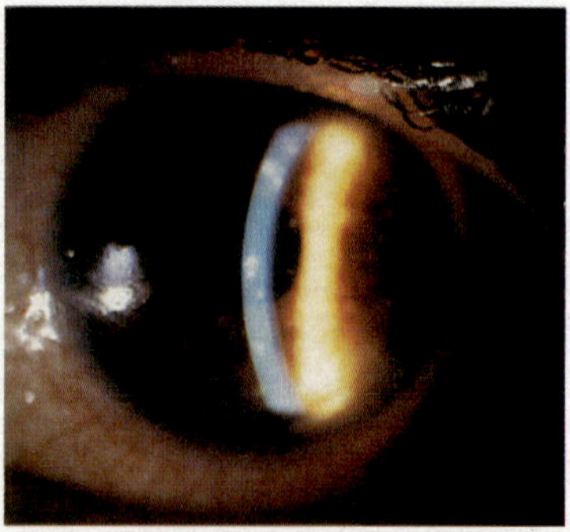

图 57　腺病毒性结膜炎的角膜浸润
Corneal infiltrates following adenoviral conjunctivitis

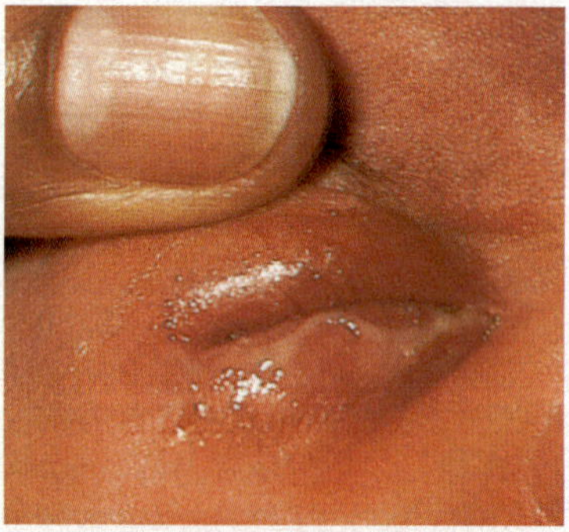

图 58　新生儿衣原体感染的粘脓性分泌物
Mucopurulent discharge in neonatal chlamydial infection

成人衣原体性结膜炎

临床特征 性接触传染，单眼亚急性发病，粘液脓性分泌物，大量的结膜滤泡（图 59）和耳前淋巴结肿大。

治疗
- 实验室检查确定诊断。
- 请生殖泌尿科专家会诊。
- 抗生素应用（如阿奇霉素）。

春季角(膜)结膜炎

临床特征 双眼慢性复发性变态反应性疾病，儿童期发病，患者常伴有遗传性过敏症（例如患哮喘症，湿疹，花粉症）。症状包括瘙痒，灼热感，畏光和粘液性分泌物。特征性的上睑结膜乳头增生（图60），有时伴角膜缘结节（图61）。角膜体征包括点状角膜上皮病变，角膜溃疡，角膜混浊（图62）和瘢痕形成，有时角膜缘出现“弓形”病变（假性老年环，图 63）。

治疗 抗过敏药物，抗组胺类药物和局部应用类固醇。

特异反应性角(膜)结膜炎

临床特征 罕见，多发病于青年男性，伴随特异性皮炎（湿疹）。类似春季角(膜)结膜炎，但预后不良。眼睑增厚，结痂，常伴发葡萄球菌感染睑缘炎（见图 1）。严重的乳头性结膜炎会导致睑球粘连（见图 75）和严重的角膜并发症。可能出现传染性单纯疱疹性角膜炎（见图 86）和细菌性角膜炎（见图 77 ~ 80）。

治疗 类似春季角(膜)结膜炎，但通常更耐药。

巨大乳头性结膜炎

异物相关性结膜炎，以上睑板巨大乳头为特征（图64）。原因主要是由于戴隐形眼镜、义眼和突出缝合。

Chronic conjunctivitis

Adult chlamydial conjunctivitis

Clinical features

Sexually transmitted infection presenting with subacute onset of typically unilateral mucopurulent discharge associated with large conjunctival follicles (Fig. 59) and preauricular lymphadenopathy.

Management

- Laboratory testing to confirm diagnosis
- Referral for assessment by a genitourinary specialist
- Treat with antibiotics (e.g. azithromycin).

Vernal keratoconjunctivitis (VKC)

Clinical features

A bilateral chronic or recurrent allergic condition that starts in childhood, usually in patients with atopy (e.g. asthma, eczema and hay fever).

Symptoms include itching, watering, photophobia and a stringy discharge. Papillary conjunctivitis particularly involves the superior tarsus (Fig. 60) and sometimes with nodules at the limbus (Fig. 61). Corneal signs include punctate epitheliopathy, ulceration, plaque formation (Fig. 62) and scarring, occasionally in the form of a limbal 'Cupid's bow' ('pseudogerontoxon' - Fig. 63).

Management

Topical mast cell stabilizers, antihistamines and topical steroids.

Atopic keratoconjunctivitis

Clinical features

A rare condition typically affecting young men with atopic dermatitis (eczema). Similar to VKC but carries a worse prognosis. The eyelids are thickened and crusted, and associated staphylococcal blepharitis (see Fig. 1) is common. Intense papillary conjunctivitis may lead to symblepharon (see Fig. 75), and corneal complications can be severe. Aggressive herpes simplex keratitis (see Fig. 86) and microbial keratitis (see Figs 77-80) may occur.

Management

Similar to VKC but frequently more resistant.

Giant papillary conjunctivitis

A foreign-body-associated conjunctivitis characterized by giant papillae on the superior tarsus (Fig. 64). Causes include contact lens wear, artificial eyes and protruding sutures.

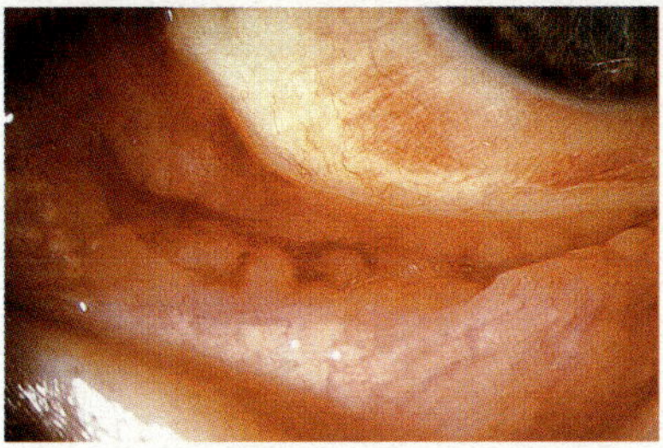

图 59　衣原体性结膜炎的大量滤泡
Large follicles in chlamydial conjunctivitis

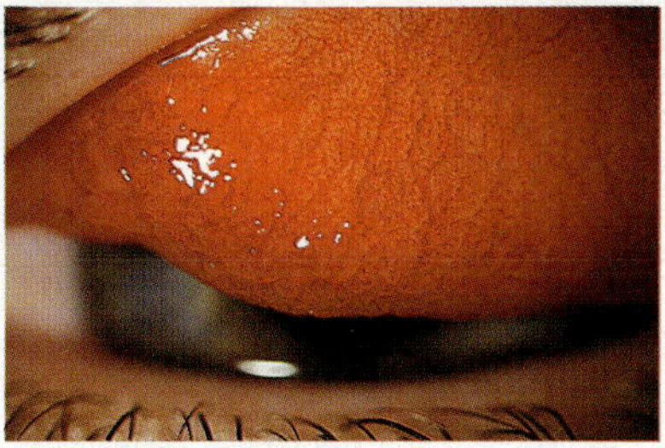

图 60　乳头结膜炎
Papillary conjunctivitis

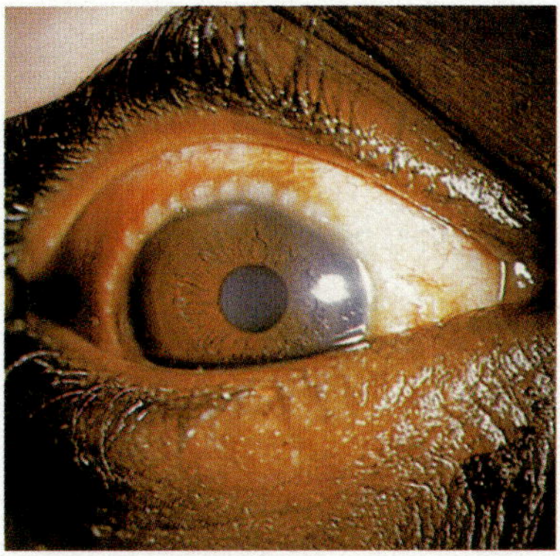

图 61　春季结膜炎
Vernal limbitis

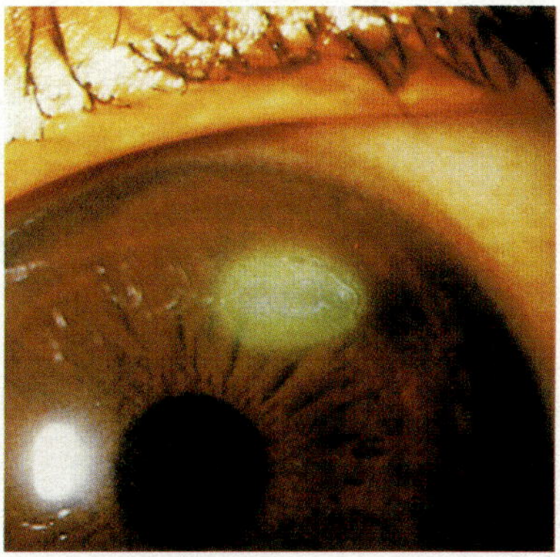

图 62　角膜浑浊
Corneal plaque

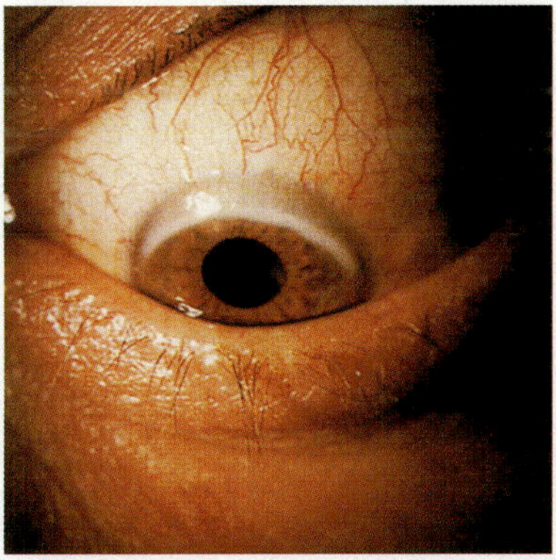

图 63　假性老年环
Pseudogerontoxon

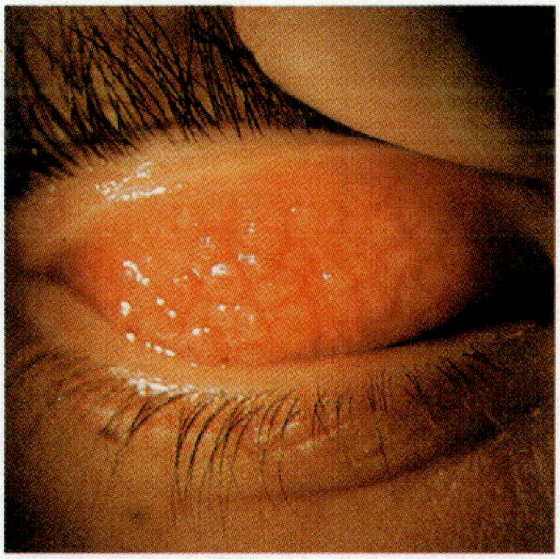

图 64　巨大乳头
Giant papillae

结膜肿瘤

乳头（状）瘤

带蒂的乳头（状）瘤 是由乳头瘤病毒引起的。多见于儿童和青少年，可为多发性乳头（状）瘤，通常位于睑结膜、穹窿或泪阜。

无蒂的乳头（状）瘤 多见于老年人。常为单个和单眼出现（图65）。位于球结膜或角膜缘上。

癌瘤

结膜和角膜上皮癌（CCIN） 微微隆起的新生血管或胶冻状肿块常出现在角膜缘（图66），有时侵犯角膜。低度恶变趋势。

浸润性癌 外观相似，但侵犯深部组织。

迷芽瘤

皮样囊肿 圆形，白色结节，多发于角膜缘（图67）。

皮脂瘤 质软，黄白色结膜下肿物，多见于外眦。

色素损害

结膜（某些种族）上皮黑色素沉着症 多见于黑肤人种。

结膜痣 发生在儿童或青少年期，少见。一般呈现单个，境界分明，扁平或轻微隆起，含色素或多或少，多发病于角膜缘（图68）；在青春期大小/色素沉着增生活跃。

原发性获得性黑色素沉着症（PAM） 罕见，主要见于老年人，上皮内的色素沉着斑生长缓慢而多变，有些有恶变倾向。

黑色素瘤 罕见肿瘤，占眼部恶性肿瘤的2%。最经常地出现在PAM内，呈结节病变（图69）。

可起源于以前存在的痣或偶尔新生，通常发生在角膜缘（图70）。

Papilloma

Pedunculated papilloma Caused by a papillomavirus. Typically affects children and young adults and may be multiple. Usually located on the palpebral conjunctiva, fornix or caruncle.

Sessile papilloma Affects older patients. Invariably single and unilateral (Fig. 65), located on the bulbar conjunctiva or at the limbus.

Carcinoma

Conjunctival and corneal intra-epithelial neoplasia (CCIN) A slightly elevated, fleshy vascular or gelatinous mobile mass, most frequently juxtalimbal (Fig. 66), sometimes with corneal extension. Low malignant potential.

Invasive carcinoma Similar in appearance but fixed to underlying tissues.

Choristoma

Dermoid A rounded, white nodule typically located at the limbus (Fig. 67).

Lipodermoid A soft yellow-white subconjunctival mass usually found at the outer canthus.

Pigmented lesions

Conjunctival (racial) epithelial melanosis A very common physiological pigmentation in dark-skinned individuals.

Conjunctival naevus An uncommon lesion presenting during childhood or early adult life. Single, well-demarcated, flat or slightly elevated, variably pigmented lesion, most commonly at the limbus (Fig. 68); size/pigmentation may increase at puberty.

Primary acquired melanosis (PAM) A rare condition presenting in old age with uni- or multifocal slowly growing patches of intraepithelial pigmentation. Some malignant potential.

Melanoma A rare tumour accounting for 2% of all ocular malignancies. Most frequently arises within PAM, as a nodular lesion (Fig. 69). May arise from a pre-existing naevus or, rarely, de novo, usually at the limbus (Fig. 70).

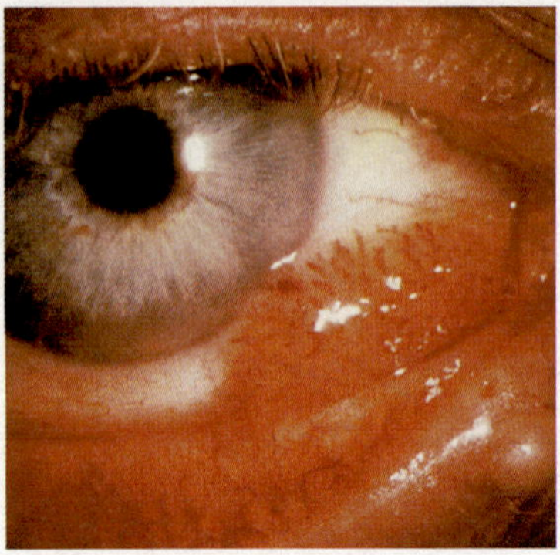

图 65 无蒂的结膜乳头状瘤
Sessile conjunctival papilloma

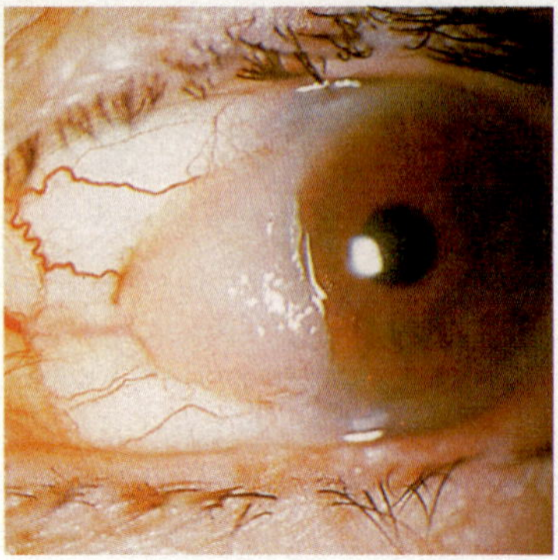

图 66 结膜和角膜上皮新生物
Conjunctival and corneal intraepithelial neoplasia

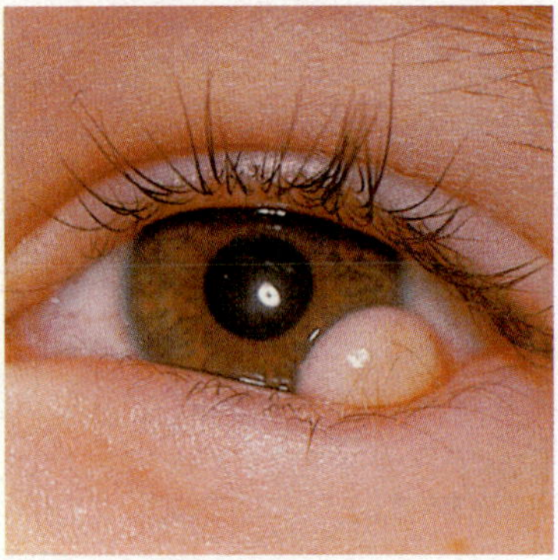

图 67 角膜缘皮样囊肿
Limbal dermoid

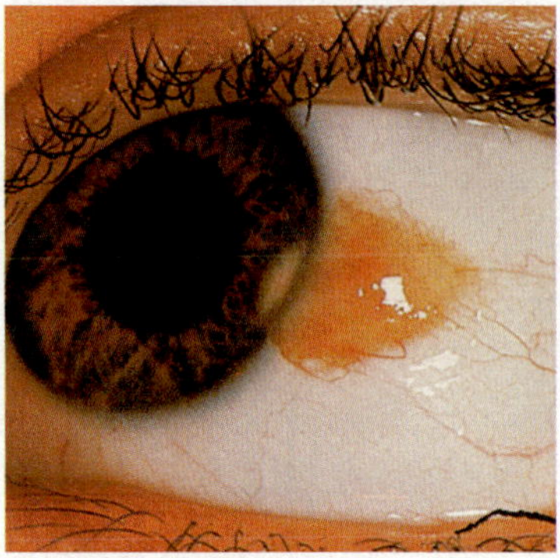

图 68 结膜痣
Conjunctival naevus

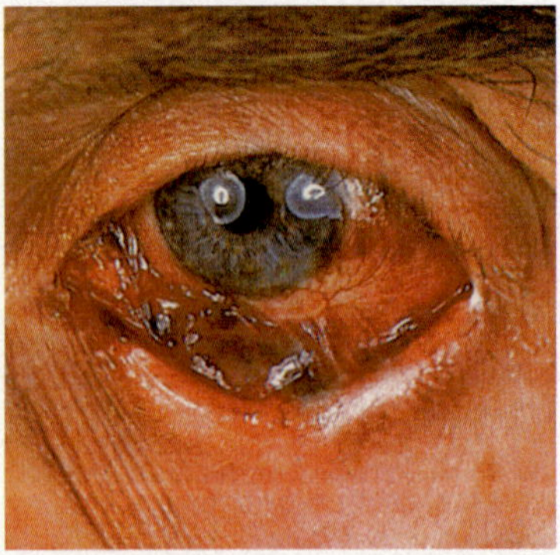

图 69 黑色素瘤出现在原发性获得性黑色素沉着症内部
Melanoma arising within an area of primary acquired melanosis

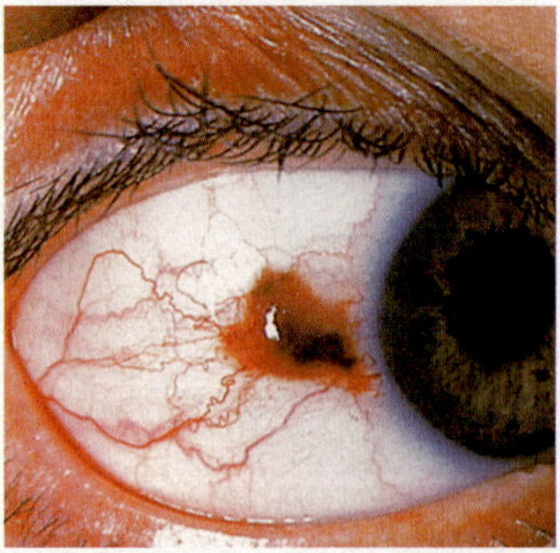

图 70 原发性结膜黑色素瘤
Primary conjunctival melanoma

干燥性角膜结膜炎和结膜瘢痕

干燥性角膜结膜炎

病因学

干燥性角膜结膜炎（KCS）或“干眼”是很常见的，任何影响泪液生成或蒸发的病变均会导致该病。年龄相关性泪腺萎缩和自身免疫疾病（Sjögren 综合征）是常见原因；继发的Sjögren综合征是KCS伴发结缔组织疾病（如类风湿性关节炎）。

临床特征

症状 包括异物感和充血，晚间加重。

体征

- 在眨眼之后泪膜很快破裂，出现不规则的干燥斑。
- 泪小管边缘可见粘液碎屑。
- 干燥的结膜和角膜用孟加拉玫瑰红染色（图 71）。
- 丝状角膜炎（图 72）。
- Schirmer 实验，滤纸条湿润程度减少。

治疗

- 规律使用人工泪液常可达到治疗效果。
- 重症患者可泪点封闭。

结膜瘢痕

病因学

双眼结膜出现免疫介导的皮肤粘膜的起疱性疾病；严重但罕见。

瘢痕性类天疱疮 慢性病，具有特征的皮肤和粘膜水疱形成。

Stevens-Johnson 综合征 为一种急性严重病变，但广泛的自身限制性血管炎常为对某一种药物和传染的超敏反应所致。表现为特异的“靶”皮肤病损和口腔粘膜的损害（图 73）。

合并症

- 结膜瘢痕（图 74）和收缩。
- 在眼球和睑结膜之间形成粘连（睑球粘连，图 75），外眦之间粘连（融合睑）。
- 干眼。
- 乱睫。
- 瘢痕性睑内翻。
- 角膜角化（图 76）。

治疗

- 局部和全身应用类固醇。
- 人工泪液。
- 手术（主要用于眼睑畸形）。

13 Keratoconjunctivitis sicca and cicatrizing conjunctivitis

Keratoconjunctivitis sicca

Aetiology

Keratoconjunctivitis sicca (KCS), or 'dry eye', is a very common condition resulting from any process that affects the production or evaporation of the tears. Age-related lacrimal gland atrophy and autoimmune damage (Sjögren's syndrome) are common causes; secondary Sjögren's syndrome is the association of KCS with a connective tissue disorder (e.g. rheumatoid arthritis).

Clinical features

Symptoms Include grittiness and redness, often worse in the evening.

Signs

- Irregular patchy tear film with rapid break-up after blinking
- Thin marginal tear strip with mucous debris
- Dry conjunctiva and cornea stains with Rose Bengal (Fig. 71)
- Corneal filaments (Fig. 72)
- Schirmer's test measures the wetting of a strip of filter paper: typically reduced.

Management

- Tear substitutes usually suffice if used regularly
- Punctal occlusion in severe cases.

Cicatrizing conjunctivitis

Aetiology

Bilateral conjunctival manifestation of immune-mediated blistering mucocutaneous diseases; serious but rare.

Cicatricial pemphigoid A chronic disease characterized by skin and mucous membrane blister formation.

Stevens-Johnson syndrome An acute, severe but generally self-limiting vasculitis most commonly caused by hypersensitivity to certain drugs and infections. Characteristic 'target' skin lesions and oral mucosal lesions (Fig. 73) are seen.

Complications

- Conjunctival scarring (Fig. 74) and shrinkage
- Adhesions between the bulbar and palpebral conjunctiva (symblepharon, Fig. 75), and of the outer canthi (ankyloblepharon)
- Dry eye
- Aberrant eyelash growth
- Cicatricial entropion
- Corneal keratinization (Fig. 76).

Management

- Topical and systemic steroids
- Tear substitutes
- Surgery (mainly for lid deformity).

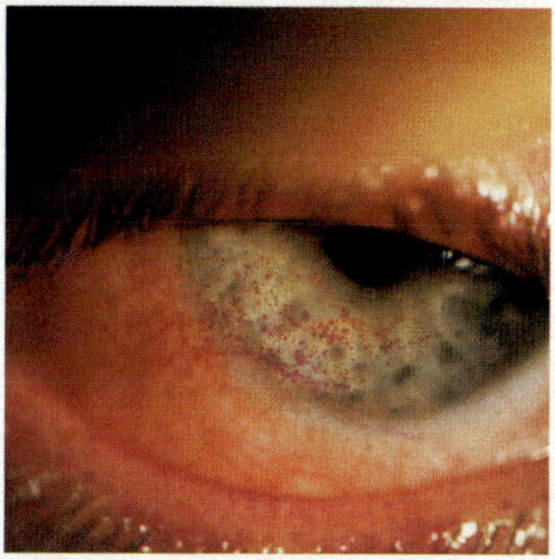

图 71　干燥的结膜和角膜用孟加拉玫瑰红染色
Dry conjunctiva and cornea stained with Rose Bengal

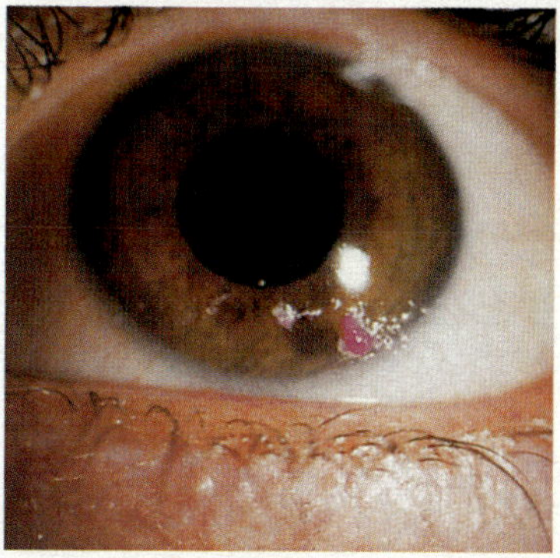

图 72　丝状角膜炎
Corneal filaments

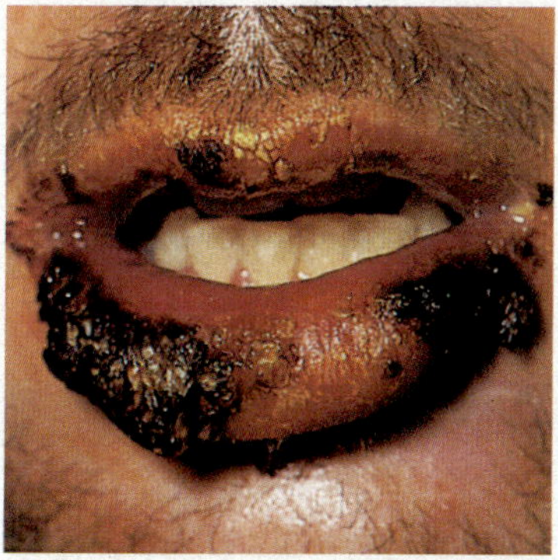

图 73　Stevens-Johnson 综合征的出血性嘴唇，有硬壳
Haemorrhagic crusting of lips in Stevens-Johnson syndrome

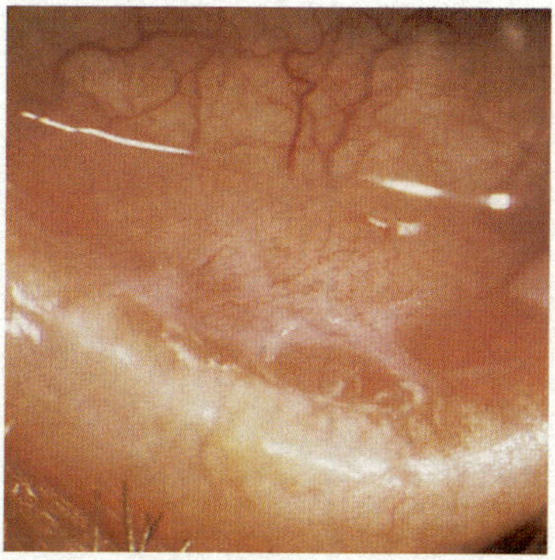

图 74　瘢痕性类天疱疮的结膜瘢痕
Conjunctival scarring in cicatricial pemphigoid

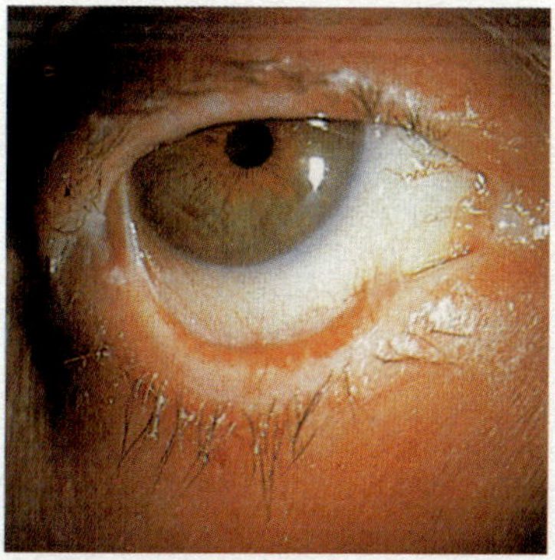

图 75　睑球粘连
Symblepharon

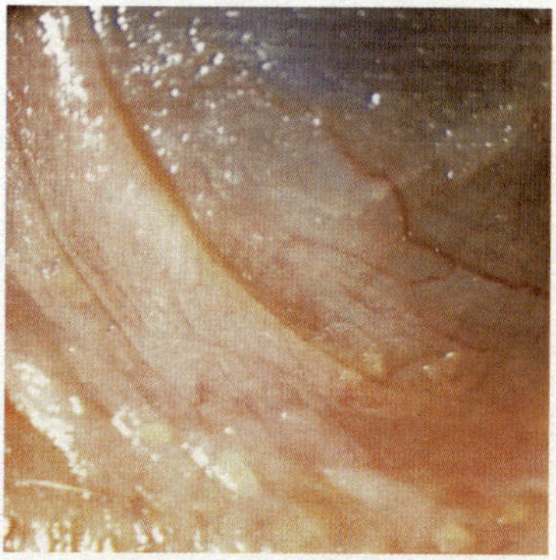

图76　瘢痕性类天疱疮的角膜角化
Corneal keratinization in cicatricial pemphigoid

细菌性角膜炎

临床特征 严重病变常起病于角膜浅层病变或由戴隐形眼镜引起。

症状 亚急性发病，单眼疼痛、发红、畏光和视力下降。

体征 角膜周围充血，基质浸润和上皮缺损。严重时可出现前房积脓。

病因学 *葡萄球菌和肺炎球菌* 典型表现为黄白色椭圆形化脓灶被相对透明角膜围绕（图 77，78）。

假单胞菌属 不规则化脓灶伴脓性粘液（图 79，80）。严重感染可能侵犯巩膜。

治疗 细菌培养（角膜刮片，结膜拭子，隐形眼镜/如果有效的情况）之前局部应用广谱抗生素（如氧氟沙星，增强的头孢呋辛 / 庆大霉素合剂）。

真菌性角膜炎

临床特征 *真菌菌丝* 多与植物引起的眼外伤有关。溃疡呈灰白色，界限不清，周围出现卫星灶（图 81）。

念珠菌属 多发生在过劳患者或以前存在角膜浅层病变者，表现和细菌性角膜炎相似。

治疗 局部应用抗真菌药。

棘阿米巴角膜炎

临床特征 患者常戴隐形眼镜。典型表现为与临床体征不符的疼痛。早期表现为树枝状角膜上皮浸润，由角膜上皮缺损发展至环形浸润，再沿角膜神经分布的放射状浸润和角膜基质层的浸润（图 82）。

治疗 局部应用抗棘阿米巴药物。

Suppurative keratitis

Bacterial keratitis

Clinical features

This serious condition is usually associated with pre-existing corneal surface disease or contact lens wear.

Symptoms Subacute onset of unilateral pain, redness, photophobia and blurred vision

Signs Circumcorneal injection, stromal infiltrate and an overlying epithelial defect. A hypopyon may be present if severe.

Aetiology

Staphylococcal and pneumococcal typically causes yellow-white, oval suppuration surrounded by relatively clear cornea (Figs 77, 78).

Pseudomonas causes irregular suppuration associated with a mucopurulent discharge (Figs 79, 80). Very severe infections may extend into the sclera.

Management

Specimens for culture (corneal scrape, conjunctival swab, contact lenses/case if available) followed by intensive topical antibiotics (e.g. ofloxacin, fortified cefuroxime/ gentamicin combination).

Fungal keratitis

Clinical features

Filamentous Frequently preceded by ocular trauma involving vegetable matter. Characterized by greyish-white ulceration with indistinct feathery margins and satellite lesions (Fig. 81).

Candida Typically occurs in debilitated patients or those with pre-existing surface disease; similar appearance to bacterial keratitis.

Management

Topical antifungal agents.

Acanthamoeba keratitis

Clinical features

Patients, usually contact lens wearers, typically experience pain disproportionate to the clinical signs. Early cases are characterized by dendritiform epithelial lesions, radial keratoneuritis and stromal keratitis followed by a central ring abscess associated with variable epithelial breakdown (Fig. 82).

Management

Topical amoebicidal agents.

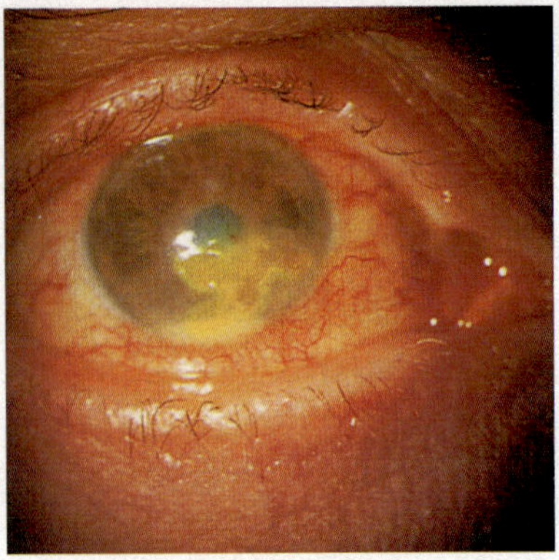

图 77　葡萄球菌性角膜炎
Staphylococcal keratitis

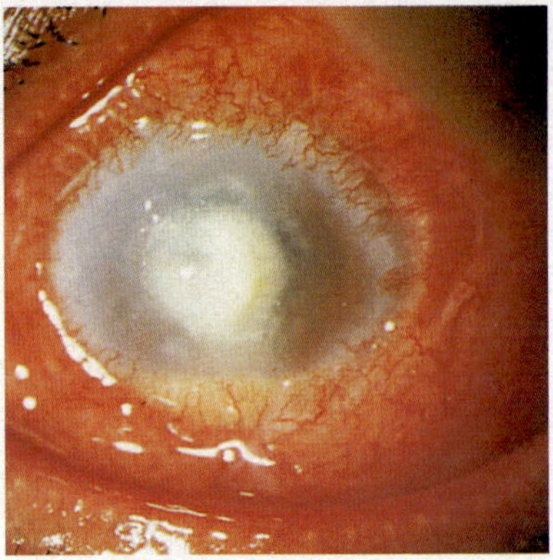

图 78　肺炎球菌性角膜炎
Pneumococcal keratitis

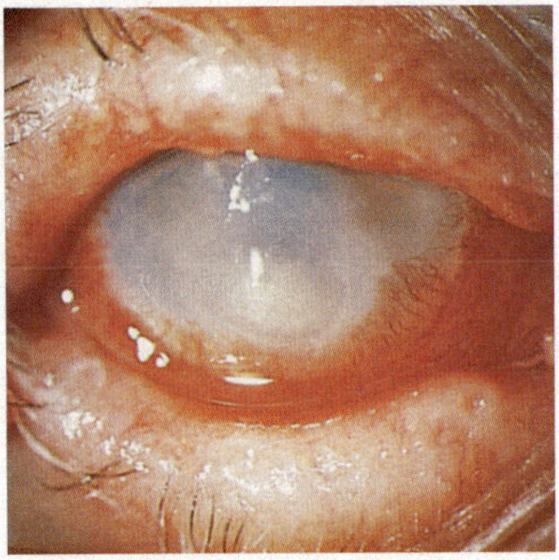

图 79　假单胞菌属性角膜炎
Pseudomonas keratitis

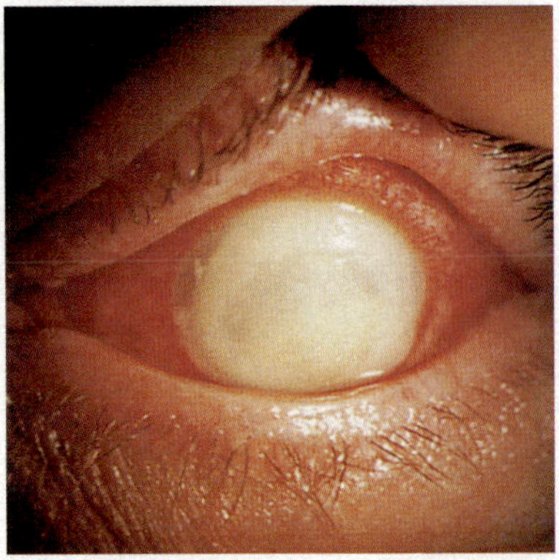

图 80　陈旧性假单胞菌属性角膜炎
Advanced pseudomonas keratitis

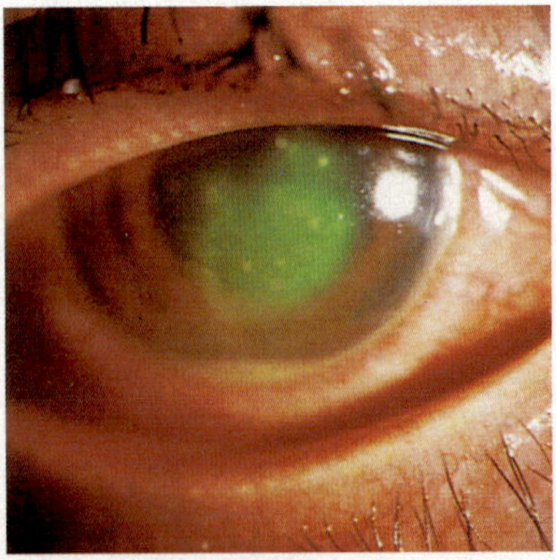

图 81　真菌性角膜炎
Fungal keratitis

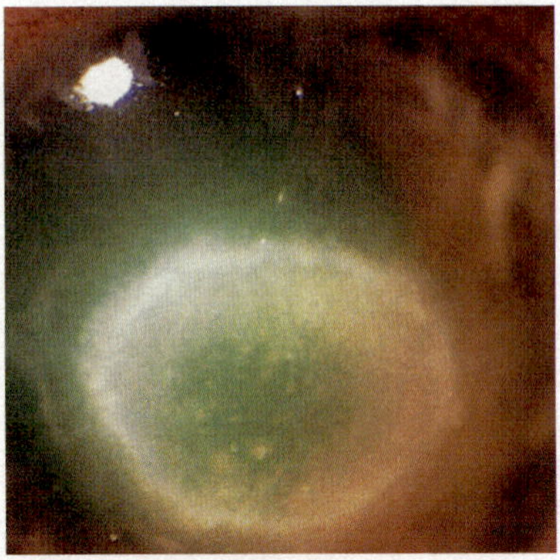

图 82　棘阿米巴角膜炎
Acanthamoeba keratitis

原发感染

由直接接触引起，病毒通过受感染的分泌物传给对本病无免疫力的患者，多为儿童。它可引起滤泡性结膜炎（见图55），睑缘炎（图83）和浅层角膜炎。

复发性角膜炎

病因学 潜伏病毒再活化，侵犯角膜上皮；常见。

临床特征 角膜的知觉减退。树枝状角膜溃疡是典型病变，荧光染色证明状况好转（图 84）。树枝状角膜溃疡未经控制或局部应用类固醇可发展扩大为地图状（虫蚀状）溃疡（图 85）。

治疗 局部抗病毒剂（如阿昔洛韦，更昔洛韦）。

基质坏死性角膜炎

病因学 少见病变，病毒直接侵入，破坏角膜基质。

临床特征 干酪样坏死的基质与细菌或真菌感染性角膜炎相似（图 86）伴随前部葡萄膜炎。
并发症包括瘢痕形成（图 87）和穿孔。

治疗
- 角膜上皮缺损的治疗。
- 对于基质角膜炎可局部应用类固醇，抗病毒和抗生素药物。

盘状角膜炎

病因学 可能是对疱疹病毒的超敏反应。

临床特征 亚急性，无痛的视力模糊伴光晕。检查可见水肿的上皮和基质区域伴有角膜后沉着物（图 88）。
其他的检查所见包括轻度虹膜炎和病灶周围的浸润环（Wessely 环）。

治疗 局部应用类固醇结合抗病毒药物。有些患者口服阿昔洛韦可减少复发。

15 Herpes simplex infection

Primary infection

This is caused by direct transmission of virus through infected secretions to a non-immune subject, usually a child. It may cause follicular conjunctivitis (see Fig. 55), blepharitis (Fig. 83) and epithelial keratitis.

Recurrent epithelial keratitis

Aetiology Invasion of the corneal epithelium by reactivated latent virus; common.

Clinical features Corneal sensation is diminished. A branching 'dendritic' ulcer is characteristic, demonstrated well with fluorescein staining (Fig. 84). A geographical (amoeboid) ulcer (Fig. 85) develops from an enlarging dendritic lesion particularly when the latter has inadvertently been treated with topical steroids.

Management Topical antiviral agents (e.g. aciclovir, ganciclovir).

Stromal necrotic keratitis

Aetiology This uncommon condition is caused by direct viral invasion and destruction of the corneal stroma.

Clinical features Cheesy, necrotic stroma appearing similar to bacterial or fungal infection (Fig. 86), with associated anterior uveitis. Complications include scarring (Fig. 87) and perforation.

Management

- Treatment of any associated epithelial defect
- Topical steroids, to reduce stromal inflammation, with antiviral and antibiotic cover.

Disciform keratitis

Aetiology Possibly a hypersensitivity reaction to herpes virus.

Clinical features Subacute, usually painless blurring of vision which may be associated with haloes around lights. Examination shows an area of epithelial and stromal oedema with associated keratic precipitates (Fig. 88). Other findings include mild iritis and a ring of infiltrates surrounding the lesion (Wessely ring).

Management Topical steroids combined with antiviral cover. In some cases, oral aciclovir may be considered to reduce recurrence.

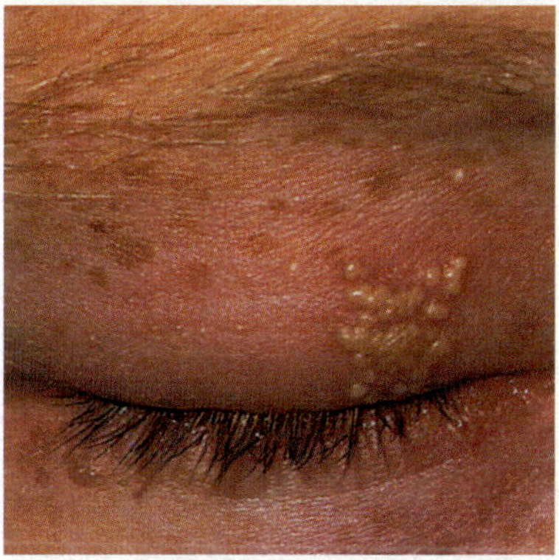

图 83　原发单纯疱疹性皮肤病损
Primary herpes simplex skin lesions

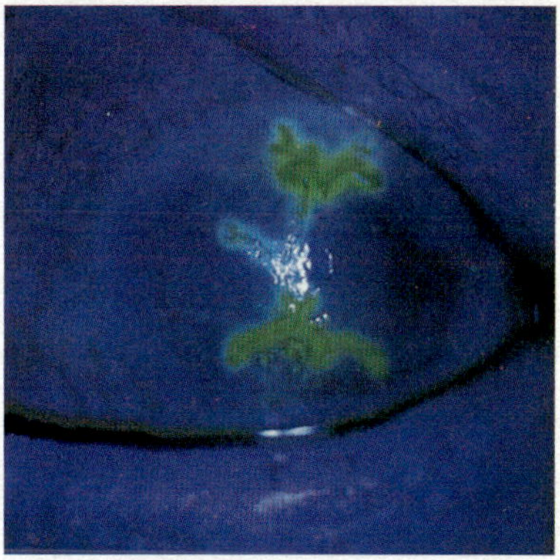

图 84　大树枝状角膜溃疡荧光素染色
Large dendritic ulcer stained with fluorescein

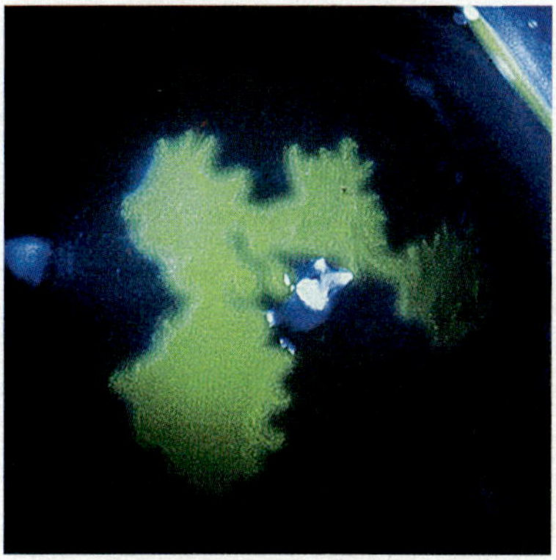

图 85　疱疹性地图状角膜溃疡荧光素染色
Geographical herpetic ulcer stained with fluorescein

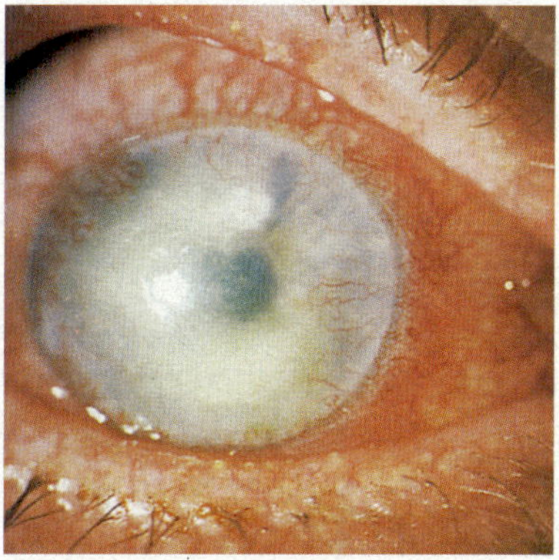

图 86　基质坏死性角膜炎
Stromal necrotic keratitis

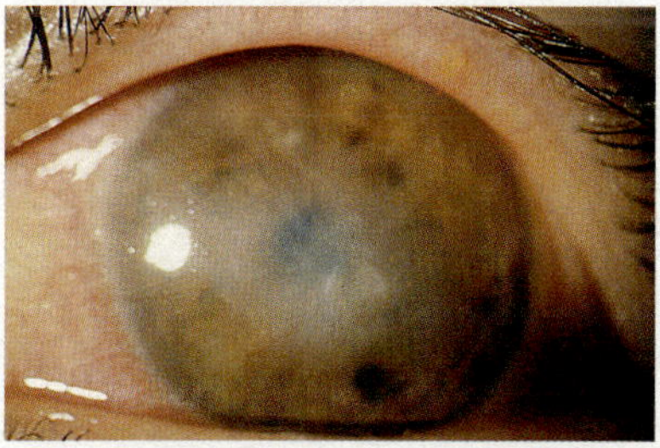

图 87　基质性角膜炎合并角膜瘢痕形成
Scarring complicating stromal keratitis

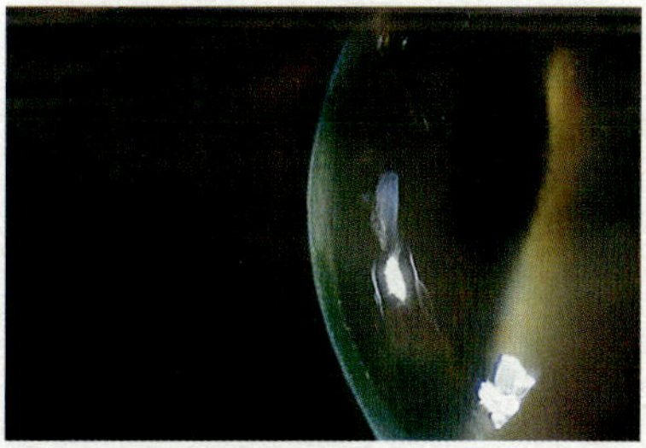

图 88　盘状角膜炎
Disciform keratitis

16 眼部带状疱疹

病因学 带状疱疹由水痘带状疱疹病毒感染所致。

定义 大约15%带状疱疹影响三叉神经眼支分布区（眼部带状疱疹）。

皮肤病损

临床特征 初期斑丘疹发展为小囊泡（小水泡），随后破裂，最终结痂。眼眶周围常出现水肿（图89）。带状疱疹后神经痛是严重，长期和痛苦的。

眼并发症

当疱疹累及以鼻为中线的一侧时，眼受累是很常见的（Hutchinson 征）。

- *结膜炎和巩膜表层炎*：很常见但很快消失。
- *急性虹膜炎*：常见，造成眼压升高和虹膜节段性萎缩（图90）。
- *急性角膜炎*：上皮点状，丝状（见图72），小树枝状，圆形（图91）和盘状（见图88）。
- *慢性角膜病损*：盘状角膜炎，继发性脂质角膜病变（图92）和神经营养性角膜炎，它可导致边缘角膜变薄（图93）和穿孔。
- *巩膜炎*（图94）：少见，常累及角膜（巩膜角膜炎）。
- *神经眼病*：视神经炎和眼肌麻痹。

治疗

- 如果早期给药，全身应用抗病毒药（如阿昔洛韦，缬昔洛韦，泛西洛韦）可减少疱疹和降低眼并发症和神经痛。
- 类固醇抗生素制剂（如氢化可的松-夫西地酸钠）适用于皮肤，对原来存在的皮肤破损是有益的。
- 治疗虹膜炎和急性角膜病变局部应用类固醇。

Herpes zoster ophthalmicus

16

Aetiology

Herpes zoster (shingles) is caused by the varicella zoster virus.

Definition

Approximately 15% of all cases of herpes zoster affect the ophthalmic division of the trigeminal nerve (herpes zoster ophthalmicus).

Clinical features

Skin lesions

An initial maculopapular rash evolves to form vesicles (small blisters), which subsequently burst to form crusting ulcers. Periorbital oedema is common (Fig. 89). Postherpetic neuralgia can be severe, chronic and very distressing.

Ocular complications

Ocular involvement is common when the rash involves the side of the nose (Hutchinson's sign).

- *Conjunctivitis and episcleritis*: very common and usually transient
- *Acute iritis*: common and may give rise to elevation of intraocular pressure and segmental iris atrophy (Fig. 90)
- *Acute keratitis*: punctate epithelial, filamentary (see Fig. 72), microdendritic, nummular (Fig. 91) and disciform (see Fig. 88)
- *Chronic corneal lesions*: mucus plaque keratitis, secondary lipid keratopathy (Fig. 92) and neurotrophic keratitis, which may lead to extreme thinning (Fig. 93) and perforation
- *Scleritis* (Fig. 94): uncommon and frequently involves the cornea (sclerokeratitis)
- *Neuro-ophthalmological*: optic neuritis and extraocular muscle palsies.

Management

- If administered early, systemic antiviral agents (e.g. aciclovir, valaciclovir, famciclovir) curtail the rash and reduce ocular complications and neuralgia
- Steroid-antibiotic preparations (e.g. hydrocortisone-fusidic acid) applied to the skin may be beneficial prior to crust separation
- Treatment of iritis and most acute corneal lesions is with topical steroids.

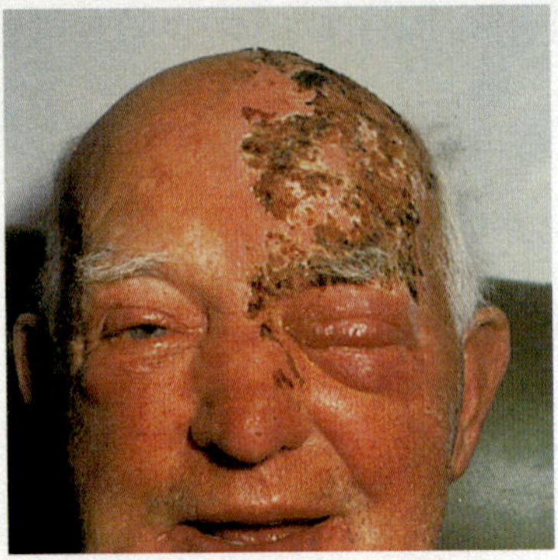

图 89　严重眼部带状疱疹
Severe herpes zoster ophthalmicus

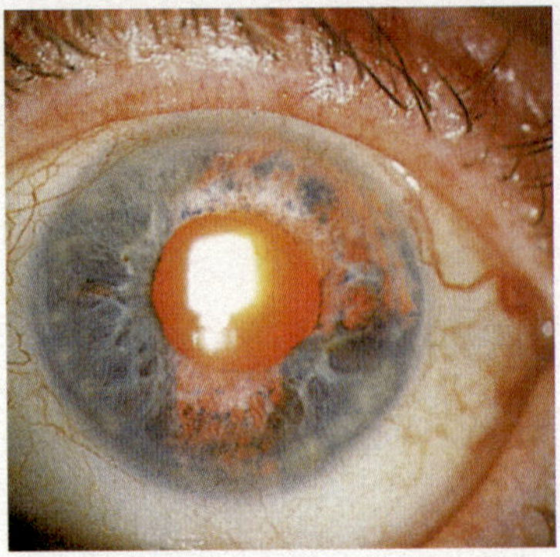

图 90　带状疱疹性虹膜炎引起虹膜节段性萎缩
Segmental iris atrophy following herpes zoster iritis

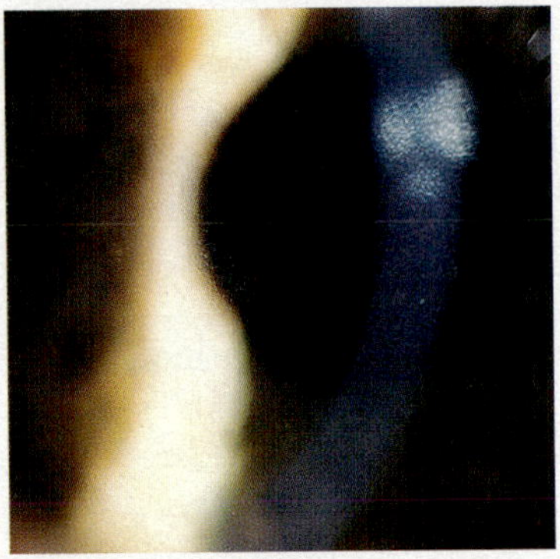

图 91　圆形角膜炎
Nummular keratitis

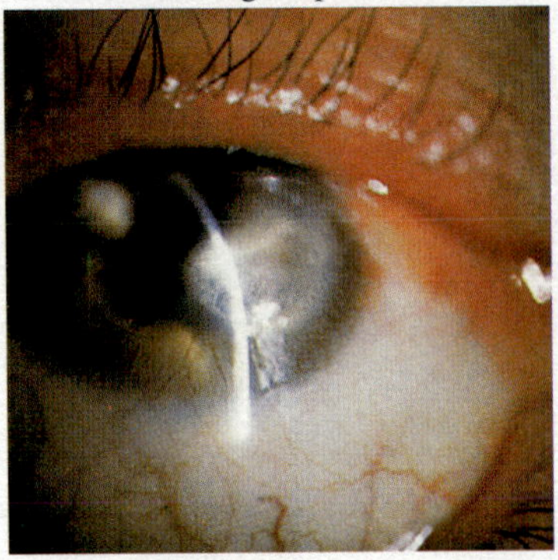

图 92　脂质角膜病
Lipid keratopathy

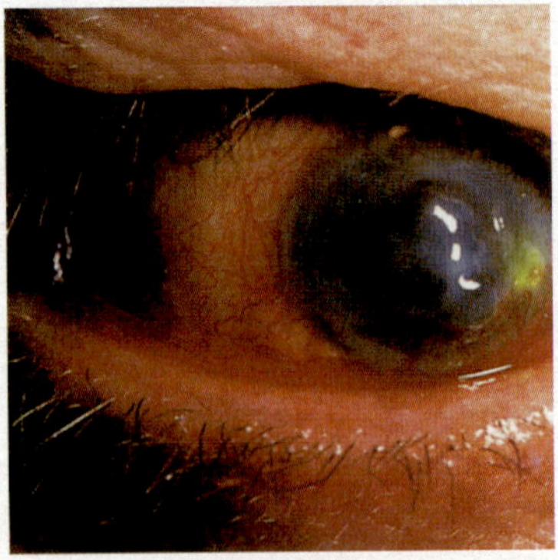

图 93　严重角膜变薄
Severe corneal thinning

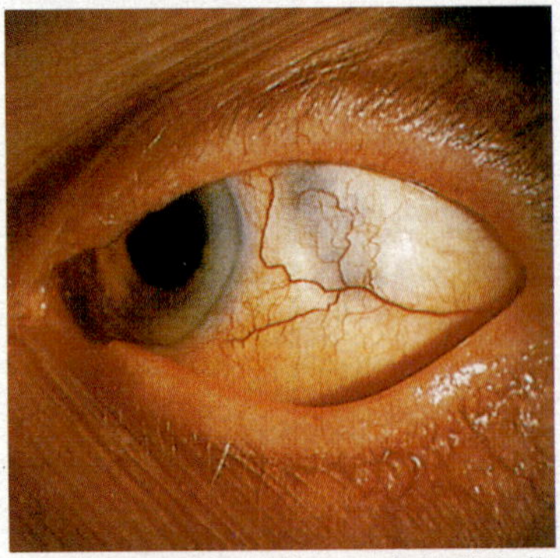

图94　陈旧性巩膜炎导致巩膜变薄
Scleral thinning due to previous scleritis

临床特征

上皮基底膜（Cogan 微囊肿性或地图状 - 点状 - 指纹状）角膜营养不良

常见，散发，无遗传表现。出现在10～30岁，复发性角膜溃疡，醒时具有异物感、流泪和畏光症状。检查可见细小的、双眼性、点状、囊状（图 95）或线状上皮损伤。

Reis-Bücklers 和 Thiel-Behnke 角膜营养不良

Bowman膜的显性遗传性营养不良，位于角膜上皮的下面，10 岁以内复发的角膜糜烂，视力逐渐下降。双眼浅表的、网状的或蜂窝状不透明浑浊（图 96）。

格子状角膜营养不良

这组（1～3型）罕见，显性遗传性营养不良，可出现在任何年龄，复发性角膜糜烂，检查可见蜘蛛网样网状构造累及基质层的前部和中部（图 97）。不同类型有不同形态。

颗粒状角膜营养不良

罕见，显性遗传，10 岁以内发病，复发性角膜糜烂。角膜基质浅层有分散的，面包渣样浑浊（图 98）。

Fuehs 内皮角膜营养不良

常散发，发病晚，初期单眼视力缺损。严重者检查可见角膜水肿——“大泡性角膜病”（图 99）。对侧眼常常出现特有的内皮变化（角膜内皮营养不良）。

治疗

- 依照角膜营养不良类型和严重程度进行多种复合治疗。
- 轻症患者应用润滑剂。
- 用绷带隐形眼镜治疗严重的角膜侵蚀和疼痛的大泡性角膜病。
- 角膜移植术（图 100）治疗重症者。

17 Corneal dystrophies

Clinical features

Epithelial basement membrane (Cogan microcystic or map-dot-fingerprint) dystrophy

Common, sporadic and non-progressive. Presents in second or third decade with recurrent corneal erosions characterized by grittiness, lacrimation and photophobia on waking. Examination shows subtle bilateral dot-like, cystic (Fig. 95) or linear epithelial lesions.

Reis-Bücklers and Thiel-Behnke dystrophies

Presentation of these dominantly inherited dystrophies of the Bowman layer, which underlies the corneal epithelium, is during the first decade of life with recurrent corneal erosions, followed later by variable blurring of vision. Bilateral superficial reticular or honeycomb-pattern opacities are seen (Fig. 96).

Lattice dystrophies

This group (types 1-3) of rare, dominantly inherited dystrophies presents at varying ages with recurrent corneal erosions. On examination a network of spidery lines involves the anterior and mid stroma (Fig. 97), the precise morphology being dependent on type.

Granular dystrophy

Rare, dominantly inherited, presenting during the first decade with recurrent erosions. Discrete, crumb-like granules are seen within the anterior stroma (Fig. 98).

Fuchs' endothelial dystrophy

Presentation of this, usually sporadic condition, is in later life with initially unilateral visual impairment. Examination shows corneal oedema - 'bullous keratopathy' if severe (Fig. 99). The fellow eye invariably shows characteristic endothelial changes (cornea guttata).

Management

- Varies according to type and severity of dystrophy
- Lubricants alone in mild cases
- Bandage contact lenses for severe erosions and painful bullous keratopathy
- Corneal grafting (Fig. 100) for advanced disease.

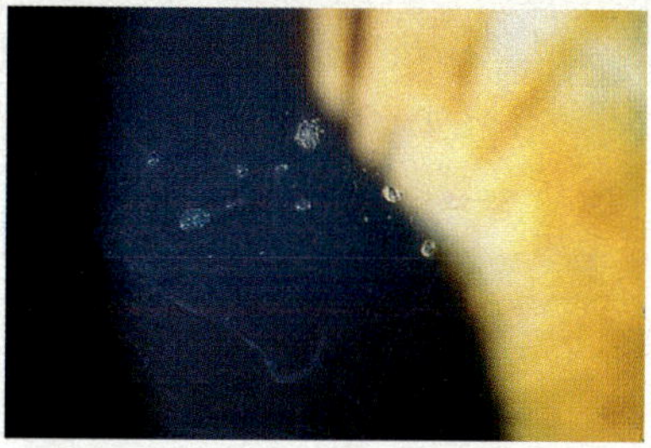

图 95　上皮基底膜营养不良
Epithelial basement membrane dystrophy

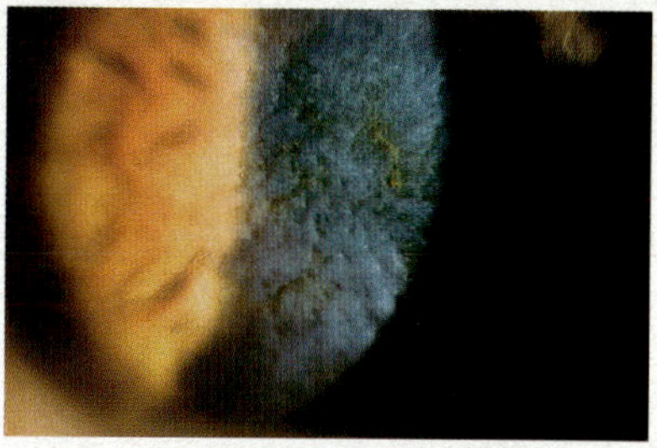

图 96　Thiel-Behnke 角膜营养不良的蜂窝状不透明浑浊
Honeycomb opacities in Thiel-Behnke dystrophy

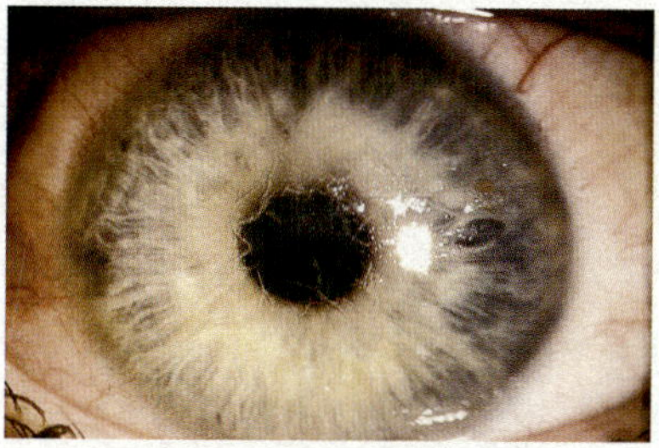

图 97　格子状角膜营养不良
Lattice dystrophy

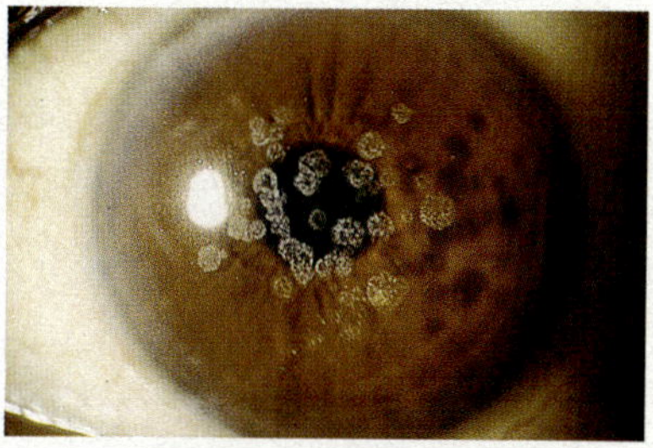

图 98　颗粒状角膜营养不良
Granular dystrophy

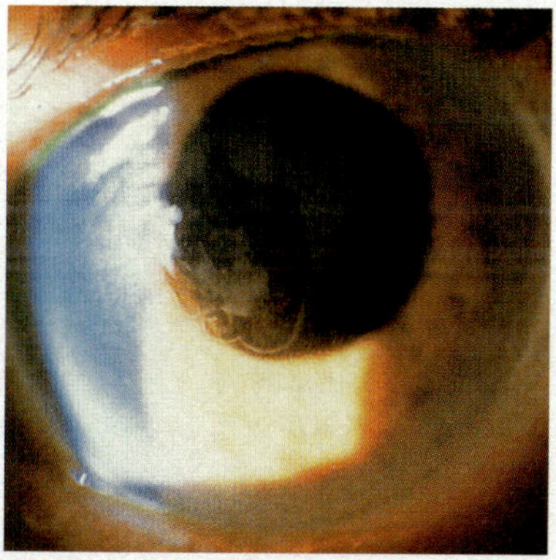

图 99　大泡性角膜病
Bullous keratopathy

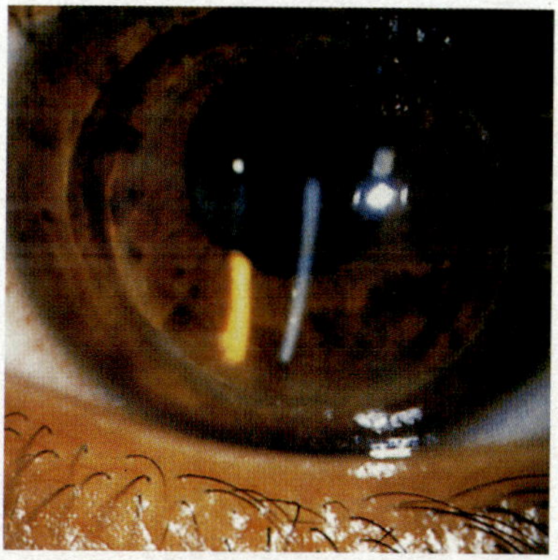

图 100　角膜移植术（穿透性角膜移植术）
Corneal graft (penetrating keratoplasty)

陷凹

临床特征 继发于局部基质脱水，常伴隆起性角膜缘损害的变薄区域（图 101）。

治疗 去除病因，促进斑片再水化作用，应用润滑剂。

边缘性角膜炎

病因学 对葡萄球菌外毒素的超敏反应。常见，常伴慢性前部睑缘炎（见图 1）。

临床特征 上皮下的浸润，将透明角膜与角膜缘分隔开（图102），常伴病变部位小的上皮缺损区域。
短时间局部应用类固醇（如 0.5% 糖皮质激素）。

酒渣鼻性角膜炎

临床特征 大约5%患者伴酒渣鼻，角膜下方上皮浸润发展为上皮下的浸润和角膜外周的血管形成（图 103）。有时会发生严重的角膜周边变薄和穿孔。

治疗
- 局部应用类固醇。
- 全身应用四环素或强力霉素。

类风湿性关节炎性角膜溃疡

临床特征 慢性，没有炎症（图104）或角膜缘急性重度炎症（图 105）。

治疗
- 润滑剂。
- 局部和全身应用类固醇。
- 另外全身应用免疫抑制剂。

Mooren 角膜溃疡

临床治疗 罕见但严重，疼痛，单眼或双眼，可向周边或中心发展（图 106）。

Peripheral corneal ulceration

Dellen

Clinical features

An area of thinning secondary to local stromal dehydration, most frequently associated with an elevated limbal lesion (Fig. 101).

Management

Eliminate the cause and promote rehydration by patching and lubricants.

Marginal keratitis

Aetiology

Hypersensitivity to staphylococcal exotoxins. Very common and frequently associated with chronic anterior blepharitis (see Fig. 1).

Clinical features

Subepithelial infiltrate, separated from the limbus by clear cornea (Fig. 102), often with an overlying smaller area of epithelial breakdown.

Management

Short course of topical steroids (e.g. fluorometholone, prednisolone 0.5%).

Rosacea keratitis

Clinical features

Occurs in about 5% of patients with acne rosacea. Inferior punctate epitheliopathy that may progress to subepithelial infiltration and peripheral vascularization (Fig. 103). Occasionally severe peripheral thinning and perforation may occur.

Management

- Topical steroids
- Systemic tetracycline or doxycycline.

Ulceration associated with rheumatoid arthritis

Clinical features

May be chronic, without inflammation (Fig.104) or acute and associated with severe inflammation at the limbus (Fig.105).

Management

- Lubricants
- Topical and systemic steroids
- Other systemic immunosuppressants.

Mooren's ulcer

Clinical features

Very rare but serious, painful condition that may be unilateral or bilateral and may spread circumferentially or centrally (Fig.106).

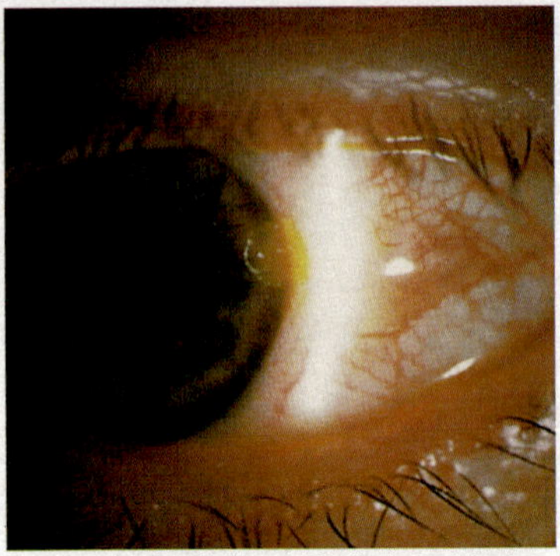

图 101　角膜陷凹的荧光素染色
Corneal dellen stained with fluorescein

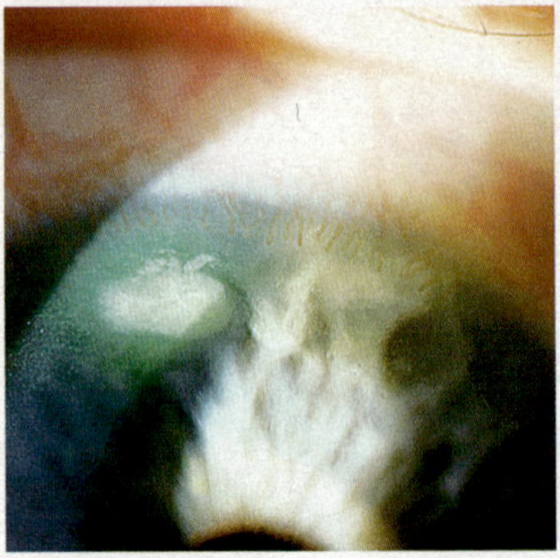

图 102　边缘性角膜炎
Marginal keratitis

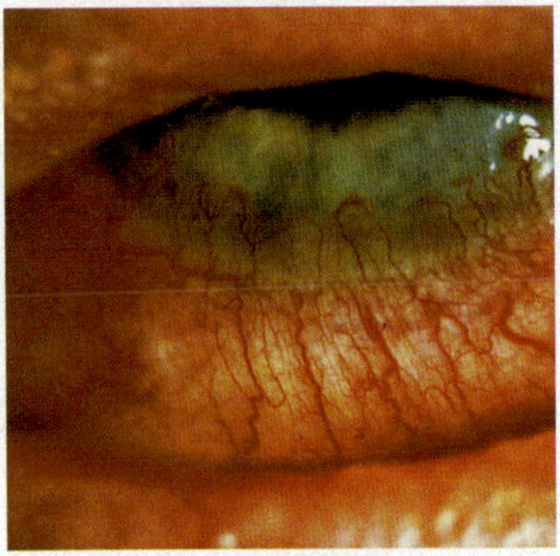

图 103　酒渣鼻性角膜炎
Rosacea keratitis

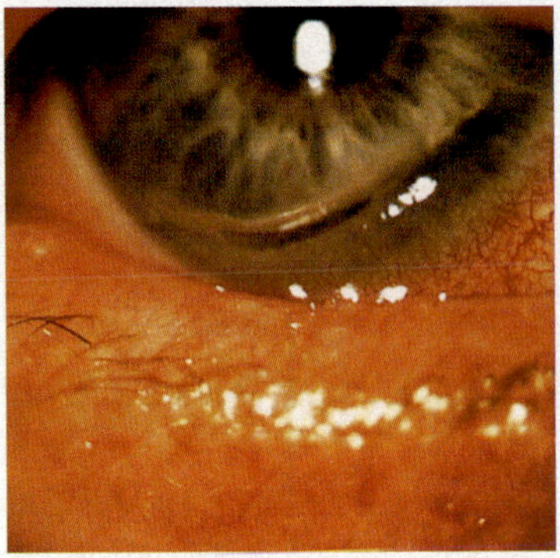

图 104　类风湿性关节炎性角膜溶解
Corneal melting in rheumatoid arthritis

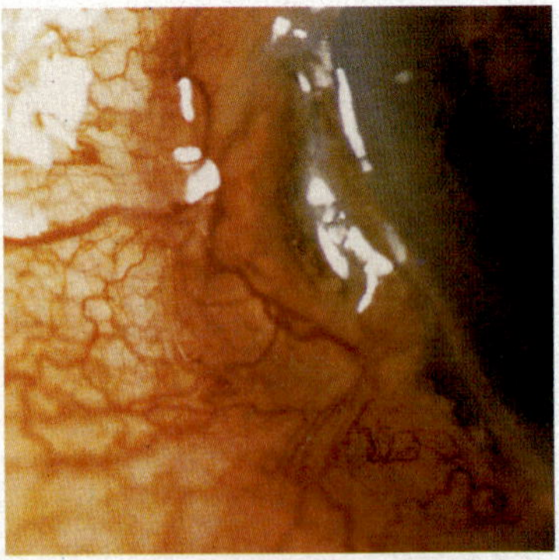

图 105　类风湿性关节炎性急性角膜溃疡
Acute corneal ulceration in rheumatoid arthritis

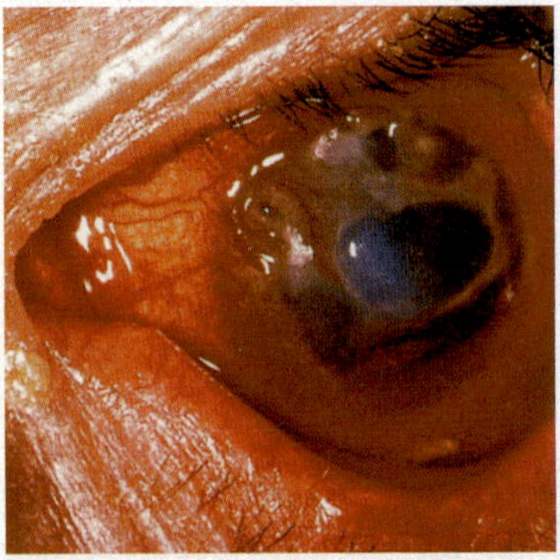

图 106　进行性蚕食性角膜溃疡
Advanced Mooren's ulcer

角膜大小和形状异常

圆锥角膜

临床特征

角膜中央锥形前凸（图 107），发病于 10 ~ 30 岁，慢性，由于不规则散光进行性视力下降。几乎所有患者双眼受累，双眼经常不对称。

早期体征 包括检眼镜检查异常，视网膜检影时瞳孔光带出现不规则的“剪刀状”表现和角膜基质层可见细的垂直线（Vogt 条纹，图 108）。

晚期体征 包括圆锥基底铁沉着物（Fleischer 环）。向下注视时，下眼睑出现一个弯曲（Munson征，图 109）。中央部突然发作角膜水肿（急性水肿，图109）和瘢痕形成。

全身影响 特发性皮炎，成骨不全；Down，Turner，Ehlers-Danlos，Marfan 综合征 。

治疗

- 早期可用眼镜进行屈光矫正。
- 进展期可用隐形眼镜矫正。
- 后期行角膜移植术。
- 急性水肿可行支持性疗法。

球形角膜

罕见，先天性颞骨变薄畸形和整个角膜突出（图 110）。所有病例均出现急性水肿。

大角膜

罕见，X 连锁隐性遗传，角膜直径超过 13 mm（图 111）。可发生晶状体半脱位。

小角膜

角膜直径小于 10 mm。

分类

- *真性小角膜*：眼球大小正常。
- *巩膜化角膜*：角膜周边被巩膜遮盖而显得小。
- *小眼球*：小畸形眼球（图 112）。
- *短眼轴*：因为眼轴短有严重的远视，在其他方面正常。

19 Disorders of corneal size and shape

Keratoconus

Clinical features

Fairly common cone-like bulging of the central cornea (Fig. 107), presenting during the second or third decades of life with slowly progressive blurring of vision from irregular astigmatism. Both eyes are affected in almost all cases, though often asymmetrically.

Early signs Include abnormal ophthalmoscopy reflex, irregular 'scissors' retinoscopy reflex and fine vertical lines in the deep stroma (Vogt striae - Fig. 108).

Late signs Include iron deposits at the base of the cone (Fleischer ring), bulging of the lower lid in downgaze (Munson sign - Fig. 109), central corneal oedema of sudden onset (acute hydrops - Fig. 109) and scarring.

Systemic associations Include atopic dermatitis, osteogenesis imperfecta; syndromes - Down's, Turner's, Ehlers-Danlos, Marfan's.

Management

- Refractive correction with spectacles is initially adequate
- As progression occurs, correction with contact lenses
- Corneal grafting in advanced cases
- Supportive treatment for acute hydrops.

Keratoglobus

Very rare congenital bilateral thinning and protrusion of the entire cornea (Fig. 110). Acute hydrops may occur in some cases.

Megalocornea

Very rare, X-linked recessive condition with corneal diameters over 13mm (Fig. 111). May develop lens subluxation.

Microcornea

Corneal diameters of less than 10mm.

Classification

- *True microcornea*: globe of normal dimensions.
- *Sclerocornea*: 'scleralization' of the peripheral cornea makes it appear small
- *Microphthalmos*: small variably malformed globe (Fig. 112)
- *Nanophthalmos*: severe hypermetropia because of short axial length, but otherwise normal.

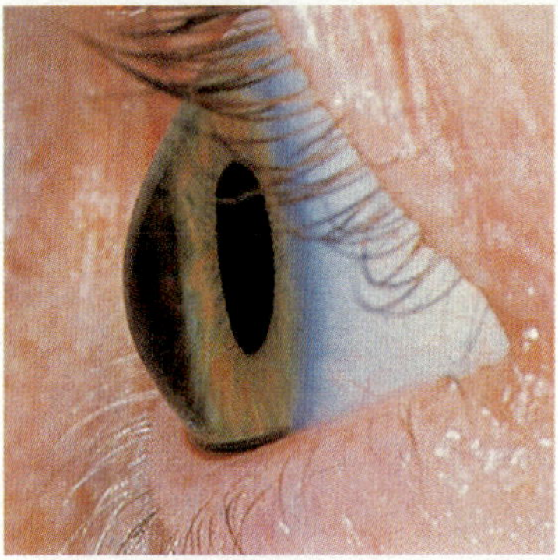

图 107 圆锥角膜
Keratoconus

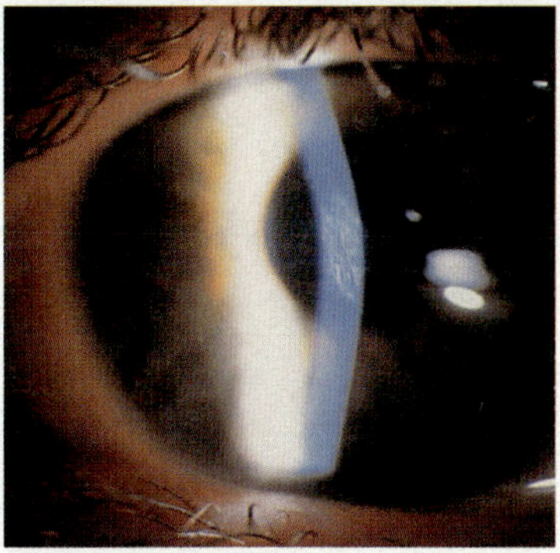

图 108 Vogt 条纹
Vogt's striae

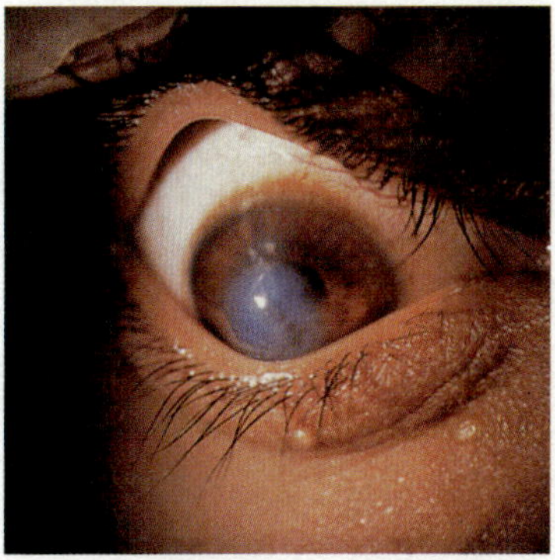

图 109 眼部 Munson 征伴随急性水肿
Munson's sign in an eye with acute hydrops

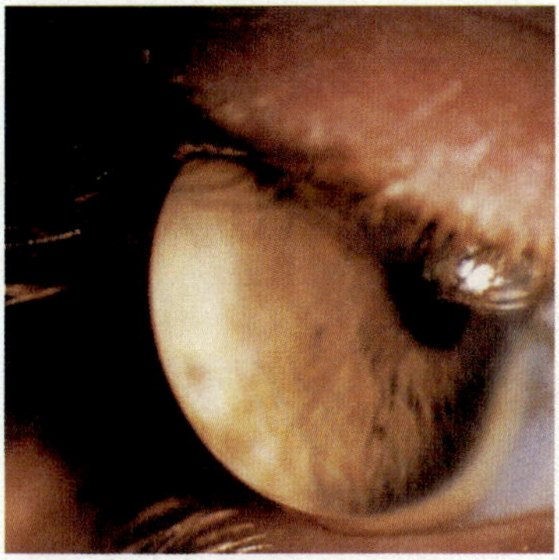

图 110 球形角膜
Keratoglobus

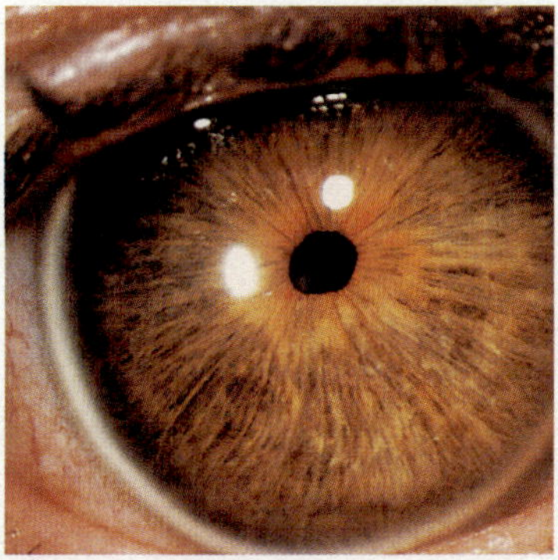

图 111 大角膜
Megalocornea

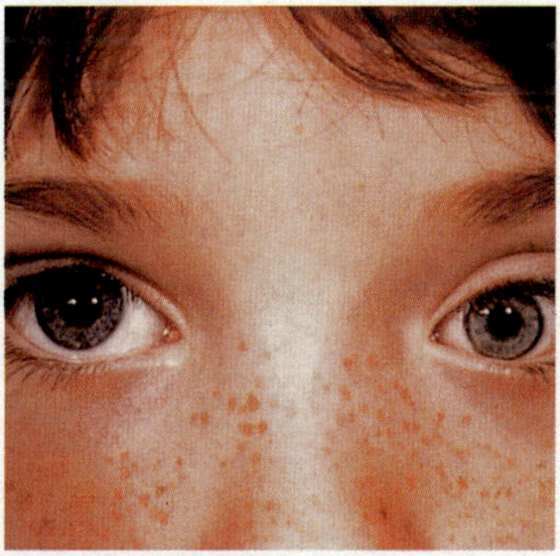

图 112 左侧小眼
Left microphthalmos

表层巩膜炎和巩膜炎

表层巩膜炎

临床特征 常见，愈后不留痕迹，单眼的充血和轻度的不适。

分类
- 结节性（图 113）。
- 弥漫性（图 114）。

治疗 治疗不是必须的。如果治疗，局部应用类固醇和全身应用其他的抗炎药。

巩膜炎

较表层巩膜炎更深层的炎症，症状更严重，常有全身病。

病因学 常为原发性的，但也可由于眼手术引起或是合并带状疱疹或全身性疾病引起，例如类风湿性关节炎、Wegener 肉芽肿和结节性多发性动脉炎。

分类 *非坏死性前巩膜炎* 这是最常见的类型，为结节性（图 115）或弥漫性。

坏死性前巩膜炎 罕见，局限性巩膜充血和坏死引起疼痛（图 116）。

穿通性巩膜软化 罕见，患者多为女性，伴有类风湿性关节炎。具有特征性的非炎性斑，巩膜坏死后暴露下面的葡萄膜（图 117）。自发性穿孔少见，但可由于外伤引发。治疗无特效疗法。

后巩膜炎

临床特征 少见，诊断困难。体征包括眼球突出，眼肌麻痹，视盘水肿，脉络膜褶（见图40）和葡萄膜的渗出（图118）。

治疗
- 全身应用非甾体抗炎剂。
- 局部和 / 或全身应用类固醇。
- 免疫抑制剂。

Episcleritis and scleritis

Episcleritis

Clinical features

This very common and innocuous condition presents with unilateral redness and slight discomfort.

Classification

- Nodular (Fig. 113)
- Diffuse (Fig. 114).

Management

Treatment is often not required. If necessary, topical steroids and systemic non-steroidal anti-inflammatory agents.

Scleritis

Deeper inflammation than episcleritis, with more severe symptoms and frequent systemic association.

Aetiology

Often idiopathic, but may follow eye surgery or be associated with herpes zoster or systemic disease such as rheumatoid arthritis, Wegener's granulomatosis and polyarteritis nodosa.

Classification

Anterior non-necrotizing The most common type may be nodular (Fig. 115) or diffuse.

Anterior necrotizing with inflammation Is a rare and painful condition characterized by local scleral injection and necrosis (Fig. 116). May be complicated by keratitis and anterior uveitis.

Scleromalacia perforans Is rare and typically occurs in women with rheumatoid arthritis. It is characterized by uninflamed patches of scleral necrosis that expose the underlying uvea (Fig. 117). Spontaneous perforation is rare but may occur as a result of trauma. No benefit has been demonstrated from treatment.

Posterior scleritis

Clinical features

Uncommon and may be difficult to diagnose. Signs include proptosis, ophthalmoplegia, optic disc swelling, choroidal folds (see Fig. 40) and uveal effusion (Fig. 118).

Management

- Systemic non-steroidal anti-inflammatory agents
- Topical and/or systemic steroids
- Other immunosuppressive agents.

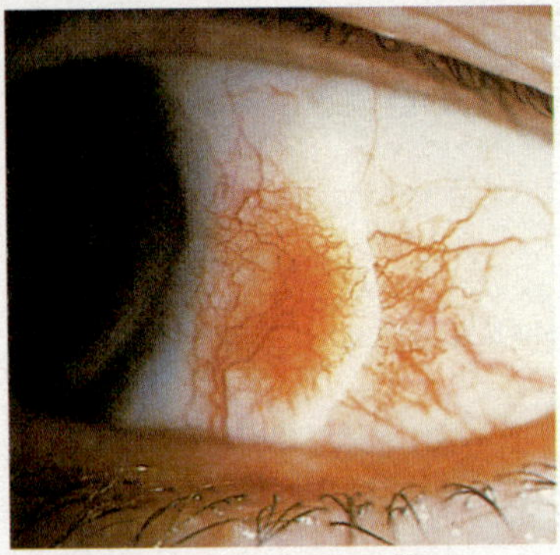

图 113　结节性表层巩膜炎
Nodular episcleritis

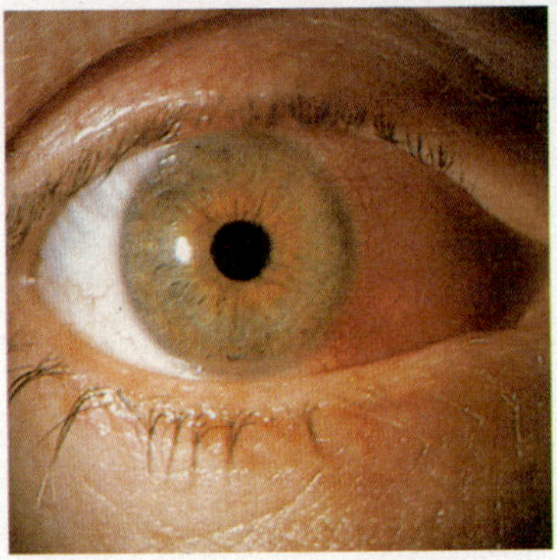

图 114　弥漫性表层巩膜炎
Diffuse episcleritis

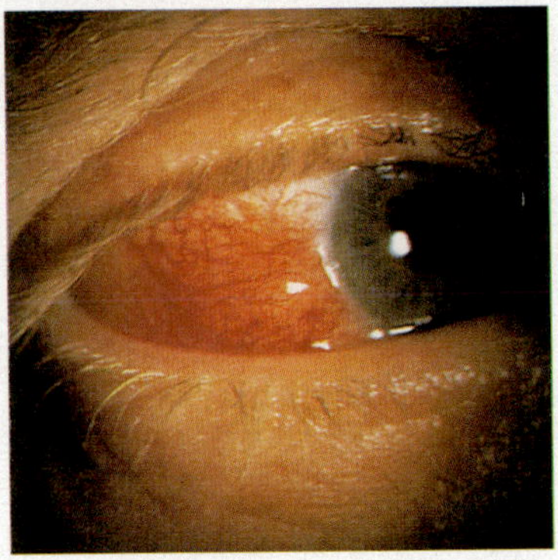

图 115　非坏死性结节性前巩膜炎
Anterior non-necrotizing nodular scleritis

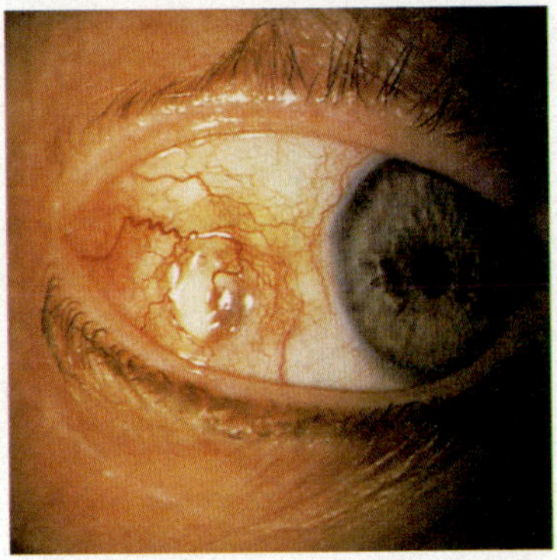

图 116　坏死性前巩膜炎合并感染
Anterior necrotizing scleritis with inflammation

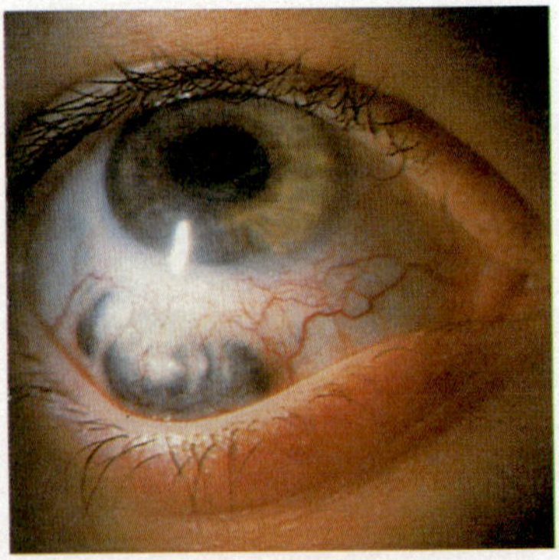

图 117　穿通性巩膜软化
Scleromalacia perforans

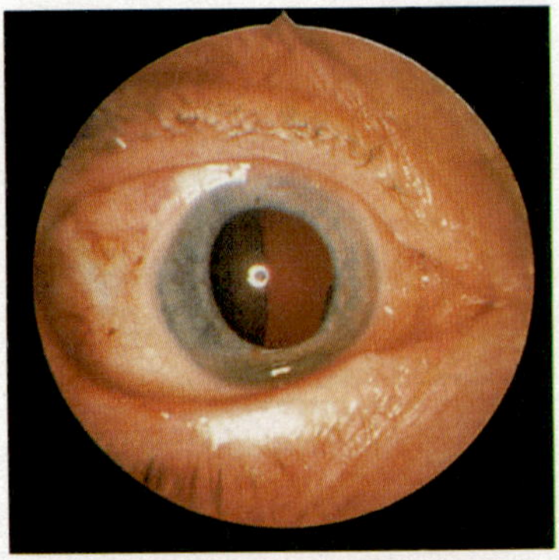

图 118　巩膜炎的葡萄膜渗出
Uveal effusion in scleritis

前葡萄膜炎

病因学

常为原发性，但是很多全身病及原因均可引起。

- *HLA-B27 阳性*：强直性脊柱炎，Reiter 综合征，牛皮癣性关节炎。
- *青少年原发性关节炎*：如果小关节发病和ANA-阳性，高危发病。
- *肠炎*：溃疡性结肠炎，Crohn 疾病。
- *非传染性的全身性疾病*：结节病，Behçet 病，Vogt-小柳 - 原田综合征。
- *传染病*：带状疱疹和单纯疱疹、梅毒、肺结核。
- *原发性*：Fuchs 虹膜异色性虹膜睫状体炎。

临床特征

症状

- 急性虹膜炎：亚急性发病，畏光、发红、疼痛和视力下降；常单眼发病。
- 慢性前葡萄膜炎：最初可能无症状或症状轻微。

体征

- *急性虹膜炎*：角膜周围（睫状）充血，小瞳孔，细小角膜后沉着物（“KP”）（图 119，120），房水闪光（图 120）和细胞，白色“液平”（眼前房积脓 图121）和重度炎症的纤维蛋白性渗出物。
- *慢性前葡萄膜炎*：常无充血或轻度充血，大量KP（“羊脂”状KP出现在肉芽肿性炎症，如伯克肉样瘤），房水闪光（图120）和细胞（常比急性虹膜炎的少），虹膜小结（在肉芽肿内）。

分类

- 虹膜 - 晶状体粘连（虹膜后粘连，图 122）。
- 角膜钙沉积（带状角膜病，图 123）。
- 白内障（图 123）。
- 青光眼。
- 视力丧失，眼球萎缩（眼球痨，图124）在慢性葡萄膜炎末期出现。

治疗

- 局部应用类固醇和散瞳剂是主要的治疗。
- 眼周的类固醇注射。
- 全身应用类固醇，免疫抑制剂和抗生素治疗传染病（如肺结核，梅毒）。

21 Anterior uveitis

Aetiology

Commonly idiopathic but numerous systemic associations/ causes:

- *HLA-B27-associated*: ankylosing spondylitis, Reiter's syndrome, psoriatic arthritis
- *Juvenile idiopathic arthritis*: especially high-risk if pauciarticular-onset and ANA-positive
- *Inflammatory bowel disease*: ulcerative colitis, Crohn's disease
- *Non-infectious systemic diseases*: sarcoidosis, Behçet's disease, Vogt-Koyanagi-Harada syndrome
- *Infections*: herpes zoster and simplex, syphilis, tuberculosis
- *Idiopathic*: Fuchs' uveitis syndrome.

Clinical features

Symptoms

- *Acute iritis*: subacute onset of photophobia, redness, pain and blurred vision; usually unilateral
- *Chronic anterior uveitis*: symptoms may initially be absent or mild.

Signs

- *Acute iritis*: circumcorneal (ciliary) injection, small pupil, fine keratic precipitates ('KPs' - Figs 119, 120), aqueous flare (Fig. 120) and cells, white 'fluid level' (hypopyon - Fig. 121) and fibrinous exudate in severe inflammation
- *Chronic anterior uveitis*: usually little or no injection, KPs typically large ('mutton fat' in granulomatous inflammation, e.g. sarcoidosis), aqueous flare (Fig. 120) and cells (often fewer than in acute iritis), iris nodules (in granulomatous).

Complications

- Iris-lens adhesions (posterior synechiae - Fig. 122)
- Corneal calcium deposition (band keratopathy - Fig. 123)
- Cataract (Fig. 123)
- Glaucoma
- A blind, soft and shrunken globe (phthisis bulbi - Fig. 124) in end stage chronic uveitis.

Management

- Topical steroids and mydriatics are the mainstay of treatment
- Periocular steroid injection
- Systemic steroids, immunosuppressive agents and antibiotics for infections (e.g. tuberculosis, syphilis).

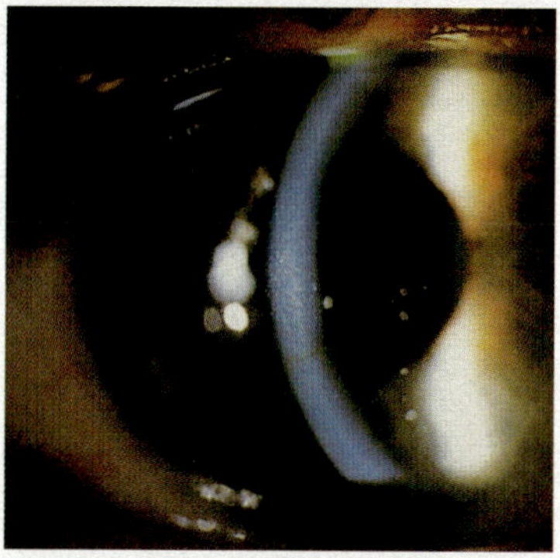

图 119　慢性前葡萄膜炎的角膜后沉着物
Keratic precipitates in chronic anterior uveitis

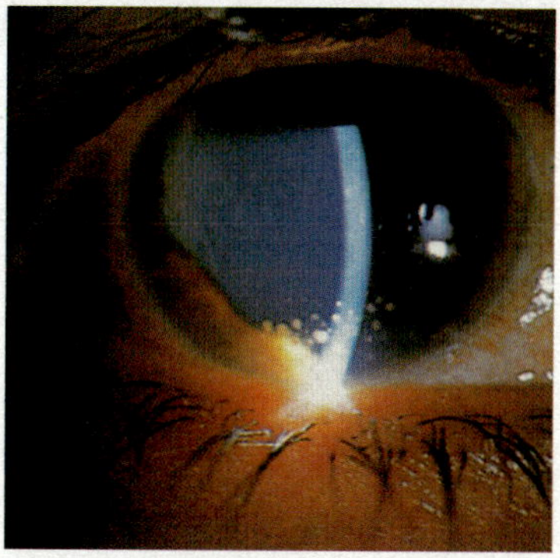

图 120　房水闪光和大角膜后大的沉着物
Aqueous flare and large keratic precipitates

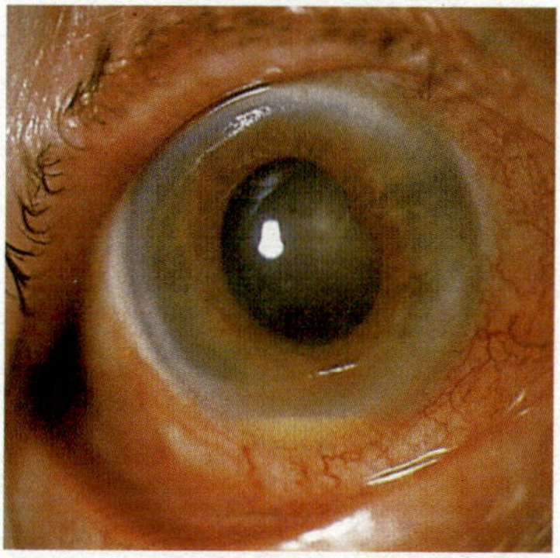

图 121　严重急性前葡萄膜炎的前房积脓
Hypopyon in severe acute anterior uveitis

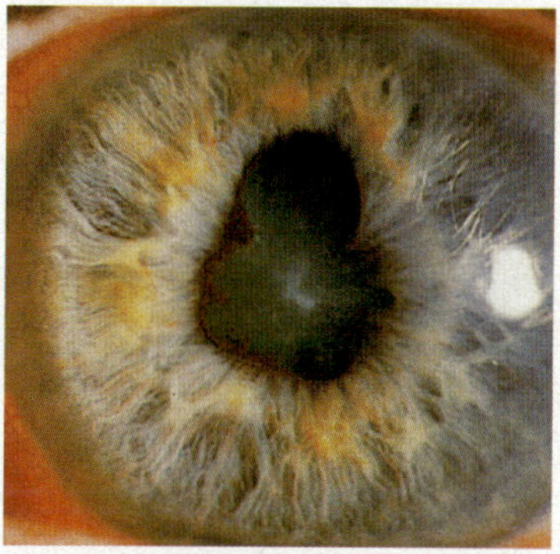

图 122　虹膜和晶状体之间粘连（虹膜后粘连）
Adhesions between the lens and iris (posterior synechiae)

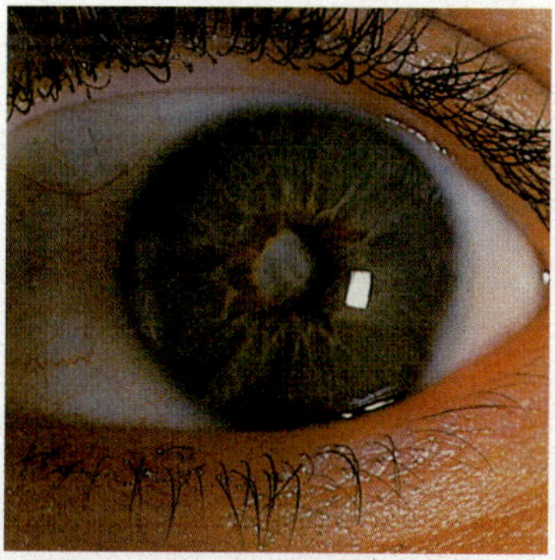

图 123　带状角膜病和白内障
Band keratopathy and cataract

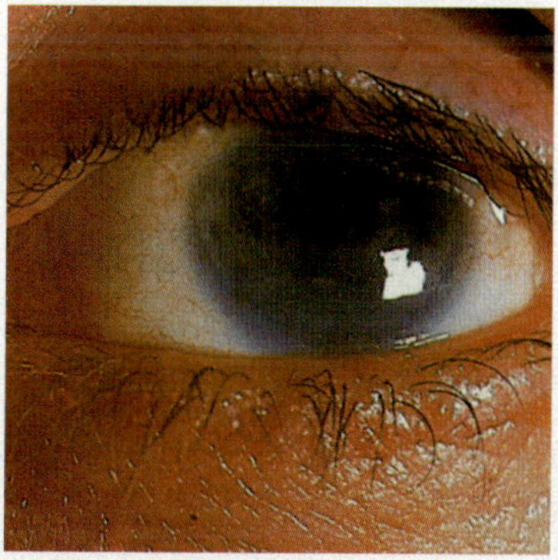

图 124　眼球痨
Phthisis bulbi

感染性后葡萄膜炎

弓形体病

病因学 出生前感染的弓形体原虫复活。

临床特征 亚急性发病，单眼玻璃体漂浮物。检查可见中等到严重的玻璃体炎伴随邻近的视网膜炎，发展至陈旧瘢痕（图125）。

治疗 用抗生素和全身应用类固醇治疗视力损害。对丧失免疫力的患者需特殊治疗。

弓蛔虫病

病因学 罕见，在肠内感染犬弓蛔虫的幼虫。

临床特征

- *后极肉芽肿*：出现一眼低视力。
- *周边肉芽肿*：出现黄斑和视盘的病变（图126）或牵引性视网膜脱离（图127）。
- *慢性眼内炎*：白瞳（见图232），斜视或视力丧失。

治疗 视网膜脱离可考虑行玻璃体切割术。

巨细胞病毒（CMV）性视网膜炎

多发于艾滋病（AIDS）患者，新药治疗较少。

临床特征 视网膜坏死的黄白色区域伴有出血和轻度玻璃体炎（图128）。病变蔓延至血管可累及视盘（图129）。

治疗 全身应用抗病毒药，玻璃体内注射或玻璃体内植入缓释片。

组织胞浆菌病

病因学 真菌夹膜组织胞浆菌的感染。

临床特征 脉络膜视网膜瘢痕（组织斑），边缘锐，视盘周围萎缩（图130）和脉络膜新生血管形成（CNV），不伴随玻璃体炎。

治疗 激光凝固或手术治疗CNV。

Toxoplasmosis

Aetiology Reactivation of prenatal infection with the protozoan *Toxoplasma gondii.*

Clinical features Subacute onset of unilateral vitreous floaters. Examination shows a moderate to severe vitreitis is associated with a solitary focus of retinitis adjacent to an old scar (Fig. 125).

Management Treatment of vision-threatening lesions is with antimicrobial agents and systemic steroids. Special considerations apply to immunocompromised patients.

Toxocariasis

Aetiology Rare infection caused by the common intestinal worm of dogs *Toxocara canis*.

Clinical features

- *Posterior pole granuloma*: presents with poor vision in one eye
- *Peripheral granuloma*: presents with distortion of the macula or disc (Fig. 126) or tractional retinal detachment (Fig. 127)
- *Chronic endophthalmitis*: presents with leukocoria (see Fig. 232), strabismus or visual loss.

Management Vitrectomy may be considered for retinal detachment.

Cytomegalovirus (CMV) retinitis

Common in patients with AIDS, though less so with the introduction of newer drug regimens.

Clinical features Yellow-white areas of retinal necrosis associated with variable haemorrhage and mild vitreitis (Fig. 128). The lesions spread along the vascular arcades and may involve the optic nerve head (Fig. 129).

Management Antiviral agents administered systemically, or intravitreally by injection or a slow-release implant.

Histoplasmosis

Aetiology Infection with the fungus *Histoplasma capsulatum*.

Clinical features Punched-out chorioretinal scars ('histo spots'), peripapillary atrophy (Fig. 130) and macular choroidal neovascularization (CNV); no associated vitreitis.

Management Laser photocoagulation or surgery may be appropriate for the CNV.

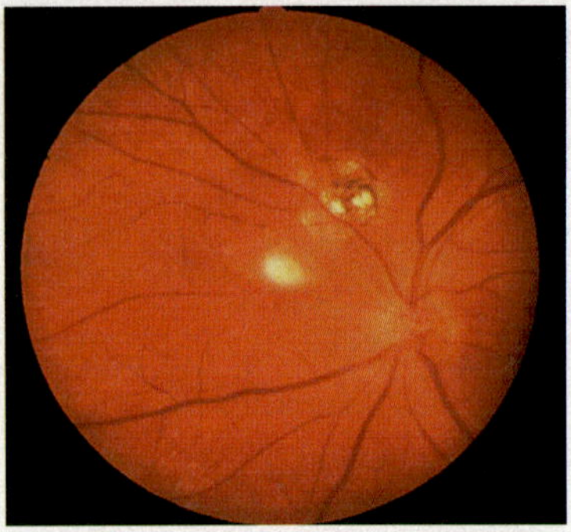

图 125　活化的视网膜弓形体病
Active retinal toxoplasmosis

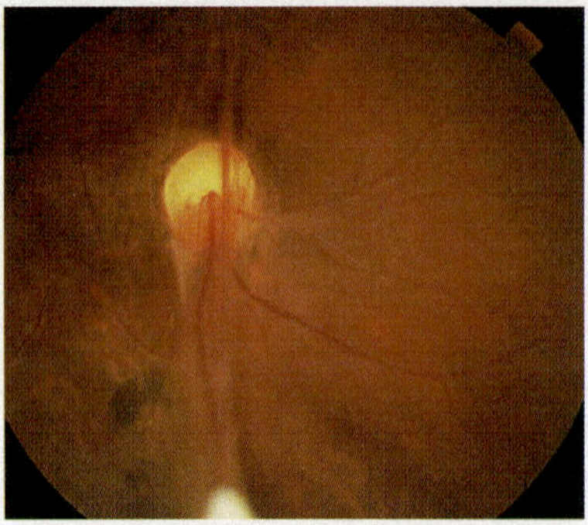

图 126　周边弓蛔虫病肉芽肿
Peripheral *Toxocara* granuloma

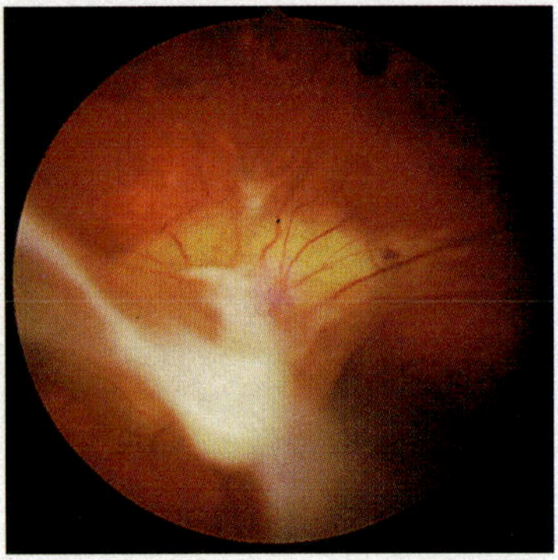

图 127　眼弓蛔虫病的牵引性视网膜脱离
Tractional retinal detachment in ocular toxocariasis

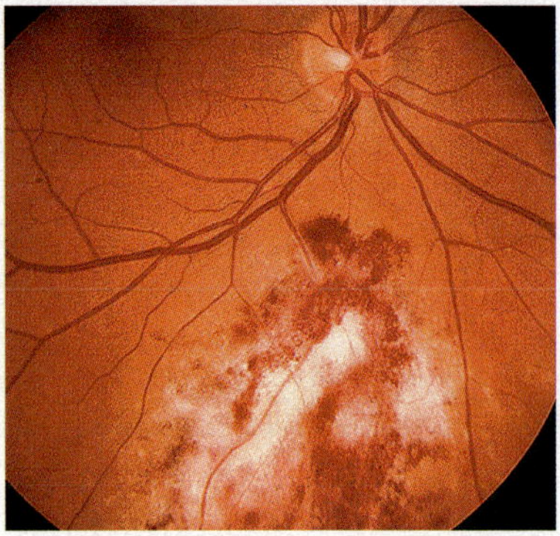

图 128　巨细胞病毒性视网膜炎
Cytomegalovirus retinitis

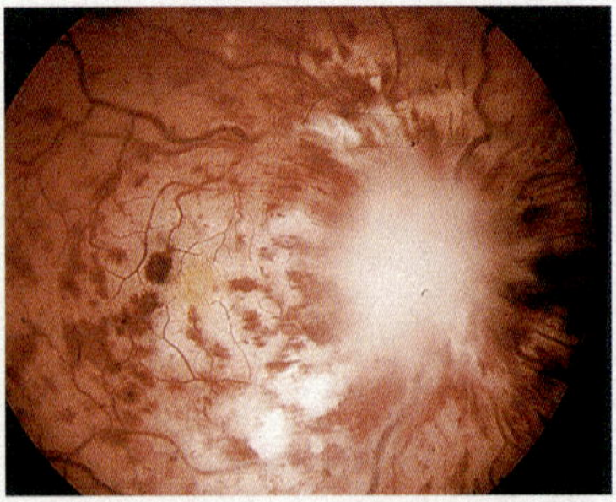

图 129　陈旧性巨细胞病毒性视网膜炎累及视神经
Advanced cytomegalovirus retinitis with optic nerve involvement

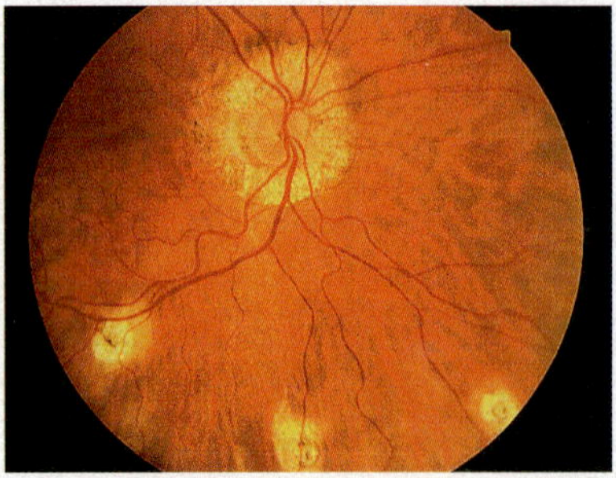

图 130　眼组织胞浆菌病
Ocular histoplasmosis

中间葡萄膜炎

临床特征 较常见，双眼发病，儿童和青少年睫状体平坦部和视网膜周边慢性原发性炎症（扁平部睫状体炎），渐增的玻璃体漂浮物。检查可见玻璃体炎（图 131），睫状体平坦部下方常见渗出（“雪堤”）。

并发症
- 慢性囊样黄斑水肿（视力下降的主要原因）。
- 白内障。

治疗 囊样黄斑水肿造成视力下降时眼周注射类固醇。

结节病

临床特征 多为特发性疾病，具有特征性的多系统肉芽肿性炎症。前葡萄膜炎常见（见 61页）；基本体征包括静脉周围炎（“烛心”，图 132），视网膜的、脉络膜的（图 133）、视神经肉芽肿（图134）和周边视网膜新生血管形成。

治疗 全身应用类固醇。

Behçet 病

临床特征 特发性的多系统疾病，具有特征性的复发性口腔粘膜溃疡，生殖器溃疡和皮肤损害。眼部特征包括静脉周围炎，它可致静脉闭塞（图135）、视网膜炎、黄斑水肿和视神经萎缩（图 136）。

治疗 全身应用类固醇和免疫抑制剂。

23 Non-infectious intermediate and posterior uveitis

Intermediate uveitis

Clinical features

Relatively common, often bilateral, chronic idiopathic inflammation of the pars plana (pars planitis) and retinal periphery of children and young adults, presenting with gradually increasing vitreous floaters. Examination shows vitreitis (Fig. 131), often accompanied by exudate on the inferior pars plana ('snowbanking').

Complications

- Chronic cystoid macular oedema (main cause of severe visual loss)
- Cataract.

Management

Periocular depot steroid injection when visual acuity is reduced by cystoid macular oedema.

Sarcoidosis

Clinical features

Common idiopathic disease characterized by multisystem granulomatous inflammation. Anterior uveitis is common (see page 62); fundus signs include periphlebitis ('candlewax drippings' - Fig. 132) and retinal, choroidal (Fig. 133) and optic nerve granulomata (Fig. 134) and peripheral retinal neovascularization.

Management

Systemic steroids.

Behçet's disease

Clinical features

Uncommon idiopathic multisystem disease characterized by aphthous oral ulceration, recurrent genital ulceration and skin lesions. Ocular features include periphlebitis, which may result in venous occlusion (Fig. 135), retinitis, macular oedema and optic atrophy (Fig. 136).

Management

Systemic steroids and immunosuppressive agents.

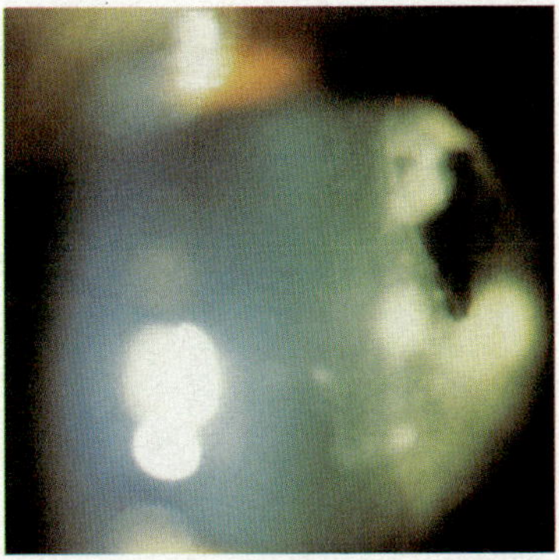

图 131 中间葡萄膜炎的严重玻璃体炎
Severe vitreitis in intermediate uveitis

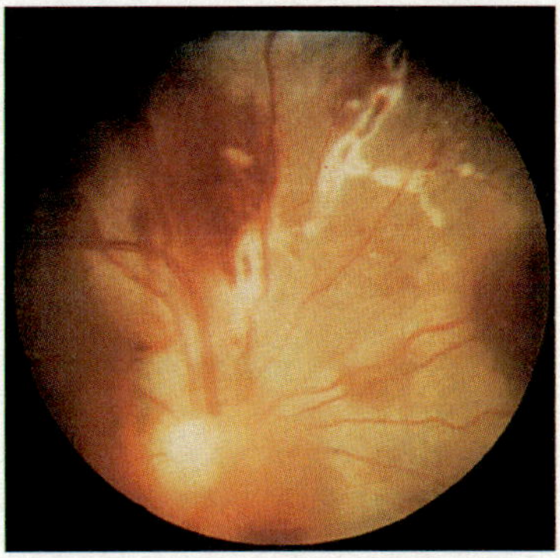

图 132 视网膜血管炎伴发“烛心”血管周围渗出
Retinal vasculitis with 'candlewax' perivascular exudates

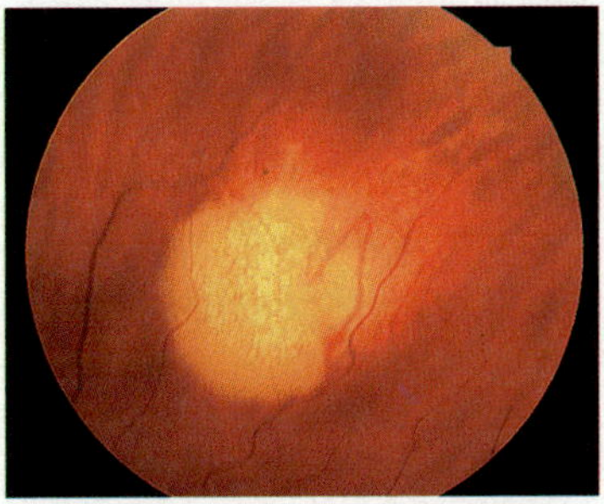

图 133 脉络膜结节性肉芽肿
Choroidal sarcoid granulomas

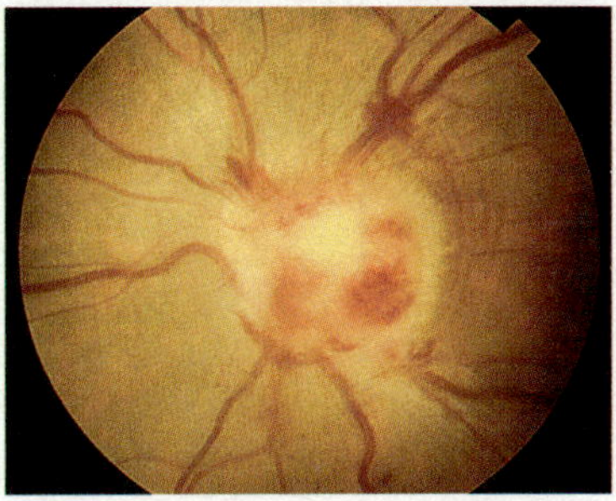

图 134 视盘结节性肉芽肿
Optic nerve head sarcoid granuloma

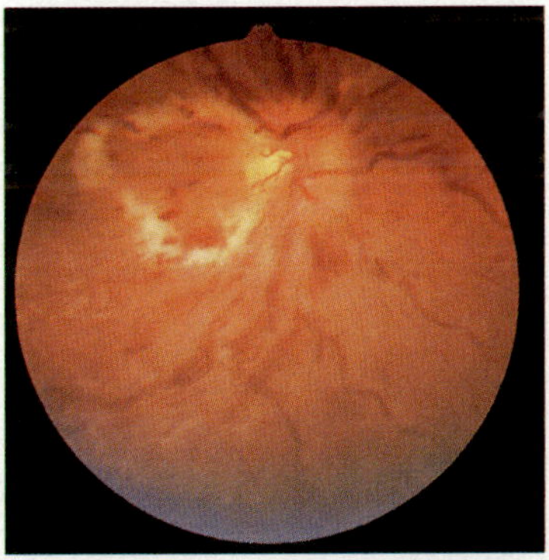

图 135 Behçet 病严重的静脉周围炎伴随静脉闭塞
Severe periphlebitis with venous occlusion in Behçet's disease

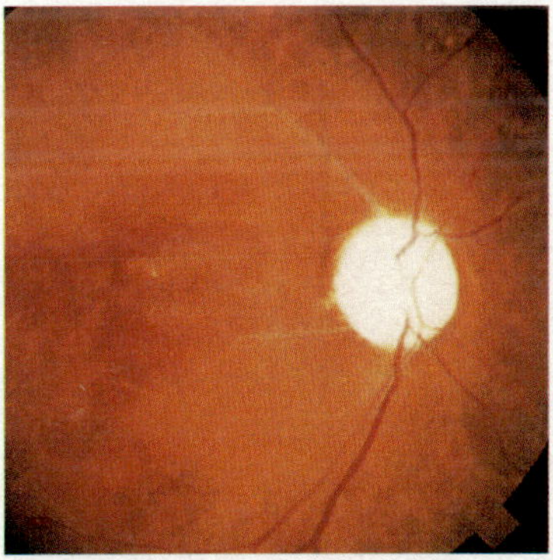

图 136 Behçet 视神经萎缩
Optic atrophy in Behçet's disease

24 原发性多病灶白色点状综合征

"白色点状综合征"是用于一组异质、罕见，原因不明的累及后节的炎症，见下面的例子。

鸟枪弹样视网膜脉络膜病

临床特征

罕见、原发的慢性双眼病变，多发于中年女性，HLA-A29遗传性。早期损害包括多发的、深的、扁平的乳脂状的斑，从视盘向外呈放射状（图 137），伴血管炎和玻璃体炎。这些可致局限的白色萎缩区（图 138）。囊样的黄斑水肿很多见，最终发展为视神经萎缩和白内障。

治疗

眼周和全身应用类固醇和免疫抑制剂是有益的，但视力预后不确定。

急性后部多发鳞状色素上皮病（AMPPPE）

临床特征

少见，原发性急性双眼病变，多见于青年。早期深的、椭圆形、淡黄色的病灶（图 139），消退后留色素瘢痕(图 140)。

治疗

虽然未经治疗视力预后通常很好。

匍行性脉络膜病变

临床特征

罕见，原发的，老年人慢性双眼发病。后极淡黄色的病变（图 141）进行性萎缩（图 142）。

治疗

类固醇和免疫抑制剂可用，预后不良。

Idiopathic multifocal white dot syndromes

24

'White dot syndromes' is the term for a heterogeneous group of rare inflammatory conditions of unknown aetiology which involve the posterior segment. Examples are presented below.

Birdshot retinochoroidopathy

Clinical features

Rare, idiopathic, chronic bilateral condition typically affecting middle-aged females who carry the genetic marker HLA-A29. Early lesions consist of multiple, deep, flat, creamy-yellow spots radiating outwards from the disc (Fig. 137), associated with variable vasculitis and vitreitis. These evolve into circumscribed, atrophic white areas (Fig. 138). Cystoid macular oedema is very common; optic atrophy and cataract may also develop.

Management

Periocular and systemic steroids and immunosuppressive agents may be beneficial but the visual prognosis is guarded.

Acute multifocal posterior placoid pigment epitheliopathy (AMPPPE)

Clinical features

Uncommon, idiopathic, acute bilateral condition typically affecting young adults. Deep, oval, cream-coloured lesions (Fig. 139) develop initially, and on resolving leave variable pigmented scars (Fig. 140).

Management

Despite the lack of treatment the visual prognosis is usually excellent.

Serpiginous choroidopathy

Clinical features

Rare, idiopathic, chronic bilateral condition of older patients. Cream-coloured lesions at the posterior pole (Fig. 141) evolve to leave atrophic areas (Fig. 142).

Management

Steroids and immunosuppressive agents may be tried but the visual prognosis is poor.

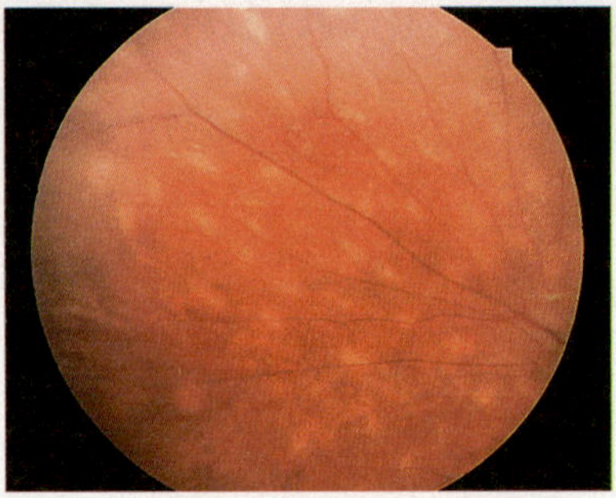

图 137 活动期的鸟枪弹样视网膜脉络膜病
Active birdshot retinochoroidopathy

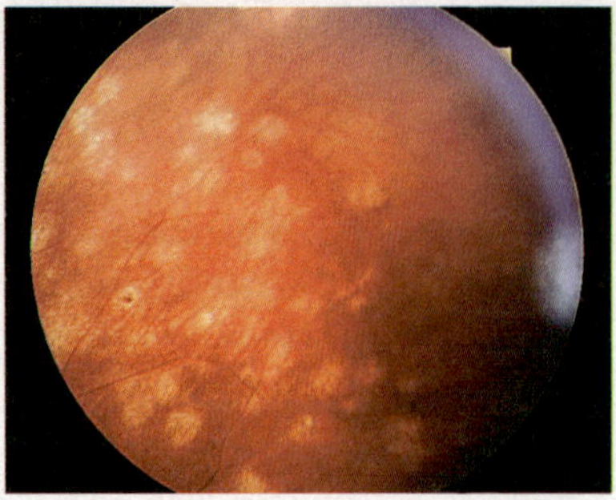

图 138 静止期鸟枪弹样视网膜脉络膜病
Inactive birdshot retinochoroidopathy

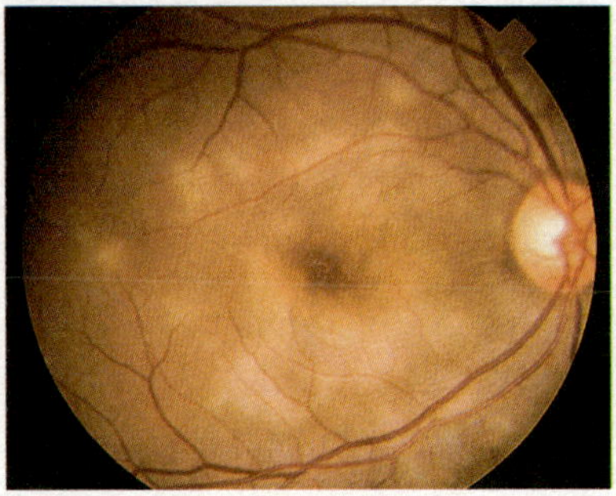

图 139 活动期 AMPPPE
Active AMPPPE

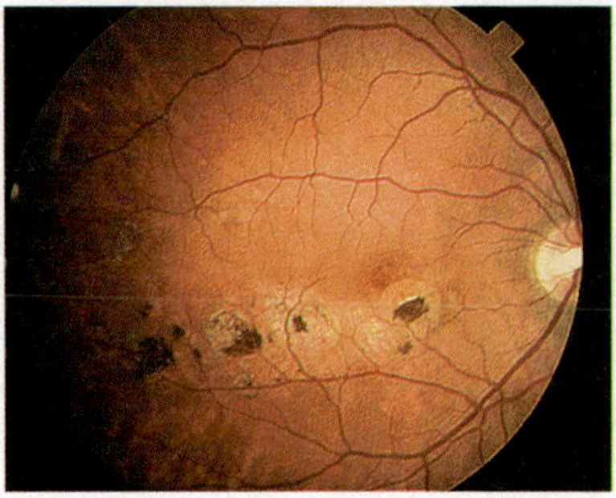

图 140 静止期 AMPPPE
Inactive AMPPPE

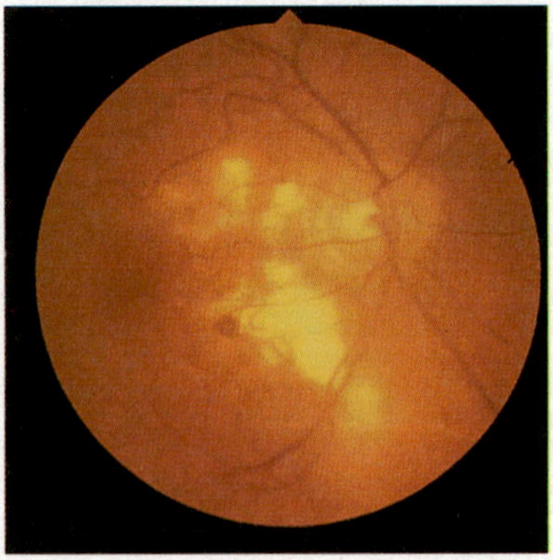

图 141 急性匍行性脉络膜病变
Active serpiginous choroidopathy

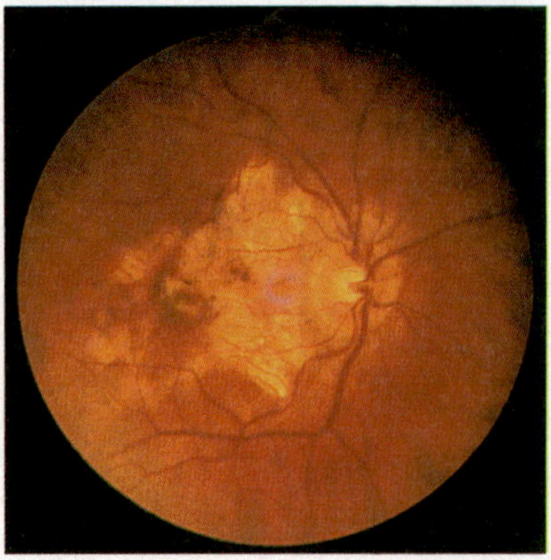

图 142 匍行性脉络膜病变的晚期瘢痕形成
Late scarring in serpiginous choroidopathy

25 原发性开角型青光眼

定义

青光眼是进展性视神经病变，眼压增高（IOP，图143）是成年人视力丧失的危险因素。原发性开角型青光眼（POAG）是最常见的青光眼，房水经由小梁网排出，逐渐减少导致眼压增高。青光眼可以出现在眼压正常的情况。

发病率

POAG在40岁以上人群发病率至少为1%。双眼受累约占受累者10%。

高发因素

- 年龄
- 黑人
- 家族史
- 近视

临床特征

常无症状，直到视野显著缺损。多为常规眼部检查时首先被发现。

体征

- 眼压升高（>21 mmHg）
- 青光眼的视神经损害（图 144 ~ 146）
- 视野缺损（图 147）
- 前房角镜检查时前房角开放

治疗

- 局部治疗（通常首选治疗）用 β- 受体阻断剂，前列腺素衍生物，碳酸酐酶抑制剂，α- 受体激动剂和缩瞳药。
- 激光小梁成形术。
- 滤过手术，如小梁切除术（图 148）。

25 Primary open-angle glaucoma

Definition

Glaucoma is a progressive optic neuropathy for which the major risk factor for visual loss is elevated intraocular pressure (IOP - Fig. 143). In primary open-angle glaucoma (POAG), the most common of the glaucomas, raised IOP occurs secondarily to a gradual reduction in the drainage of aqueous humour via the trabecular meshwork. Glaucoma can be present, however, in the presence of normal IOP ('normal-tension' glaucoma).

Incidence

POAG affects at least 1% of the population over the age of 40 years. Both eyes are usually affected. The risk to siblings of affected individuals is approximately 10%.

Important risk factors

- Age
- Black race
- Family history
- Myopia

Clinical features

Usually asymptomatic until significant loss of visual field has occurred. Frequently the condition is first suspected at a routine eye examination.

Signs

- Elevated IOP (>21mmHg)
- Glaucomatous optic nerve damage (Figs 144-146)
- Visual field loss (Fig. 147)
- Open anterior chamber angle on gonioscopy.

Management

- Topical treatment (usually first-line) with beta-blockers, prostaglandin derivatives, carbonic anhydrase inhibitors, alpha-agonists and miotics
- Laser trabeculoplasty
- Filtration surgery, e.g. trabeculectomy (Fig. 148).

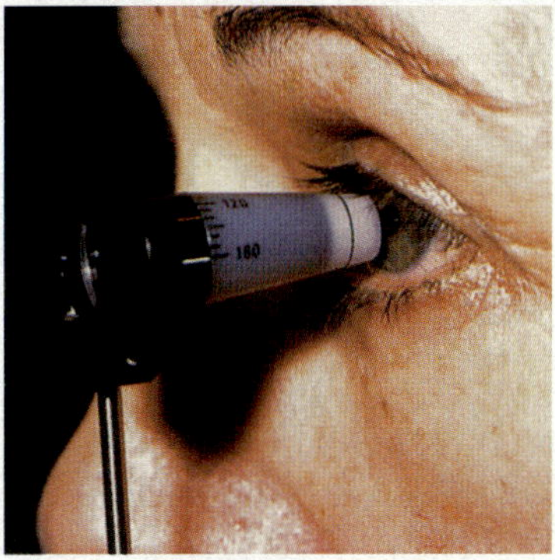

图 143　测量眼压
Measurement of intraocular pressure

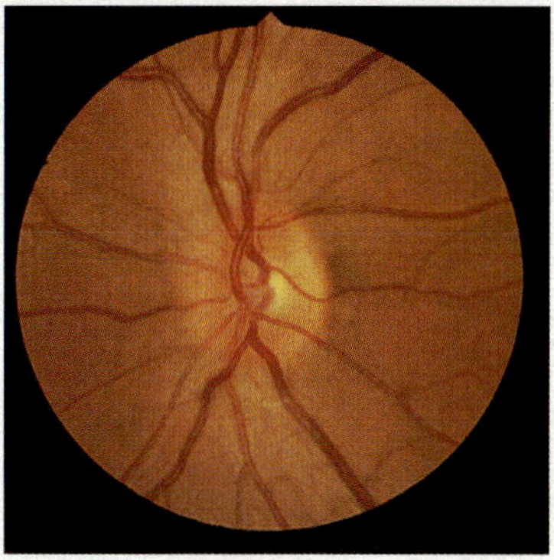

图 144　正常视盘
Normal optic disc

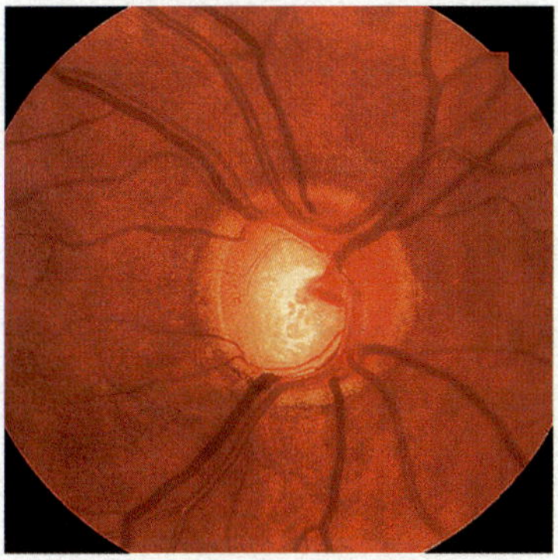

图 145　中度视杯下方凹陷
Moderate cupping with an inferior notching

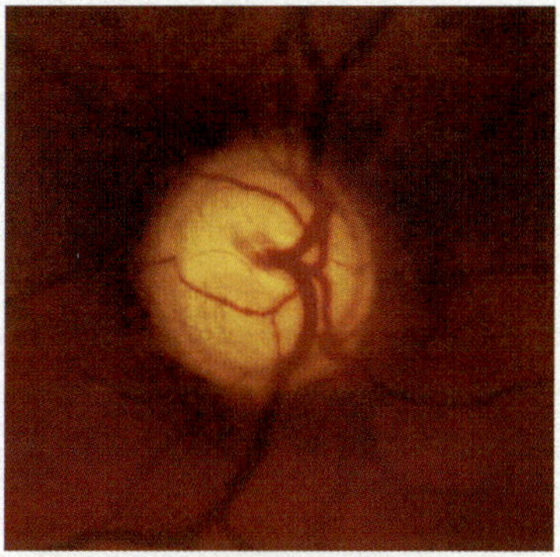

图 146　陈旧性视杯凹陷
Advanced cupping

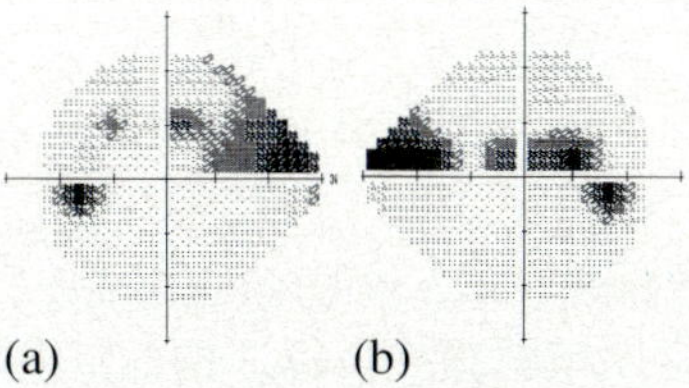

图 147　青光眼患者视野缺损（a）左眼（b）右眼
Visual field loss in a glaucoma patient (a) left eye (b) right eye

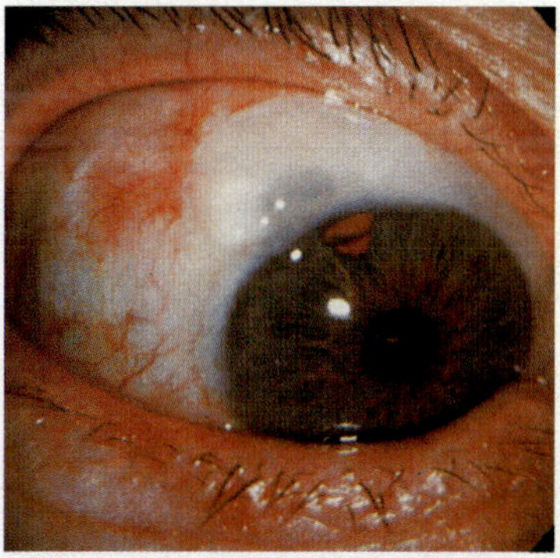

图 148　小梁切除术后结膜滤泡
Conjunctival filtration bleb following trabeculectomy

26 继发性开角型青光眼

色素性青光眼

病因学 来自于虹膜的色素颗粒造成房水流出阻滞和继发的小梁网损伤。

临床特征 常见：大多数患者是年轻的近视男性。

体征

- 在角膜内皮呈垂直梭形分布的色素颗粒（克鲁肯贝格梭，图 149）。
- 透照法在虹膜中周边部轮辐状缺损（图 150）。
- 前房角镜检查：宽前房角伴小梁网的大量色素（图151）。
- 其他特点：前房深，虹膜表面有色素颗粒。
- 如果没有青光眼损伤：色素播散综合征。

治疗 同POAG。

假性剥脱性青光眼

病因学 假性剥脱性物质致房水流出阻滞。

临床特征 常见：中年以上的人发病为其特征。

体征

- 假性剥脱性物质位于晶状体前囊膜（图152）和瞳孔缘（图 153）。
- 前房角镜检查：小梁色素沉着和假性剥脱性物质沉着。

治疗 同 POAG，但对药物治疗的反应比 POAG 差。

房角退缩性青光眼

病因 钝挫伤致小梁的损伤。

临床特征 罕见。通常于受伤后数月或数年，单眼的IOP升高。对诊断有意义的检查包括以前的损伤体征，例如虹膜括约肌的撕裂或虹膜根部断离（见图 264），比对侧眼有轻度的前房加深，前房角镜检查可见房角退缩及不规则（图 154）。

治疗 最初采用药物治疗，最后经常需要做滤过手术。

Secondary open-angle glaucomas

Pigmentary glaucoma

Aetiology

Blockage of aqueous outflow and secondary trabecular meshwork damage is caused by pigment granules derived from the iris.

Clinical features

Common: most patients are young myopic males.

Signs

- Vertical strip of pigment granules on the corneal endothelium (Krukenberg spindle - Fig. 149)
- Spoke-like transillumination defects in the mid-peripheral iris (Fig. 150)
- Gonioscopy: wide anterior chamber angle with heavily pigmented trabecular meshwork (Fig. 151)
- Other features: deep anterior chamber, pigment granules on the iris surface
- If no glaucomatous damage: 'pigment dispersion syndrome'.

Management

As for POAG.

Pseudoexfoliation glaucoma

Aetiology

Blockage of aqueous outflow by pseudoexfoliative material.

Clinical features

Common: typically affects the elderly.

Signs

- Pseudoexfoliative material on anterior lens surface (Fig. 152) and pupillary border (Fig. 153)
- Gonioscopy: trabecular hyperpigmentation and deposits of pseudoexfoliative material.

Management

As for POAG but may be more resistant to treatment.

Angle-recession glaucoma

Aetiology

Blunt traumatic trabecular damage.

Clinical features

Uncommon. Uniocular elevation of IOP, usually months or years after the initial injury. Examination clues to the diagnosis include signs of previous damage such as tears in the iris sphincter or iridodialysis (see Fig. 264), a slightly deeper anterior chamber than in the fellow eye, and a recessed and irregular angle on gonioscopy (Fig. 154).

Management

Treatment is initially medical although filtration surgery is often required eventually.

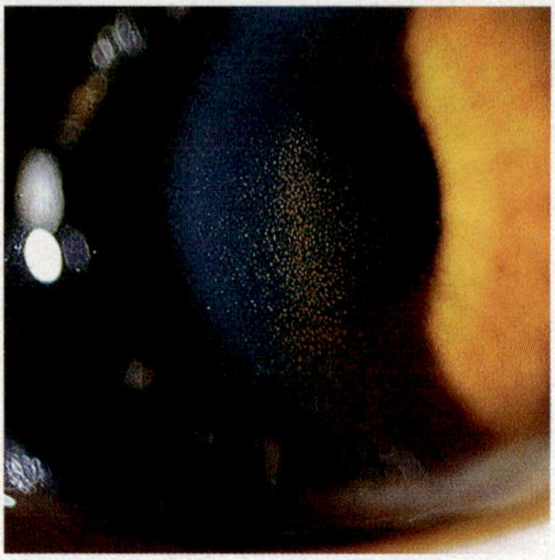

图 149 克鲁肯贝格梭
Krukenberg spindle

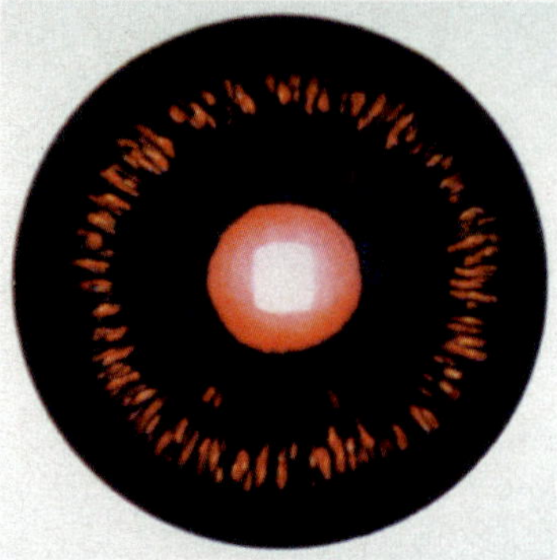

图 150 虹膜透照缺损
Iris transillumination defects

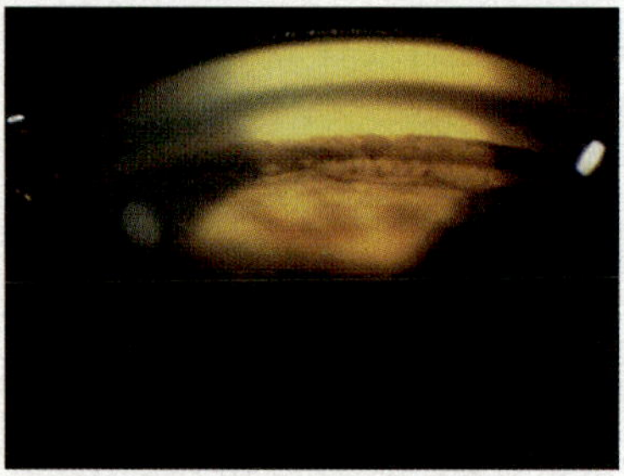

图 151 小梁色素沉着过度
Trabecular hyperpigmentation

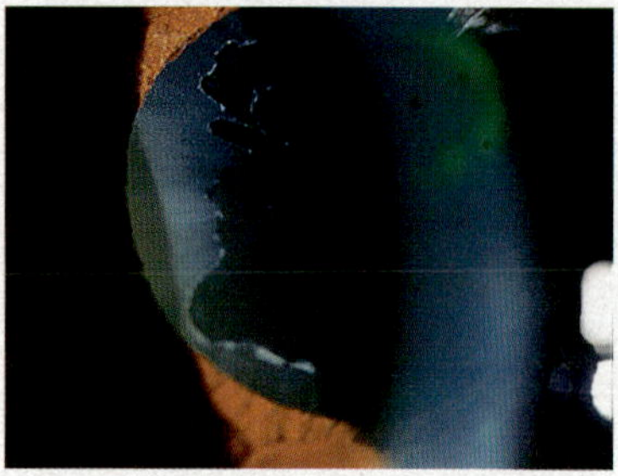

图 152 假性剥脱性物质位于晶状体前囊膜
Pseudoexfoliative material on the anterior lens capsule

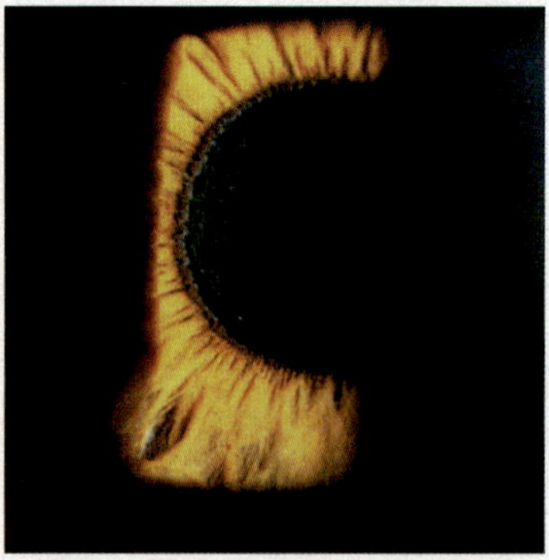

图 153 假性剥脱性物质位于晶状体和瞳孔缘
Pseudoexfoliative material on the lens and pupil edge

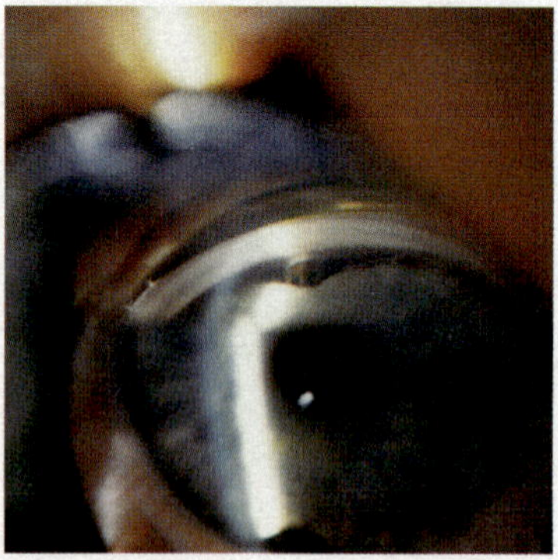

图 154 严重的房角退缩
Severe angle recession

原发性闭角型青光眼

定义 由于周边的虹膜膨隆，前房角闭塞导致眼压升高。

病因学 晶状体增厚和老化导致前房角狭窄。在解剖学上易感眼可发展至前房角闭塞。

高发因素
- 年龄增大（常大于 60 岁）。
- 女性。
- 远视，浅前房和房角狭窄。

分类 *亚急性闭角* 间断的房角闭塞导致暂时的视力下降和虹视伴随疼痛和 / 或充血，可自然地缓解。

慢性闭角 逐渐的隐匿的房角狭窄，没有急性症状，常见进行眼压升高。

急性闭角 突然发作全房角闭塞（图 155），导致急性和非常严重的眼压升高与视力丧失、眼痛和充血，经常伴发恶心和呕吐。

临床特征 急性闭角型青光眼体征包括：
- 眼压非常高。
- 角膜周围的（睫状）充血。
- 角膜水肿（图 156）。
- 固定的椭圆形瞳孔，中度散大（图 157）。
- 前房极浅。

急性发作缓解后体征：

- 虹膜萎缩（图 158）。
- 前部晶状体混浊（*青光眼性白内障*，图 159）。

治疗
- 治疗急性青光眼时全身应用碳酸酐酶抑制剂和局部应用 β- 受体阻滞剂、缩瞳剂和类固醇；全身应用高渗剂。
- 角膜透明时可行激光周边虹膜切开术（图 160）。

27 Primary angle-closure glaucoma

Definition

Elevation of IOP as a result of obstruction of the anterior chamber angle by the peripheral iris.

Aetiology

The normal increase in size of the lens with ageing may lead to narrowing of the anterior chamber angle. In an anatomically predisposed eye this can progress to obstruction.

Risk factors

- Increasing age (usually over 60)
- Female gender
- Hypermetropia, shallow anterior chamber and narrow angle.

Classification

Subacute angle-closure Episodic transient blurring of vision and haloes around lights associated with aching and/or redness of the eye caused by intermittent angle closure that resolves spontaneously.

Chronic angle-closure Gradual and insidious narrowing of the angle without acute symptoms, usually with gradual elevation of IOP.

Acute angle-closure Sudden onset of total angle occlusion (Fig. 155) results in an acute and very severe increase in IOP with corresponding visual loss, ocular pain and redness, frequently accompanied by nausea and vomiting.

Clinical features

Signs of acute angle-closure glaucoma include:

- Very high IOP
- Circumcorneal ('ciliary') injection
- Corneal oedema (Fig. 156)
- Fixed, mid-dilated, oval pupil (Fig. 157)
- Very shallow anterior chamber.

Signs following resolution of the acute attack:

- Iris atrophy (Fig. 158)
- Anterior lens opacity (*Glaukomflecken* - Fig. 159)

Management

- Treatment of acute glaucoma is with systemic carbonic anhydrase inhibitors and topical beta blockers, miotics and steroids; systemic osmotic agents may also be required
- Laser peripheral iridotomies (Fig. 160) once the cornea has cleared.

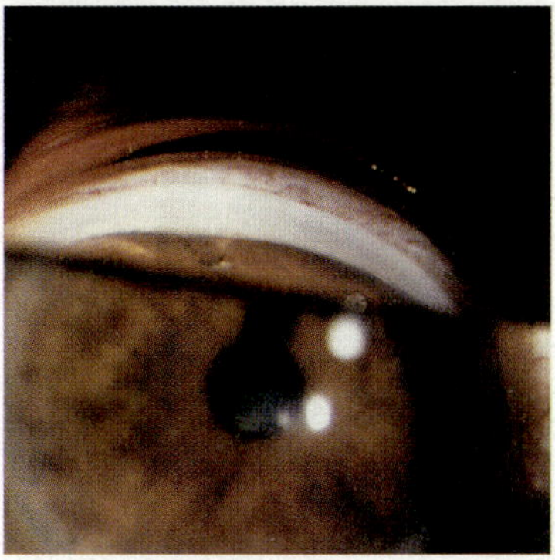

图 155 周边虹膜膨隆导致全房角闭塞
Total angle occlusion by peripheral iris

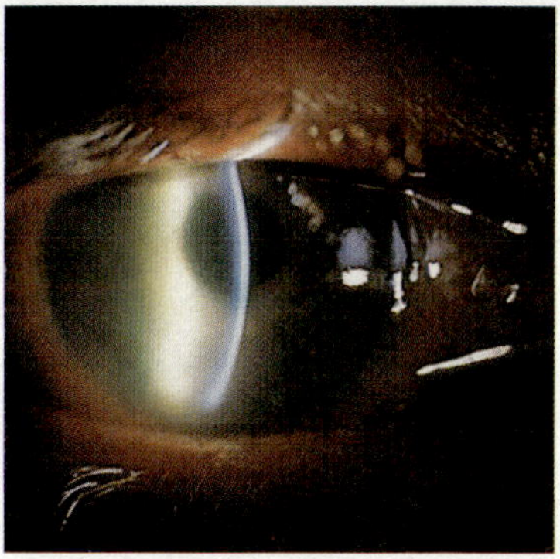

图 156 急性闭角型青光眼角膜水肿
Corneal oedema in acute angle-closure

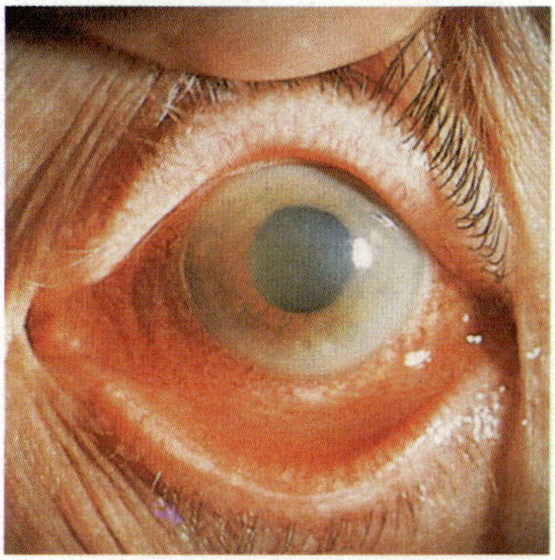

图 157 急性闭角型青光眼的固定的中度散大的椭圆形瞳孔
Fixed mid-dilated pupil in acute angle-closure

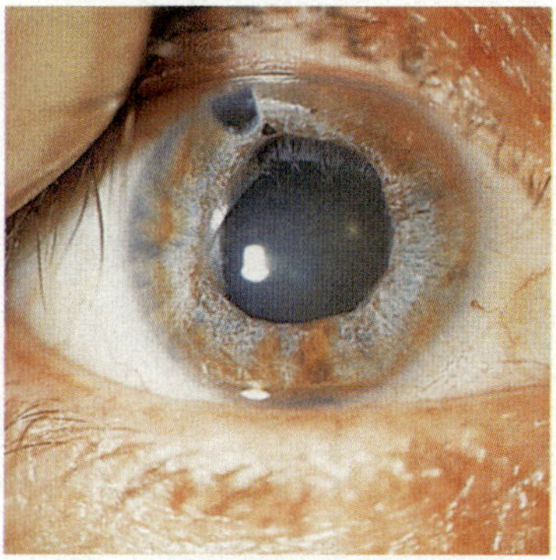

图 158 急性闭角型青光眼缓解后的虹膜萎缩
Iris atrophy following resolution of acute angle-closure

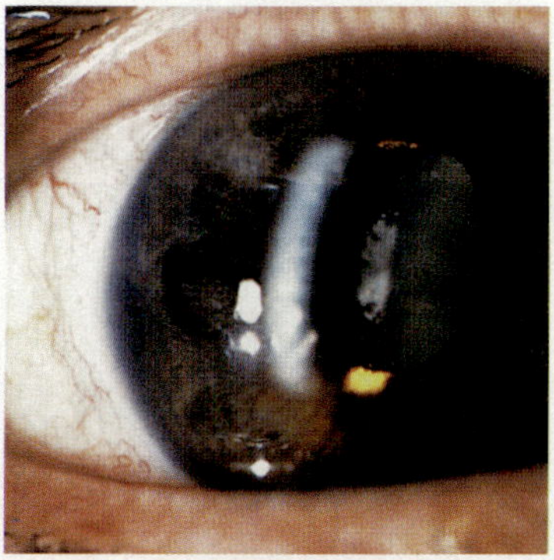

图 159 青光眼性白内障
Glaukomflecken

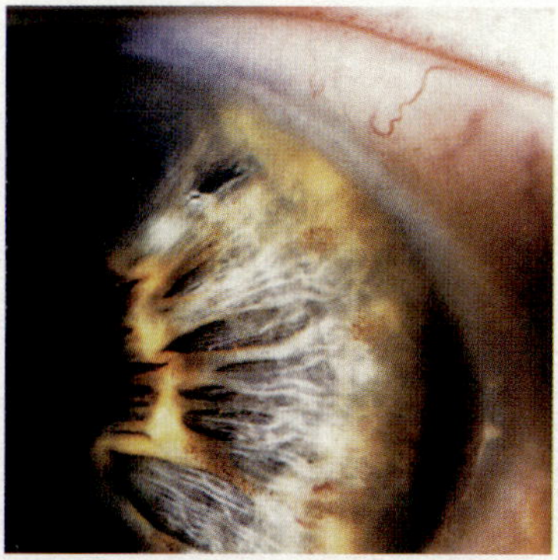

图 160 激光周边虹膜切除术
Laser peripheral iridotomy

继发性闭角型青光眼

新生血管性青光眼

病因学

慢性视网膜的局部缺血导致虹膜和前房角新生血管形成（虹膜红变）。新生血管组织收缩（周边前粘连，PAS）导致房角关闭。常见于局部缺血，视网膜中央静脉阻塞 （见图 196）（于血栓形成后 3 个月左右出现）和严重增殖型糖尿病视网膜病变。

临床特征

疼痛，视力减低，前段充血，极高的眼压伴角膜水肿和严重的虹膜红变（图 161，162）。

治疗

- 眼底若可见、行全视网膜光凝，不可见行周边视网膜冷冻疗法。
- 局部应用阿托品和类固醇减少炎症。
- 滤过手术（小梁切除术辅以抗代谢药或植入引流装置，图 163）。
- 激光局部的睫状体切除（“睫状体光凝术”）。

炎症性的闭角型青光眼

病因学

前葡萄膜炎导致闭角型青光眼的两种机制：

- 360° 虹膜后粘连（瞳孔闭锁，图 164）致虹膜膨隆，浅前房和房角关闭。
- 房角炎症性的碎屑收缩导致周边前粘连形成，没有瞳孔阻滞。

虹膜角膜内皮（ICE）综合征

病因学

由于异常角膜内皮细胞增殖和收缩致虹膜粘连，房角关闭。

临床特征

罕见。常发病于中年女性，单眼受累。体征包括虹膜萎缩（图 165，166），虹膜痣或结节和/或严重的角膜内皮变化。

治疗

常植入引流装置。

Secondary angle-closure glaucomas

Neovascular glaucoma

Aetiology

Chronic retinal ischaemia leads to neovascularization on the iris (rubeosis iridis) and in the anterior chamber angle. Contraction of fibrovascular tissue (peripheral anterior synechiae - PAS) causes angle closure. Common causes are ischaemic central retinal vein occlusion (see Fig. 196), typically about 3 months after the thrombosis, and severe proliferative diabetic retinopathy.

Clinical features

Pain, decreased vision, anterior segment congestion, a very high IOP with corneal oedema, and severe rubeosis iridis (Figs 161, 162).

Management

- Panretinal photocoagulation if the fundus is visible, or peripheral retinal cryotherapy if not
- Topical atropine and steroids to decrease inflammation
- Filtration surgery (trabeculectomy with adjunctive antimetabolite, or drainage implant - Fig. 163)
- Partial ablation of the ciliary body with laser ('cyclodiode').

Inflammatory angle-closure glaucomas

Aetiology

Anterior uveitis may lead to angle-closure glaucoma via two mechanisms:

- 360° posterior synechiae (seclusio pupillae- Fig. 164) causes iris bombé, a shallow anterior chamber and angle closure
- Without pupil block due to contraction of inflammatory debris in the angle with consequent PAS formation.

Iridocorneal endothelial (ICE) syndrome

Aetiology

Synechial angle closure by proliferation and contraction of abnormal corneal endothelial cells.

Clinical features

Rare. Typically affects one eye of a middle-aged woman. Signs include iris atrophy (Figs 165, 166), iris naevus or nodules and/or severe corneal endothelial changes.

Management

A drainage implant is often required.

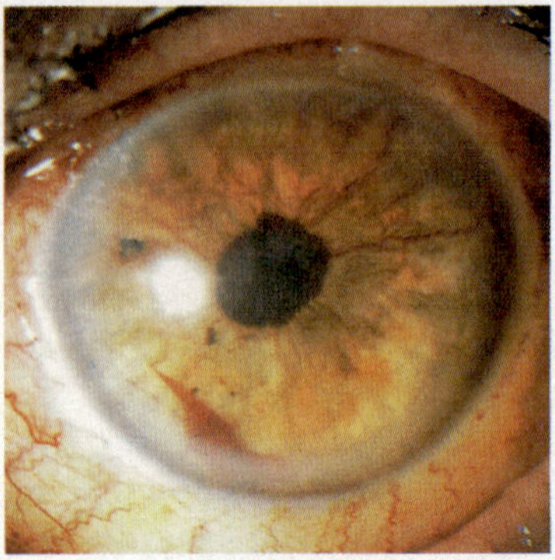

图 161 虹膜红变伴新生血管出血
Rubeosis iridis with bleeding from new vessels

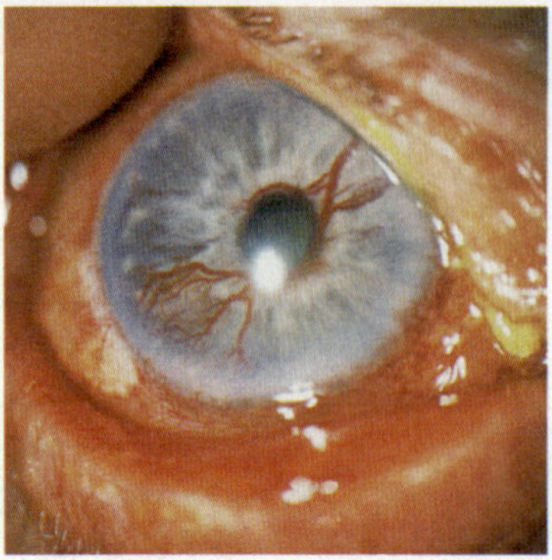

图 162 陈旧性虹膜红变
Advanced rubeosis iridis

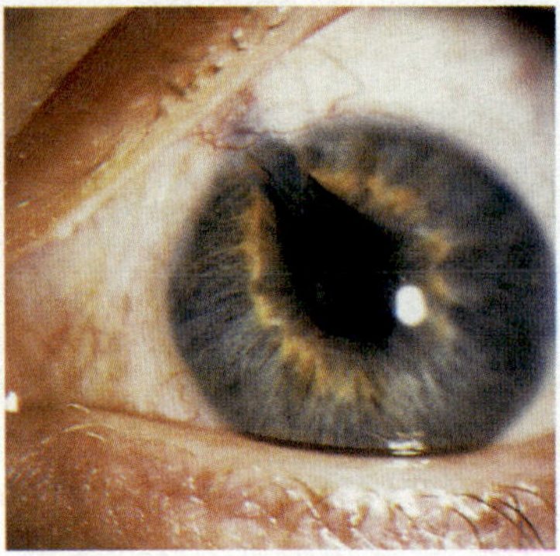

图 163 植入引流装置
Drainage implant

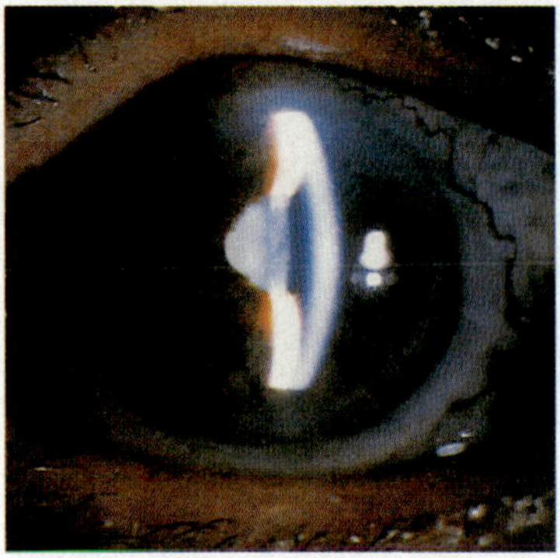

图 164 瞳孔闭锁伴浅前房
Seclusio pupillae with shallow anterior chamber

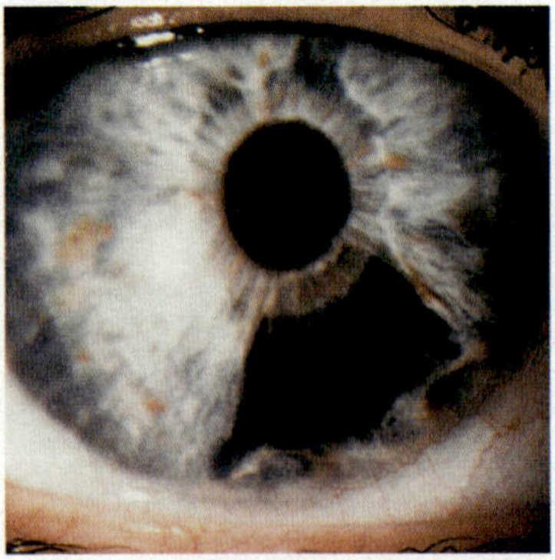

图 165 虹膜角膜内皮综合征的虹膜萎缩
Iris atrophy in ICE syndrome

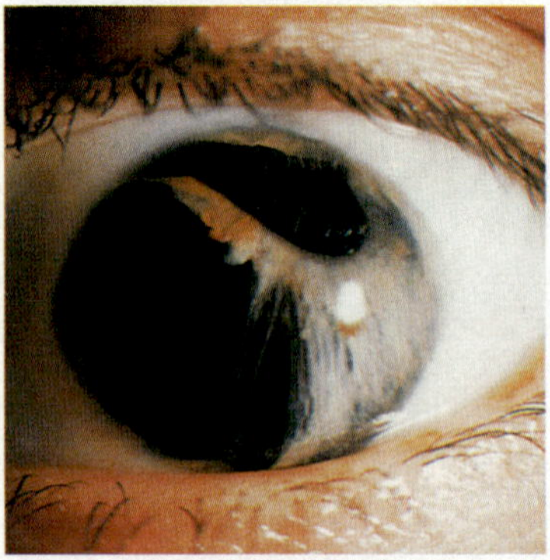

图 166 陈旧性虹膜萎缩
Very advanced iris atrophy

原发性先天性青光眼

发病率 于产后存活者中占1/10 000；65%是男孩。75%双眼受累，通常不对称。

临床特征

- 大眼（牛眼，图167），如果3岁以前发病，IOP升高。
- 后弹力层断裂（哈布纹，图 168）。
- 前房角异常。

治疗

- 小梁网切开（前房角切开术）。
- 较少行小梁切开术或小梁切除术。

虹膜角膜的畸形

定义 罕见的，包括眼球前段的一系列先天性疾病，有时合并先天性或儿童期青光眼。

分类 *Axenfeld-Rieger综合征* 角膜后胚胎环伴随广泛的PAS，虹膜发育不良，裂孔，眼色素层外翻和瞳孔移位（图169）。

Peters异常 非常罕见，具有特征的角膜瘢痕合并虹膜或晶状体粘连（图 170）。

无虹膜 可能完全或部分缺损（图 171）。分三型：

- *AN-1（~66%）*：孤立的眼部缺损，常染色体显性遗传。
- *AN-2（~33%）*：散发；在 5 岁以前发病者 30% 发生于 Wilms 肿瘤（Miller 综合征）。
- *AN-3（1%~2%）*：精神残疾和小脑共济失调（Gillespie 综合征）。

斑痣性错构瘤病

多器官的一系列具有特征的错构瘤。先天性青光眼可能发生在：

- Sturge-Weber 综合征（图 172）；由于房角畸形或浅层巩膜静脉压升高，30% 有青光眼。
- 多发性神经纤维瘤 -1 型；罕有青光眼。

29 Developmental glaucomas

Primary congenital glaucoma

Incidence

1/10 000 live births; 65% are boys. Both eyes involved in 75% of cases, usually asymmetrically.

Clinical features

- Large eye (buphthalmos - Fig.167) if IOP becomes elevated before age 3 years
- Breaks in Descemet's membrane (Haab striae - Fig. 168)
- Anterior chamber angle anomaly.

Management

- Incision of the trabecular meshwork (goniotomy)
- Less commonly trabeculotomy or trabeculectomy.

Iridocorneal dysgenesis

Definition

A spectrum of rare congenital disorders involving the anterior segment, sometimes associated with congenital or childhood glaucoma.

Classification

Axenfeld-Rieger syndrome Posterior embryotoxon associated with extensive PAS, iris hypoplasia, holes, ectropion uveae and displaced pupil (Fig. 169).

Peters anomaly Extremely rare condition characterized by a corneal scar associated with iris or lens adhesions (Fig. 170).

Aniridia May be complete or partial (Fig. 171). Three phenotypes:

- *AN-1 (~66%)*: isolated ocular defect with autosomal dominant inheritance
- *AN-2 (~33%)*: sporadic; 30% chance of Wilms' tumour by age 5 years (Miller's syndrome)
- *AN-3 (1-2%)*: mental handicap and cerebellar ataxia (Gillespie's syndrome).

Phacomatoses

A group of conditions characterized by hamartomas in multiple organs. Congenital glaucoma may occur in:

- Sturge-Weber syndrome (Fig. 172); glaucoma in 30% of cases, due to either an angle anomaly or elevation of episcleral venous pressure.
- Neurofibromatosis-1; glaucoma is uncommon.

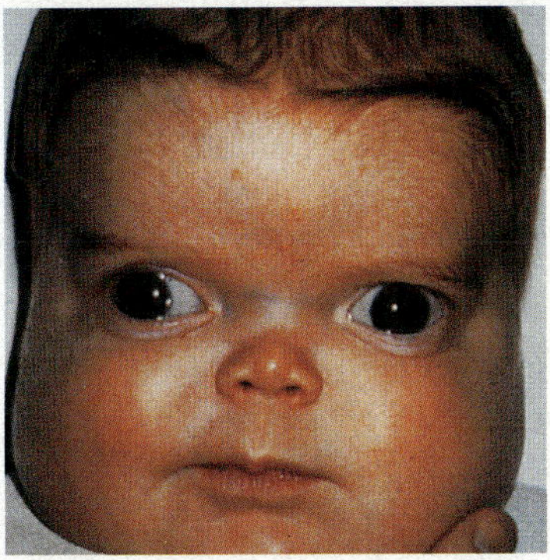

图 167　双侧牛眼
Bilateral buphthalmos

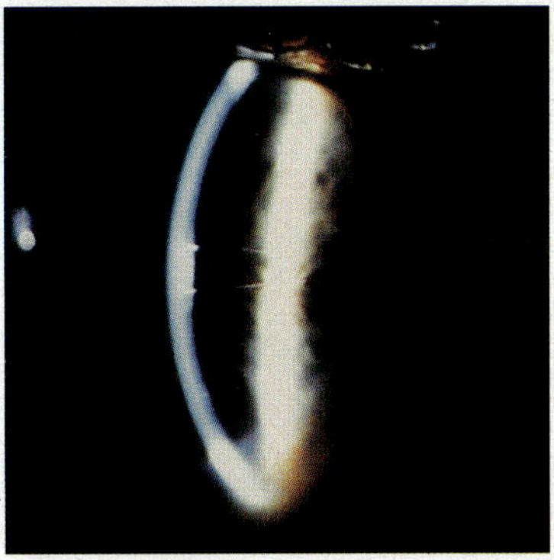

图 168　哈布纹
Haab striae

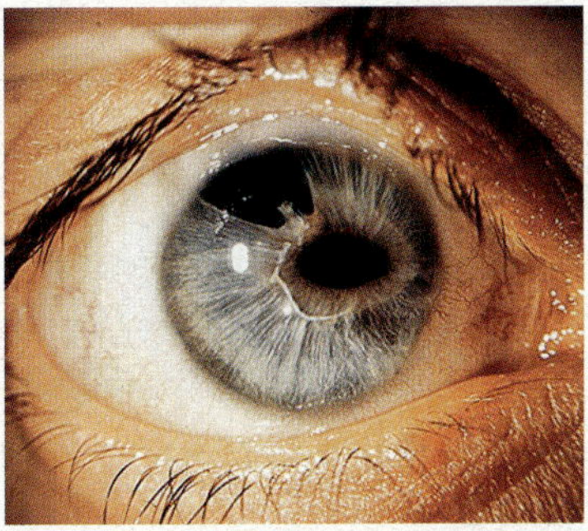

图 169　Axenfeld-Rieger 综合征
Axenfeld-Rieger syndrome

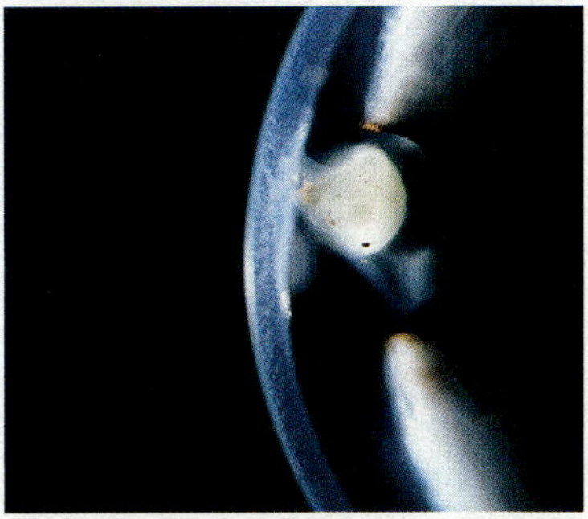

图 170　Peters 异常
Peters anomaly

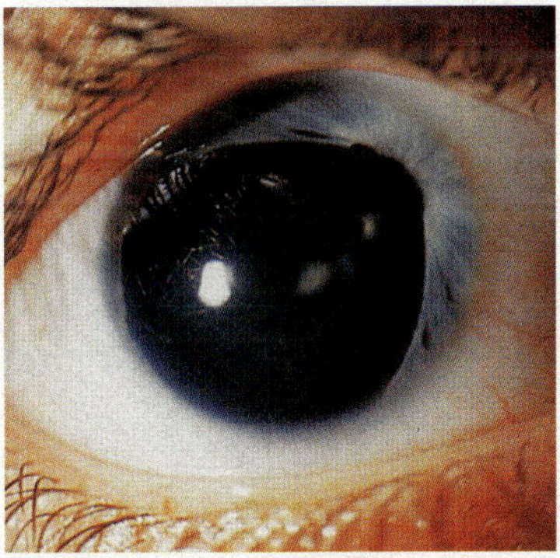

图 171　不完全无虹膜
Incomplete aniridia

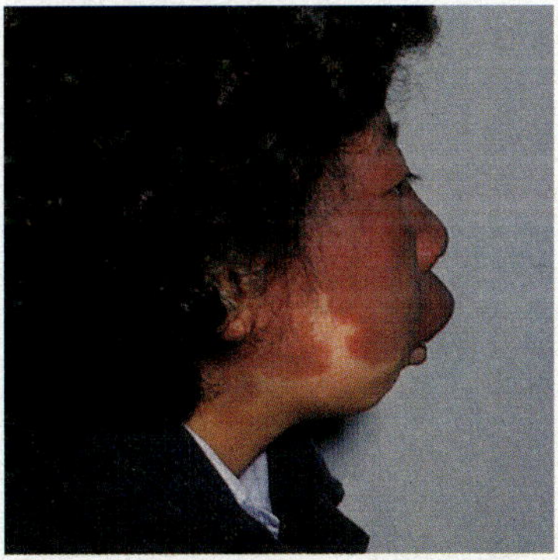

图 172　Stuge-Weber 综合征的鲜红斑痣
Naevus flammeus in Sturge-Weber syndrome

年龄相关性白内障

定义 白内障是晶状体混浊。它是老年患者视力下降最常见的原因。

分类 *囊下白内障* 可出现在晶状体前端或后端（图 173）。患者感到眩光，近视力较远视力下降明显。

核性白内障（“核硬化”） 主要是晶状体核颜色加深（图 174）。可使近视加重，远视力受累较近视力明显。

皮质性白内障 辐轮状混浊（图 175）。

成熟期白内障 完全混浊晶状体伴白瞳孔（图 176）。

治疗 手术摘除术是白内障的最佳的治疗方式。大多数的现代白内障手术是使用白内障超声乳化仪，晶状体通过小切口用小口径的超声探针取出。人工晶状体（IOL，图177）植入代替原来的晶状体。在特殊的环境或没有白内障超声乳化仪时，可行“囊外摘出术”，其需要缝合大角膜切口。

并发症

- 晶状体后囊膜浑浊（图 178）发生率大约为20%；可行 YAG 激光晶状体囊切开术。
- 急性或慢性的细菌性眼内炎罕见但严重。
- 驱逐性（脉络膜）出血罕见，却是最严重的手术并发症。
- 视网膜脱离少见，近视者多发。

Age-related cataract

Definition

Cataract is an opacity of the natural crystalline lens. It is an extremely common cause of visual impairment in older patients.

Classification

Subcapsular cataract May be anterior or posterior (Fig. 173). Patients experience glare and typically have more problems with reading than distance vision.

Nuclear cataract ('nuclear sclerosis') Consists of a central darkening of the lens (Fig. 174). It may cause an increase in myopia so that distance vision is affected more than near.

Cortical cataract - spoke-like opacities (Fig. 175).

Mature cataract - completely opaque lens with a white pupil (Fig. 176).

Management

Surgical extraction is the only treatment for cataract. The majority of modern cataract surgery is now carried out by means of phacoemulsification, in which the lens is removed through a narrow incision using a small-bore ultrasonic probe. The natural lens is replaced by an artificial intraocular lens implant (IOL - Fig. 177). Under special circumstances or where phacoemulsification equipment is not available, 'extracapsular' extraction is carried out, involving a larger corneal incision requiring sutures.

Complications

- Posterior lens capsular opacification (Fig. 178) occurs eventually in about 20% of cases; can be treated by YAG laser capsulotomy
- Acute or chronic bacterial endophthalmitis is rare but serious
- Expulsive (suprachoroidal) haemorrhage is a rare but potentially disastrous operative complication
- Retinal detachment is rare; myopes are particularly at risk.

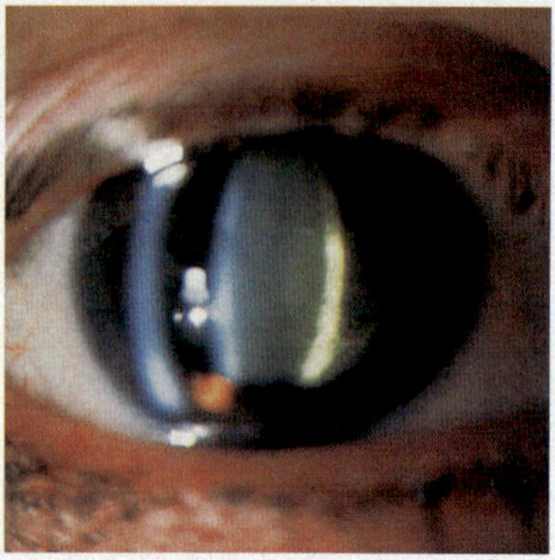

图 173　前囊下白内障
Posterior subcapsular cataract

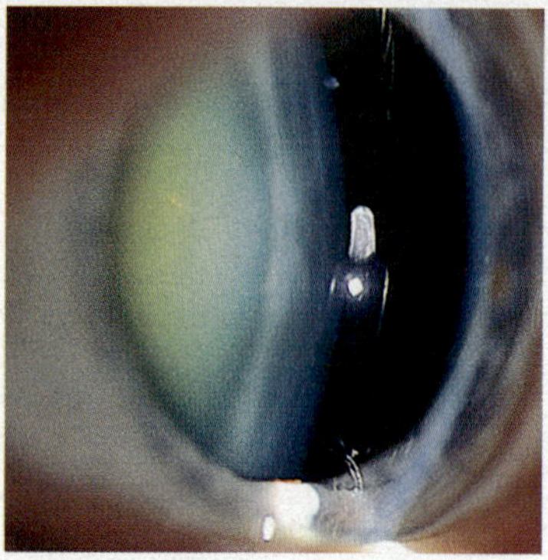

图 174　核性白内障（核硬化）
Nuclear cataract (nuclear sclerosis)

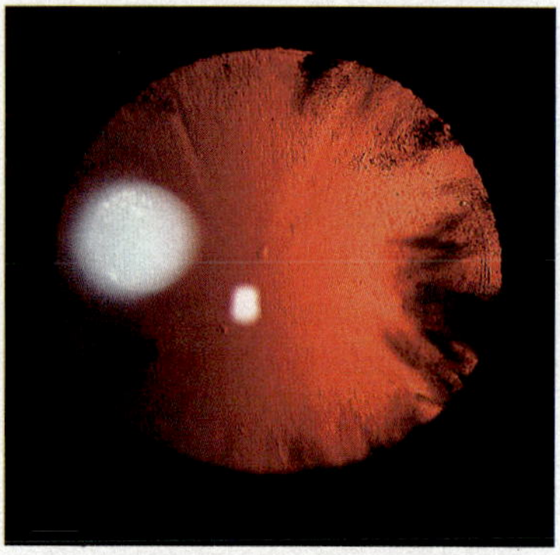

图 175　皮质性白内障的红光反射
Cortical cataract seen against the red reflex

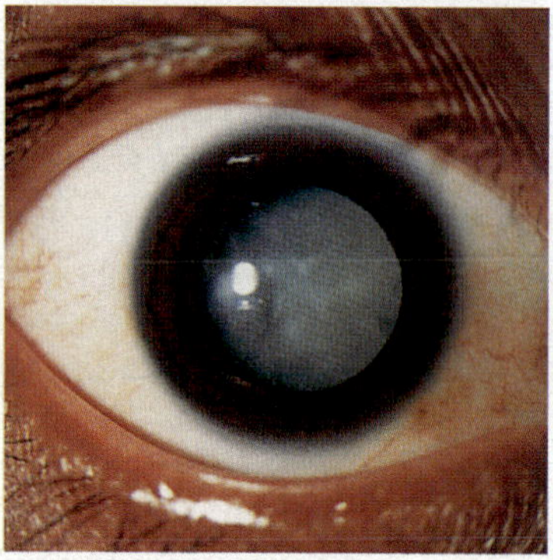

图 176　成熟期白内障
Mature cataract

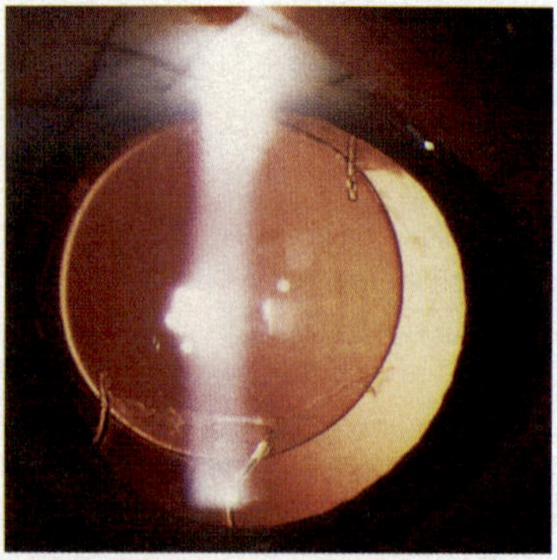

图 177　人工晶状体
Intraocular lens implant

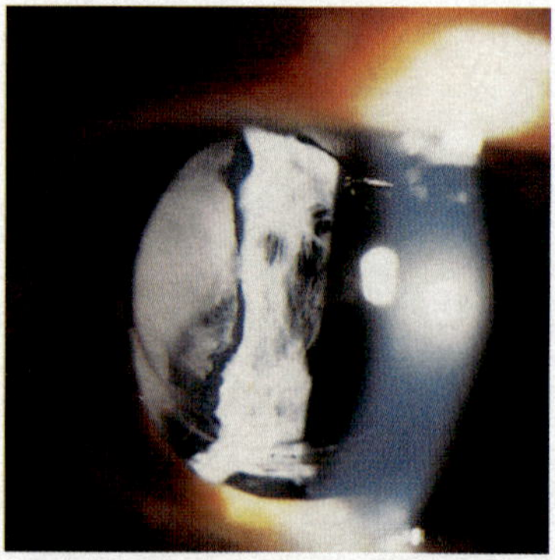

图 178　严重的晶状体后囊膜浑浊
Severe posterior capsular opacification

其他晶状体疾病

继发性白内障

病因学

- *外伤*：穿透伤、钝挫伤、辐射伤和电击伤。
- *合并眼部疾病*：慢性前葡萄膜炎（见图123）、高度近视、急性闭角型青光眼（见图159）、遗传性视网膜营养不良。
- *合并全身性疾病*：糖尿病、肌强直性营养不良和特发性皮炎。
- *药物造成*：多见于全身使用类固醇。

婴儿性（白）内障

病因学

- *原发性散发*：单眼。
- *遗传性*：多为常染色体显性遗传。
- *合并其他的眼部畸形*：永存增生原始玻璃体、早产儿视网膜病、虹膜缺失（见图 171）、Peters异常（见图 170）。
- *胚胎病*：子宫内感染（如风疹病毒、弓形体病）。
- *代谢病*：半乳糖激酶缺乏、半乳糖血症和低钙血症。
- *综合征*：Lowe综合征、Down综合征、Turner综合征和猫叫样哭泣综合征。

临床特征

婴儿性白内障的形态多态性（图 179，180）。

晶状体异位

定义

晶状体移位；部分的（半脱位）或完全的。

病因学

- *外伤*（图 181）。
- *家族性晶状体异位*：可合并异位的瞳孔（图 182）。
- *合并其他的眼病*：虹膜缺失（见图171）和牛眼（见图 167）。
- *综合征*：Marfan综合征(图 183)和Weill-Marchesani综合征。
- *代谢病*：高胱氨酸尿症和高赖氨酸血症。

晶状体大小和形状异常

- *小晶状体*：小型的晶状体。
- *小球形晶状体*：小型的球面晶状体。
- *晶状体缺损*：（图 184）可伴虹膜和脉络膜缺损和巨大视网膜撕裂。
- *圆锥形晶状体*：圆锥体形晶状体外观（如Alport综合征的前圆锥形晶状体）。

Miscellaneous disorders of the lens

Secondary cataract

Aetiology

- *Trauma*: penetrating, concussion, radiation and electric shock
- *Associated with ocular disease*: chronic anterior uveitis (see Fig. 123), high myopia, acute angle-closure glaucoma (see Fig. 159), hereditary retinal dystrophies
- *Associated with systemic disease*: diabetes, myotonic dystrophy and atopic dermatitis
- *Drug-induced*: most commonly systemic steroids.

Infantile cataract

Aetiology

- *Idiopathic sporadic*: may be unilateral
- *Hereditary*: most frequently autosomal dominant
- *Associated with other ocular malformations*: persistent hyperplastic primary vitreous, retinopathy of prematurity, aniridia (see Fig. 171), Peters anomaly (see Fig. 170)
- *Embryopathies*: intrauterine infections (e.g. rubella, toxoplasmosis)
- *Metabolic*: galactokinase deficiency, galactosaemia and hypocalcaemia
- *Syndromes*: Lowe's, Down's, Turner's and *cri du chat*.

Clinical features

Appearance of infantile cataract is variable (Figs 179, 180).

Ectopia lentis

Definition

Displacement of the lens; may be partial (subluxation) or complete.

Aetiology

- *Trauma* (Fig. 181)
- *Familial ectopia lentis*: may be associated with ectopic pupil (Fig. 182)
- *Associated with other ocular disorders*: aniridia (see Fig. 171) and buphthalmos (see Fig. 167)
- *Syndromes*: Marfan's (Fig. 183) and Weill-Marchesani
- *Metabolic*: homocystinuria and hyperlysinaemia.

Abnormalities of lens size and shape

- *Microphakia*: small lens
- *Microspherophakia*: small spherical lens
- *Coloboma*: (Fig. 184) may be associated with colobomas of the iris and choroid, and giant retinal tears
- *Lenticonus*: cone-shaped lens surface (e.g. anterior lenticonus in Alport syndrome).

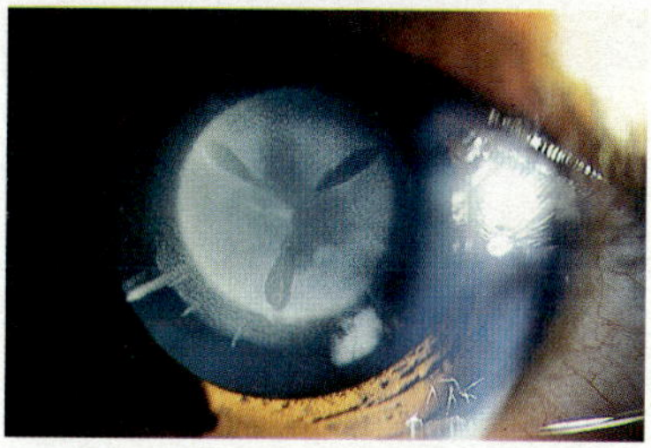
图 179　层状先天性白内障
Lamellar congenital cataract

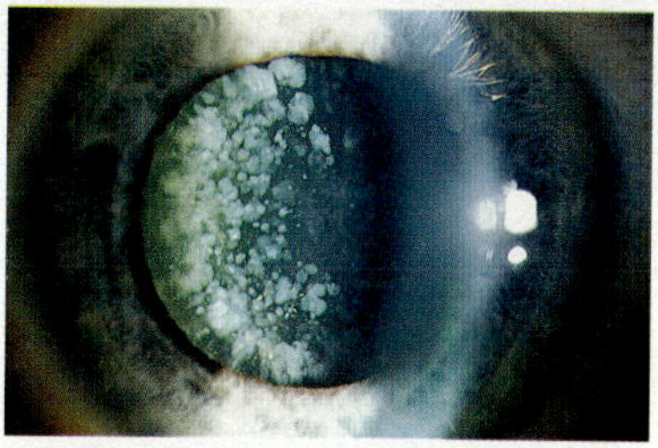
图 180　点状先天性晶状体浑浊
Punctate congenital lens opacities

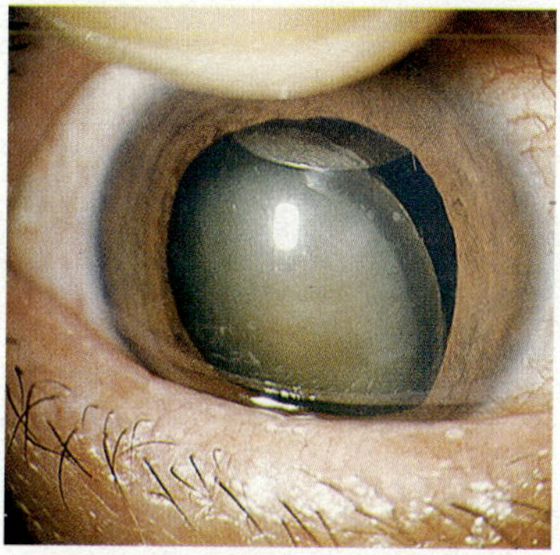
图 181　钝挫伤致晶状体半脱位
Lens subluxation due to blunt trauma

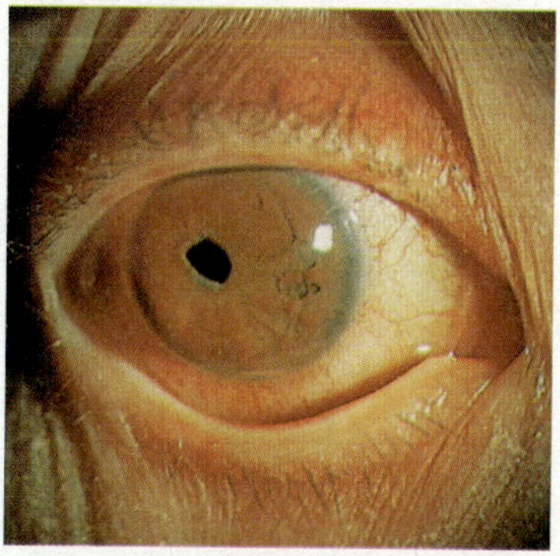
图 182　先天性瞳孔移位伴晶状体半脱位
Congenital ectopic pupil with associated lens subluxation

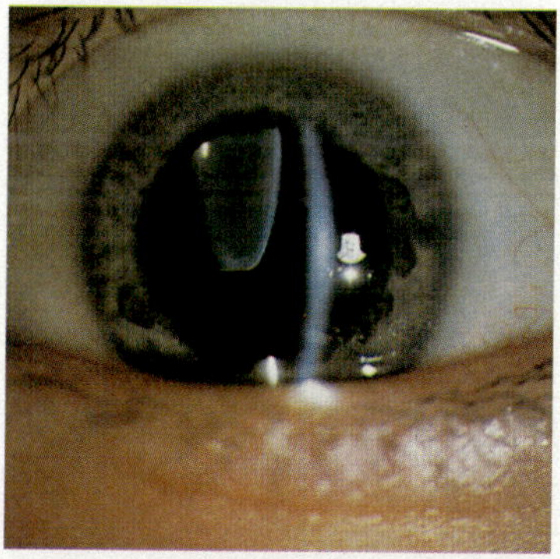
图 183　Marfan 综合征晶状体向上半脱位
Upward lens subluxation in Marfan's syndrome

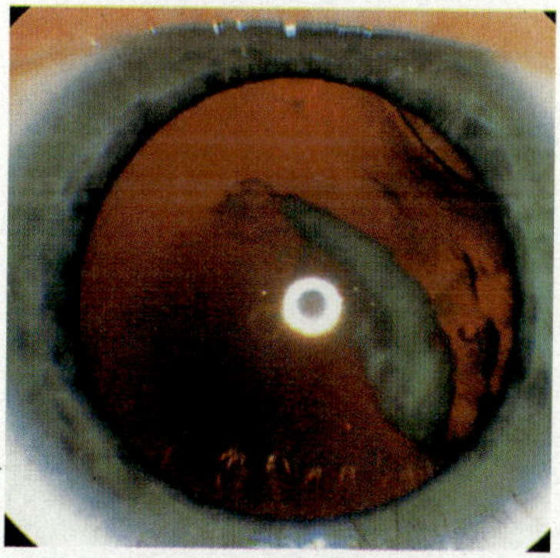
图 184　晶状体缺损和浑浊
Lens coloboma and opacity

32 糖尿病性视网膜病变

发病率

糖尿病性视网膜病变（DR）是青壮年最常见的致盲原因。DR的高发病率和严重性在于糖尿病持续时间；控制好血糖和高血压是重要的。

临床特征

背景性（单纯型）DR 微动脉瘤、圆点和污点状出血，硬性渗出(图 185，186)。

增殖前期DR 棉絮状斑，视网膜内微血管异常（IRMA），静脉的变化（串珠状、环状和节段状）和黑色污点状出血（图 187）。

增殖型糖尿病性视网膜病变 视盘新生血管形成（NVD，图188）或视网膜其他位置的新生血管形成（NVE，图189）。严重的视力丧失是由于玻璃体出血或纤维血管组织收缩导致的牵引性视网膜脱离（见图 224）。

糖尿病性黄斑病变 黄斑病变是引起糖尿病患者视力缺损最常见的原因。视功能下降通常是黄斑渗出水肿造成。如果黄斑出现局部缺血，常导致中心视力严重下降。

治疗

- 如果没有治疗指征，需定期检查，其频率取决于 DR 的严重度。
- 增殖型糖尿病性视网膜病变可行全视网膜的激光光凝（图 190）。
- 黄斑水肿（临床上明显的黄斑水肿）行格子样或病灶的激光光凝。
- 玻璃体切割术用于治疗长期玻璃体出血或包括黄斑中心的牵引性视网膜脱离。

Diabetic retinopathy

Incidence

Diabetic retinopathy (DR) is the most common cause of blindness in the working-age population. The incidence and severity of DR are strongly related to duration of diabetes; good control of blood glucose and hypertension are very important.

Clinical features

Background DR Microaneurysms, dot and blot haemorrhages and hard exudates (Figs 185, 186).

Preproliferative DR Cotton-wool spots, intraretinal microvascular anomalies (IRMA), venous changes (beading, looping and segmentation) and dark blot haemorrhages (Fig. 187).

Proliferative diabetic retinopathy New vessel formation at the optic disc (NVD - Fig. 188) or elsewhere on the retina (NVE - Fig. 189). Severe visual loss may occur as a result of vitreous haemorrhage or tractional retinal detachment due to contraction of fibrovascular tissue (see Fig. 224).

Diabetic maculopathy Maculopathy is the most common cause of visual impairment in patients with diabetes. Loss of visual function is usually caused by oedema, typically accompanied by exudates. Less commonly, the macula becomes ischaemic, often with severe deterioration in central vision.

Management

- Regular review if treatment is not indicated, frequency dependent on severity of DR
- Panretinal laser photocoagulation for proliferative DR (Fig. 190)
- Grid or focal laser photocoagulation for macular oedema fitting certain criteria ('clinically significant macular oedema')
- Vitrectomy for persistent vitreous haemorrhage or tractional retinal detachment involving the centre of the macula.

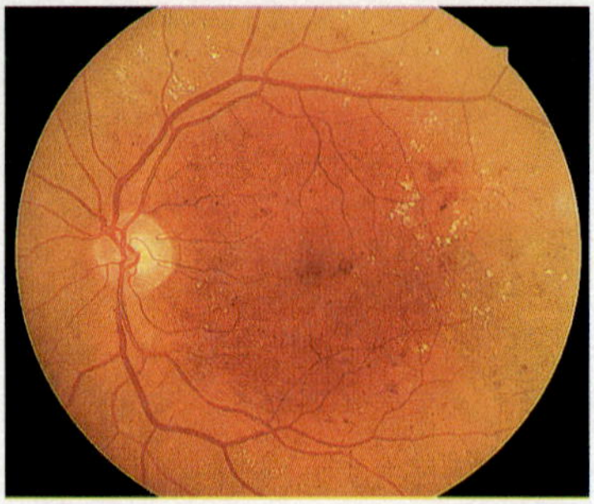

图 185 轻度单纯型糖尿病性视网膜病变
Mild background diabetic retinopathy

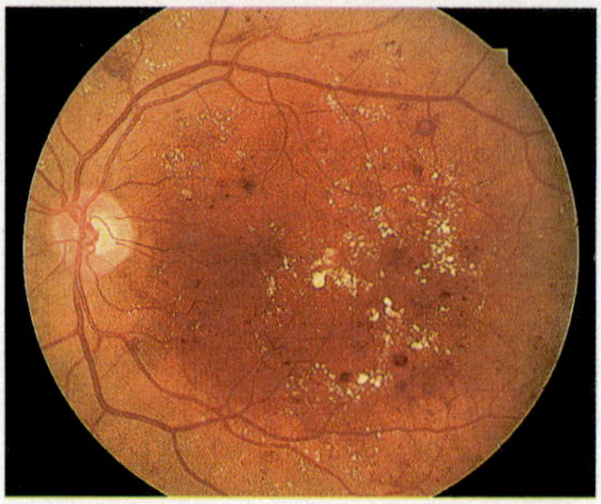

图 186 严重的单纯型糖尿病性视网膜病变
Severe background diabetic retinopathy

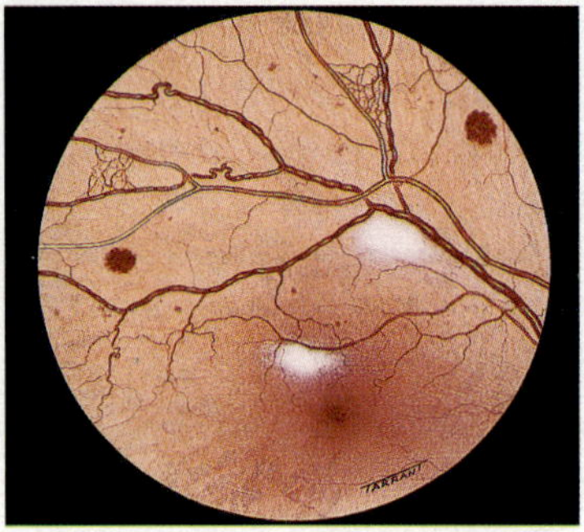

图 187 增殖前期糖尿病性视网膜病变
Pre-proliferative diabetic retinopathy

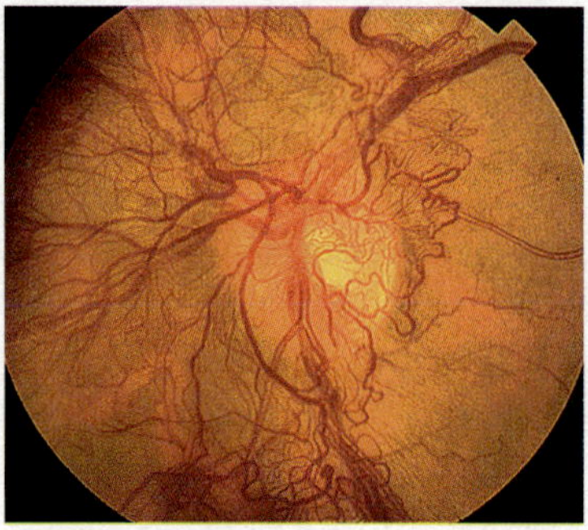

图 188 严重的视盘新生血管形成
Severe NVD

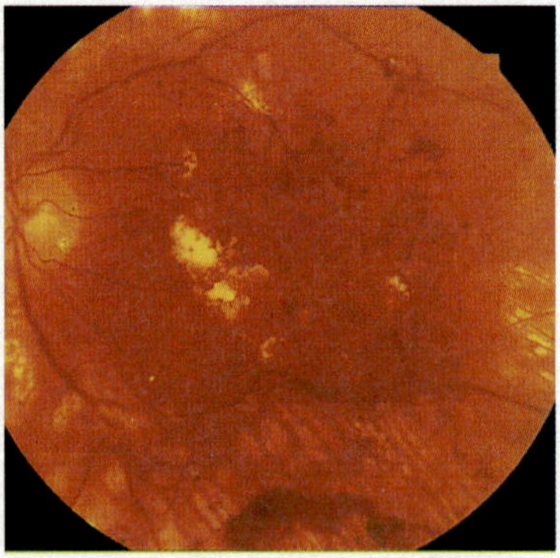

图 189 严重的视网膜新生血管形成
Severe NVE

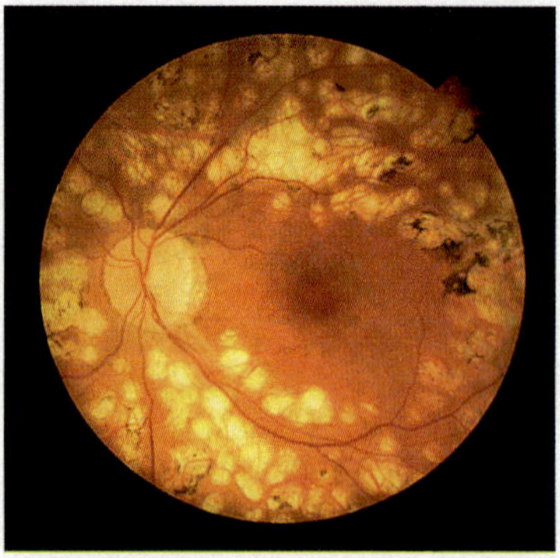

图 190 全视网膜光凝后的激光斑
Laser scars following panretinal photocoagulation

视网膜血管阻塞

视网膜静脉阻塞（RVO）

病因学

易感因素包括老年人、高血压、高血粘度、血管炎、血栓形成和高眼压。

临床特征

单眼突然出现由轻到重的视力下降。急性体征包括出血、棉絮状斑、静脉迂曲、视盘和视网膜水肿。

分类

- *视网膜分支静脉阻塞*（图191）：常累及视网膜一个象限。
- *半侧视网膜静脉阻塞*（图 192）。
- *视网膜中央静脉阻塞*：局部缺血或全部缺血（图193）。

并发症

- 视网膜新生血管形成，尤其是视网膜分支静脉阻塞，可行激光光凝。
- 黄斑水肿可行格子样激光光凝。
- 局部缺血的视网膜中央静脉阻塞可发生新生血管性青光眼（见图 161）。

视网膜动脉阻塞（RAO）

病因学

来源于颈动脉或心脏的栓塞，动脉粥样化或动脉炎导致的血管闭塞。

临床特征

突然视力丧失；永久或暂时的（一过性黑矇）。相关区域（中央动脉或分支动脉）可见视网膜苍白（图 194）和黄斑中心凹的“樱桃红斑”是视网膜中央动脉阻塞的特征性表现（图 195）。可见小动脉的节段状血流。晚期小动脉变细和视盘苍白。

治疗

- 急检红细胞沉降率（ESR），排除巨细胞性动脉炎和其他的危险度因素。
- 一过性黑矇：阿司匹林；严重的狭窄行颈动脉内膜剥离术。
- 急性的 RAO 可用按摩眼球法，静脉注射乙酰唑胺，行前房穿刺术降低眼压。

33 Retinal vascular occlusion

Retinal vein occlusion (RVO)

Aetiology

Predisposing factors include increasing age, hypertension, hyperviscosity, vasculitis, thrombophilic disorders and raised IOP.

Clinical features

Presents with sudden mild to severe loss of vision in one eye. Acute signs include haemorrhages, cotton wool spots, venous tortuosity, optic disc and retinal oedema.

Classification

- *Branch RVO* (Fig. 191): usually involves a retinal quadrant
- *Hemiretinal vein occlusion* (Fig. 192)
- *Central RVO*: ischaemic or non-ischaemic (Fig. 193).

Complications

- Retinal neovascularization, especially in BRVO, is treated with laser photocoagulation
- Macular oedema is treated with grid laser photocoagulation to the macula in selected cases
- Neovascular glaucoma (see Fig. 161) in ischaemic CRVO.

Retinal artery occlusion (RAO)

Aetiology

Embolization from a carotid or cardiac source, or vaso-obliteration by atheroma or arteritis.

Clinical features

Acute loss of vision; may be permanent or transient (amaurosis fugax). Retinal pallor corresponding to the involved area (central or branch) is seen (Fig. 194), and in central RAO a 'cherry red spot' at the fovea is typically present (Fig. 195). Segmentation of the arteriolar blood column ('cattle trucking') may be seen. Later the arterioles become attenuated and the optic disc pale.

Management

- Urgent erythrocyte sedimentation rate (ESR) to exclude giant cell arteritis and investigation of other risk factors
- Amaurosis fugax: aspirin; carotid endarterectomy for severe stenosis
- Acute RAO may be relieved by lowering IOP by massage, intravenous acetazolamide, anterior chamber paracentesis.

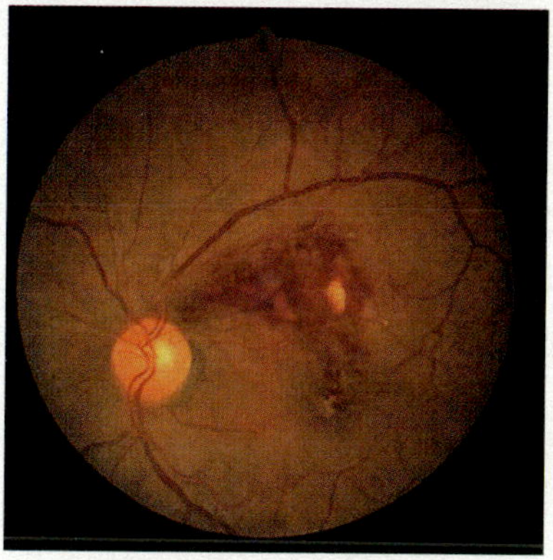

图 191 视网膜分支静脉阻塞
Branch retinal vein occlusion

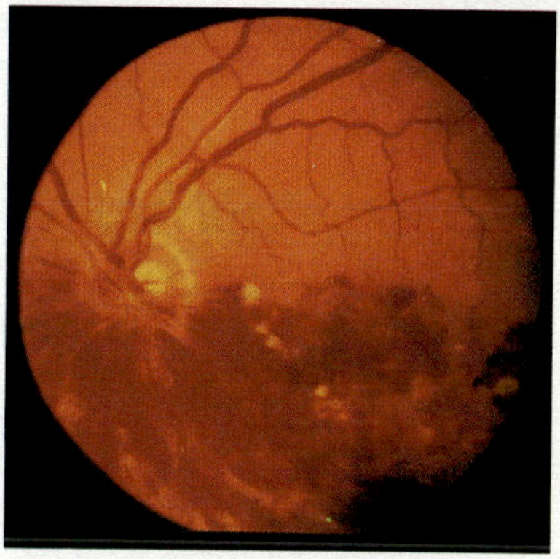

图 192 半侧视网膜静脉阻塞
Inferior hemiretinal vein occlusion

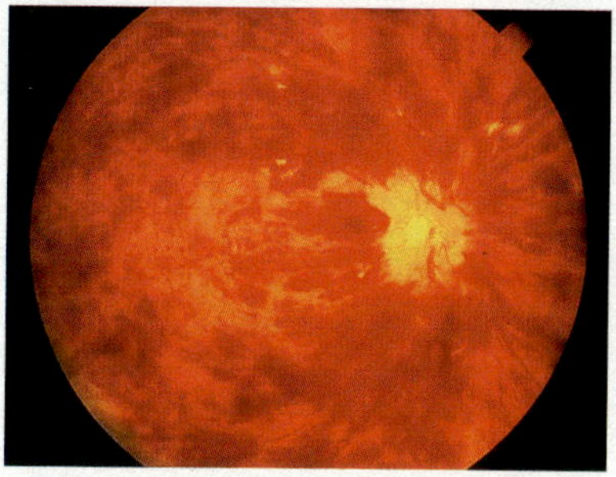

图 193 视网膜中央静脉阻塞
Central retinal vein occlusion

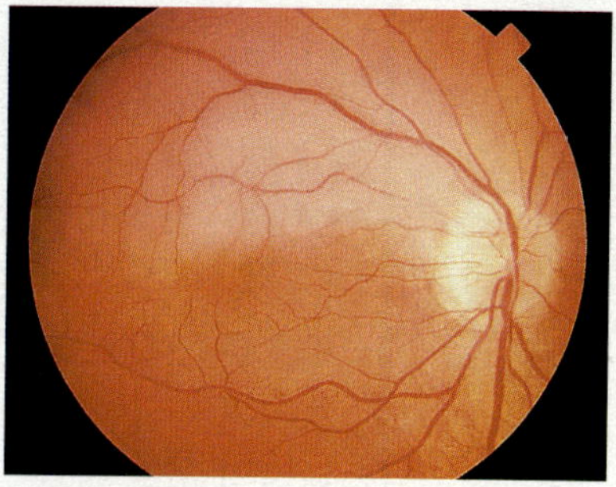

图 194 视网膜分支动脉阻塞
Branch retinal artery occlusion

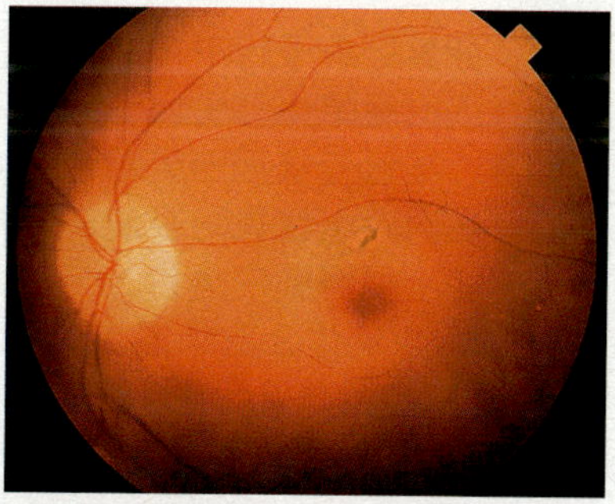

图 195 视网膜中央动脉阻塞伴“樱桃红斑”
Central retinal artery occlusion with 'cherry-red spot'

其他视网膜病变

高血压性视网膜病变

分类

- *1 期*：轻度的广泛小动脉收缩（图 196）。
- *2 期*：视网膜小动脉广泛的、明显的局限性狭窄（图 197）。
- *3 期*：2 期加上视网膜出血、棉絮状斑和硬性渗出物（图 198）。
- *4 期*：3 期加上视盘水肿（图 199）。

镰状红细胞视网膜病变

患者具有典型的镰状细胞或镰状细胞性地中海贫血。

分类

- *1 期*：末梢小动脉阻塞。
- *2 期*：末梢动静脉吻合。
- *3 期*：视网膜外的新生血管从动静脉吻合处生长。
- *4 期*：玻璃体出血（图 200）。
- *5 期*：牵引性视网膜脱离。

治疗

局部缺血区域多自发形成梗死，光凝固法很难成功，但玻璃体切割术对 4 期和 5 期需要的。

早产儿视网膜病变（ROP）

定义

低出生体重早产儿吸入高浓度氧气出现的增殖性视网膜病变。

分类

- *1 期*：分界标志平行于视网膜锯齿缘。
- *2 期*：视网膜嵴伴新生血管丛。
- *3 期*：纤维血管从视网膜嵴增殖（图 201）。
- *4 期*：次全牵引性视网膜脱离。
- *5 期*：完全视网膜脱离。
- *Plus 病*：玻璃体云雾状混浊，后极血管迂曲。
- *瘢痕性 ROP*：并发症由于急性期进入纤维化。

治疗

- 高危婴儿有组织的筛选。
- 冷冻疗法或激光光凝治疗周边视网膜病变分界线。

Miscellaneous retinopathies

Hypertensive retinopathy

Classification

- *Grade 1*: mild generalized arteriolar narrowing (Fig. 196)
- *Grade 2*: focal as well as marked generalized arteriolar constriction (Fig. 197)
- *Grade 3*: as Grade 2 plus retinal haemorrhages, cotton wool spots and hard exudates (Fig. 198)
- *Grade 4*: as Grade 3 plus optic disc swelling (Fig. 199).

Sickle-cell retinopathy

Patients typically have SC or SThal disease.

Classification

- *Stage 1*: peripheral arteriolar occlusion
- *Stage 2*: peripheral arteriovenous anastomoses
- *Stage 3*: growth of extraretinal new vessels from anastomoses
- *Stage 4*: vitreous haemorrhage (Fig. 200)
- *Stage 5*: tractional retinal detachment.

Management

A high rate of spontaneous infarction of ischaemic areas means that photocoagulation is rarely performed but vitrectomy may be required for stage 4 and 5 disease.

Retinopathy of prematurity (ROP)

Definition

Proliferative retinopathy affecting low-birth-weight preterm infants exposed to high ambient levels of oxygen.

Classification

- *Stage 1*: demarcation mark parallel to the ora serrata
- *Stage 2*: ridge with associated neovascular tufts
- *Stage 3*: fibrovascular proliferation from the ridge (Fig. 201)
- *Stage 4*: subtotal tractional retinal detachment
- *Stage 5*: total retinal detachment
- *'Plus' disease*: vitreous haze, posterior pole vascular tortuosity
- *Cicatricial ROP*: complications due to fibrosis following involution of acute disease.

Management

- Structured screening of at-risk infants
- Treatment with peripheral retinal cryotherapy or laser photocoagulation for 'threshold' disease.

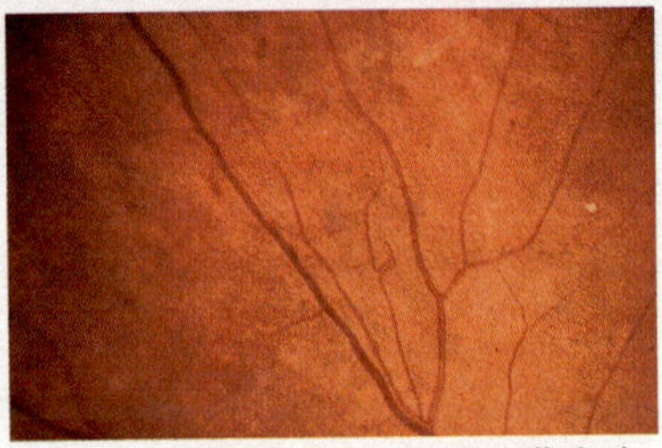

图 196 1 期高血压性视网膜病变的泛发性小动脉收缩
Generalized arteriolar constriction in Grade 1 hypertensive retinopathy

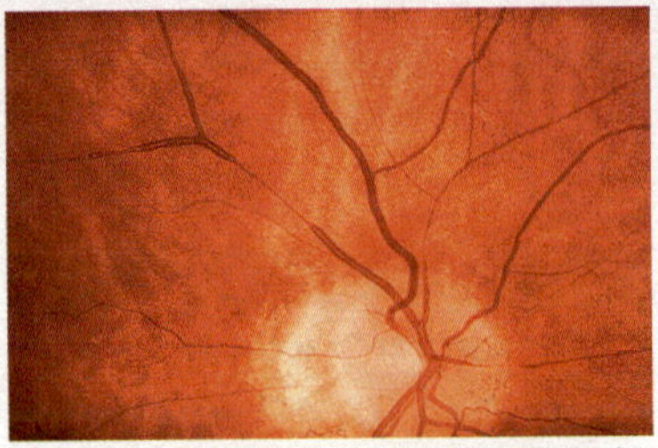

图 197 2 期高血压性视网膜病变的局部小动脉收缩
Focal arteriolar constriction in Grade 2 hypertensive retinopathy

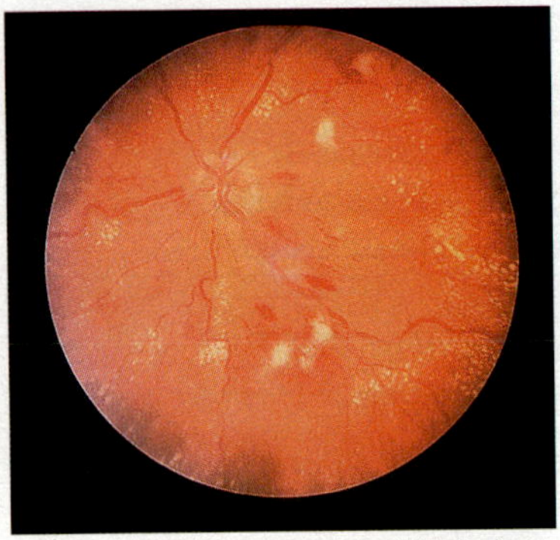

图 198 3 期高血压视网膜病变的出血、棉絮斑和硬性渗出
Haemorrhages, cotton wool spots and hard exudates in Grade 3 hypertensive retinopathy

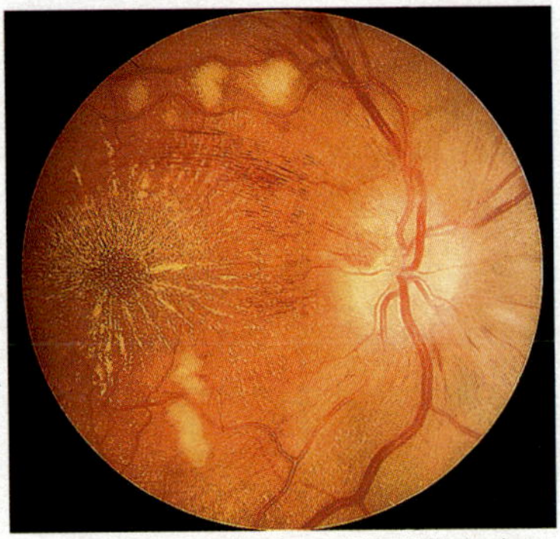

图 199 4 期高血压视网膜病变：3 期病变加上视盘水肿和黄斑星状水肿
Grade 3 changes plus optic disc swelling and a macular star in Grade 4 hypertensive retinopathy

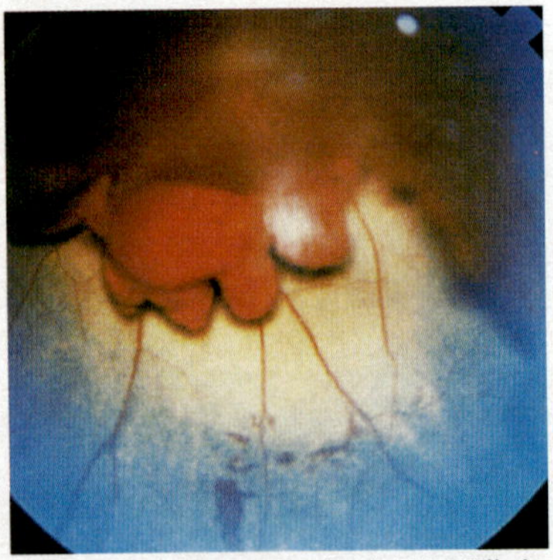

图 200 4 期镰状红细胞视网膜病变玻璃体出血
Vitreous haemorrhage in Stage 4 sickle-cell retinopathy

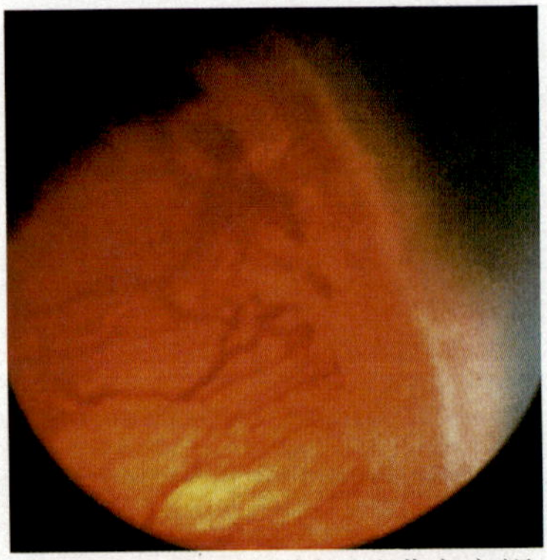

图 201 3 期早产儿视网膜病变视网膜嵴伴纤维血管增殖
Ridge with fibrovascular proliferation in Stage 3 ROP

年龄相关性黄斑退行性改变

发病率

年龄相关性黄斑退行性改变（AMD）是工业化社会最常见的致盲疾病。患者多为65岁以上；常双眼受累且多不对称。

临床特征

硬玻璃疣 小的、圆形、分散的、黄白色，常位于黄斑区（图 202）。

软玻璃疣 大的，边界不清的病变（图203）伴渗出性的 AMD。

非渗出性（"干性"）黄斑变性 视网膜色素上皮（RPE）萎缩和增生性改变伴随视神经视网膜和下面的脉络膜毛细血管层慢性进展性退变（图 204）。

渗出性（"湿性"）黄斑变性 脉络膜的新生血管向内生长穿过Bruch膜：脉络膜新生血管（CNV）。出现单眼中央视觉变形。检查可见黄斑一个区域由于视网膜下渗液或出血而隆起（图 205），常伴片状渗出（图 206）。大多数病变进展为视网膜下"盘状"瘢痕形成伴中心视力永久性缺失（图 207）。

RPE脱离（PED） RPE圆顶形渗出性脱离。可进展为上面描述的渗出性 AMD，有时可自然复位。

息肉的脉络膜血管病变（PCV） 这是最近描述的AMD，其表现像CNV。治疗效果明显，仍有明确的定义。

治疗

- 治疗常常无用或暂时有用，因此只能有选择的治疗。
- 抗氧化维生素和矿物的补充可能延缓 AMD 发展。
- 常规的激光消除 CNV 是有效的，可防止侵犯黄斑中心。
- 光动力疗法（PDT）是一项新技术，可用激光，使被 CNV 吸收的光敏染料活化。

35 Age-related macular degeneration

Incidence

Age-related macular degeneration (AMD) is the most common cause of legal blindness in industrialized societies. Patients are typically over the age of 65 years; both eyes are usually affected, frequently asymmetrically.

Clinical features

Hard drusen Small, round, discrete, yellow-white lesions, usually located at the macula (Fig. 202).

Soft drusen Larger lesions with ill-defined edges (Fig. 203) associated with exudative AMD.

Non-exudative ('dry') macular degeneration Atrophic and hyperplastic changes of the retinal pigment epithelium (RPE) associated with slowly progressive degeneration of the overlying neuroretina and underlying choriocapillaris (Fig. 204).

Exudative ('wet') macular degeneration The ingrowth of choroidal new vessels through Bruch membrane: choroidal neovascularization (CNV). Presents with unilateral distortion of central vision. On examination, an area of the macula is elevated by subretinal fluid or blood (Fig. 205), often with associated clumps of exudates (Fig. 206). The lesion evolves in most cases to leave subretinal 'disciform' scarring with permanent loss of central vision (Fig.207).

RPE detachment (PED) Fluid elevates the RPE in a dome configuration. This may progress to exudative AMD described above or may occasionally settle spontaneously.

Polypoidal choroidal vasculopathy (PCV) This recently-described form of AMD may masquerade as CNV. Its behaviour, particularly the response to treatment, has yet to be clearly defined.

Management

- Often of negligible or temporary benefit and therefore only used in selected cases
- Antioxidant vitamin and mineral supplements may retard the progression of AMD
- Conventional laser may be effective at destroying CNV that does not encroach on the central macula
- Photodynamic therapy (PDT) is a newer technique using a laser to activate a light-sensitive dye preferentially taken up by CNV.

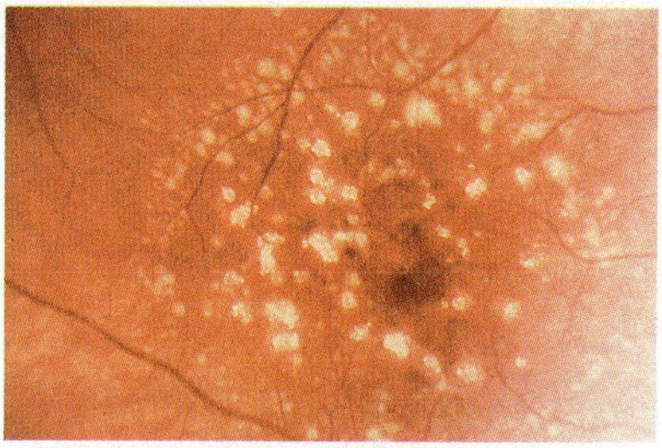

图 202　黄斑区的硬玻璃疣
Macular hard drusen

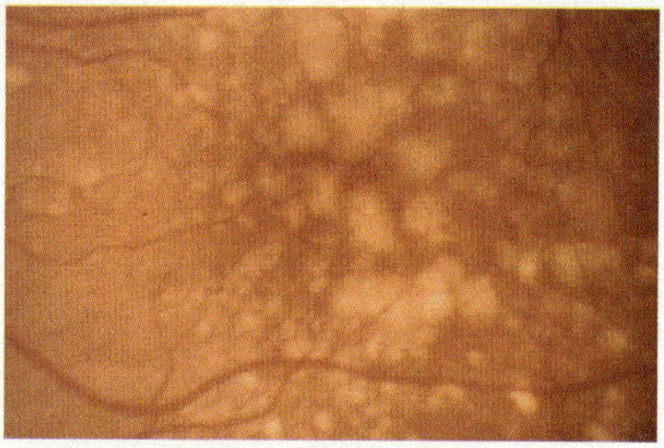

图 203　黄斑区的软玻璃疣
Macular soft drusen

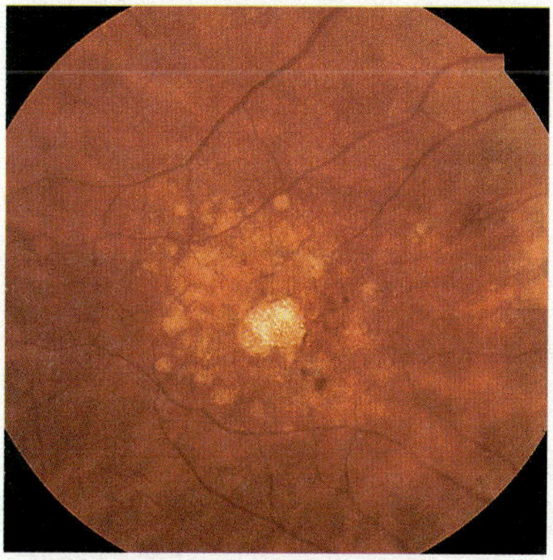

图 204　早期干性黄斑变性
Early 'dry' macular degeneration

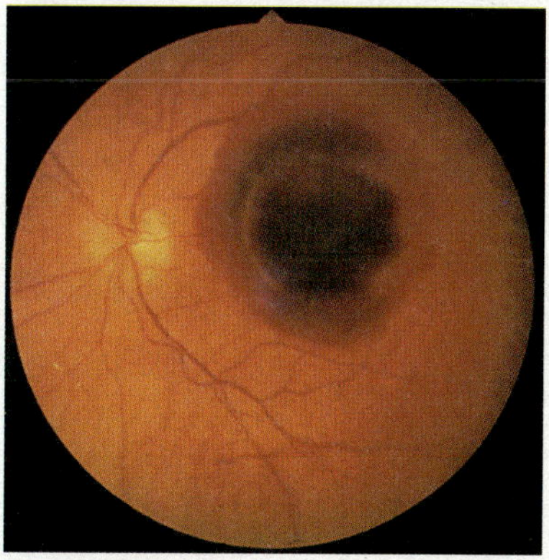

图 205　视网膜下出血伴脉络膜新生血管
Subretinal haemorrhage associated with CNV

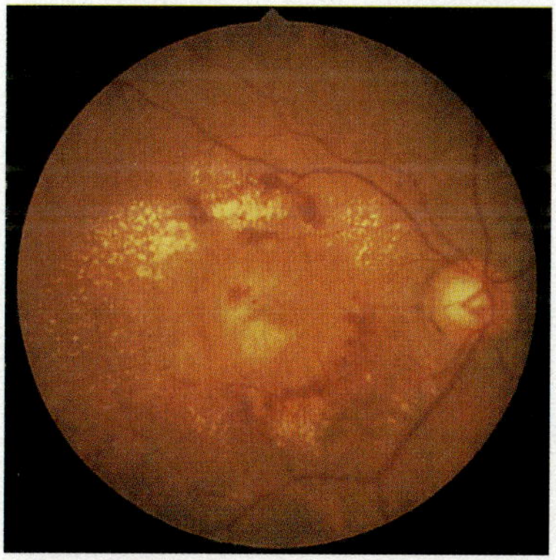

图 206　视网膜内部和下面渗出伴脉络膜新生血管
Intra- and subretinal exudation associated with CNV

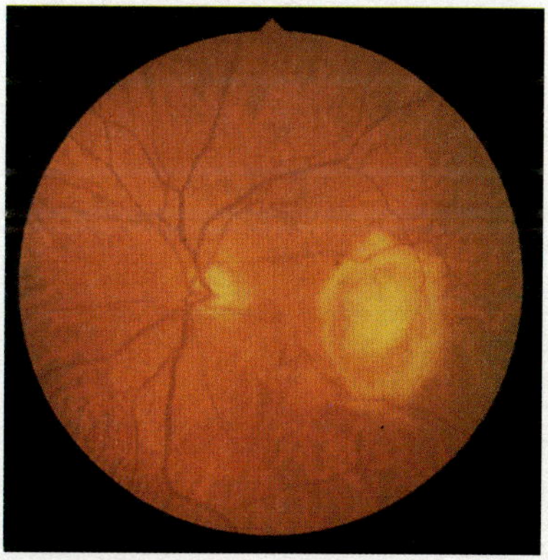

图 207　陈旧性盘状瘢痕
Advanced disciform scarring

36 后天性黄斑病变

黄斑裂孔

临床特征

当一眼闭上时偶然发现另一眼视力缺损。检查可见中心凹圆形缺损区域，测量为1/3视盘直径，周围有一圈灰白色的视网膜隆起（图 208）。早期病例治疗可行玻璃体切割术和眼球内注气。

近视性黄斑病变

临床特征

常见疾病表现为一眼视物变形或视力下降。检查可见多种变化：色素增殖（Fuchs斑，图209），黄斑萎缩（图210），Bruch 膜裂隙（“漆器裂缝”）和黄斑出血。

黄斑视网膜前膜

临床特征

神经胶质细胞增殖伴随纤维组织穿过视网膜表面，常为特发性，也可为视网膜疾病、震荡或创伤造成。表现为一眼视物变形和逐渐发生的视物模糊。早期前膜较薄（“玻璃纸样黄斑病变”），出现轻度视网膜皱纹和血管迂曲。前膜变厚和收缩，病变变得明显（黄斑皱褶，图 211）。

血管样纹

罕见的双眼病变，可见自视盘发出线形条纹（图 212）。视力较CNV受累明显。大约50%的血管样纹患者有弹性（纤维）假黄瘤。

“靶心”状黄斑病变

黄斑中心凹色素沉着被无色素的区域围绕，依次再被色素沉着环环绕（图 213）。原因包括抗疟药，锥体营养不良，Stargardt病（眼底黄色斑点症，见图215）和少年型家族性黑矇性痴呆。

Macular hole

Clinical features

The visual deficit is often noticed by chance when one eye is closed. On examination a rounded punched-out area measuring one-third of a disc diameter is seen at the fovea, surrounded by a grey halo of retinal elevation (Fig. 208). Treatment in early cases is by vitrectomy and intraocular gas.

Myopic maculopathy

Clinical features

Presentation of this common disorder is with either unilateral metamorphopsia or impaired visual acuity. On examination, a variety of changes may be seen: pigment proliferation (Fuchs spot - Fig. 209), atrophic maculopathy (Fig. 210), breaks in the Bruch membrane ('lacquer cracks') and macular haemorrhage.

Macular epiretinal membrane

Clinical features

This proliferation of glial cells and associated fibrous tissue across the retinal surface is often idiopathic but may occur following retinal disease, surgery or trauma. Presentation is with unilateral distortion and blurring of gradual onset. An early membrane may be subtle ('cellophane maculopathy') and manifest mild retinal wrinkling and vascular tortuosity. As a membrane thickens and contracts, the changes become more evident ('macular pucker' - Fig. 211).

Angioid streaks

In this rare binocular condition, linear streaks are seen radiating from the optic disc (Fig. 212). Vision can be affected, particularly by CNV. About 50% of individuals with angioid streaks have pseudoxanthoma elasticum.

Bull's eye maculopathy

Central foveolar hyperpigmentation surrounded by a depigmented zone encircled in turn by a hyperpigmented ring (Fig. 213). Causes include antimalarial drugs, cone dystrophy, Stargardt disease (see Fig. 215) and Batten disease.

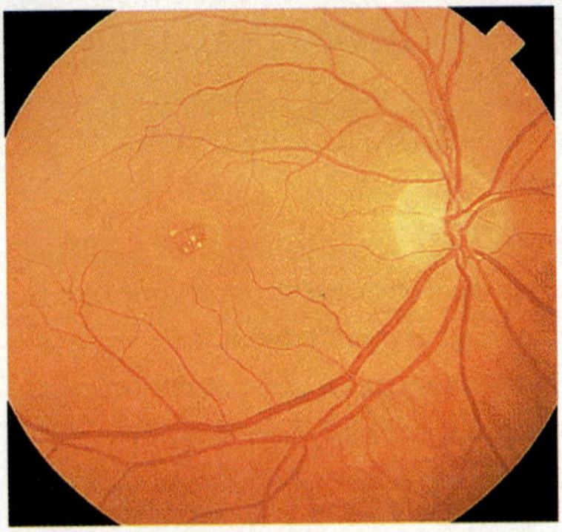

图 208　黄斑裂孔
Macular hole

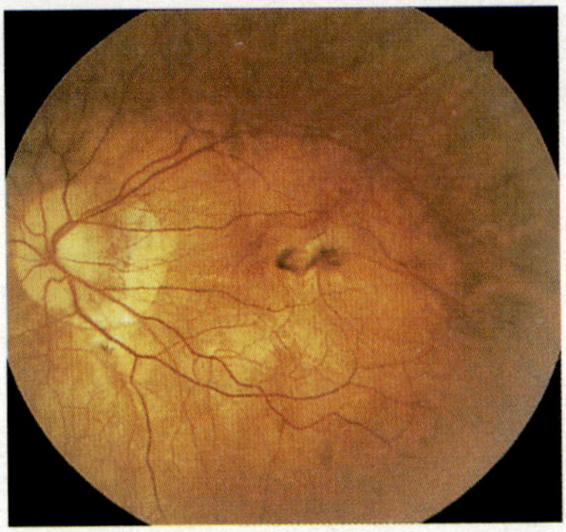

图 209　近视性黄斑病变：Fuchs 斑
Myopic maculopathy: Fuchs spot

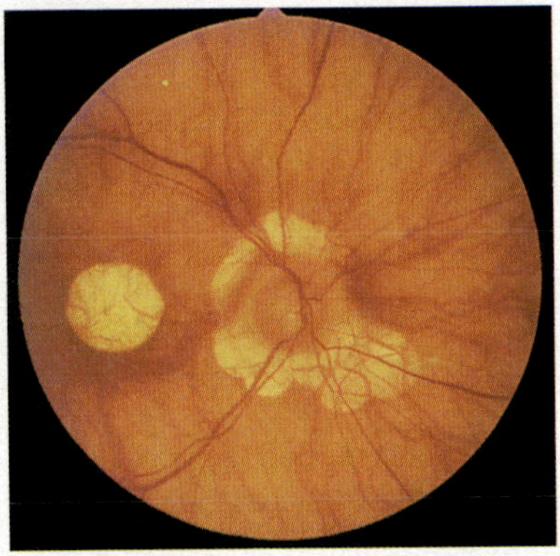

图 210　黄斑萎缩
Atrophic maculopathy

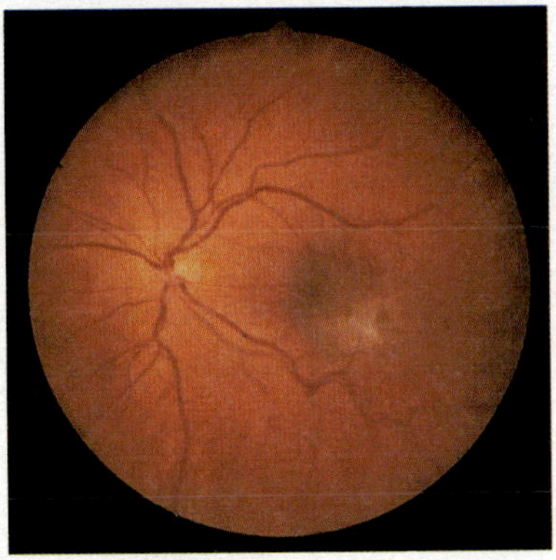

图 211　黄斑皱褶
Macular pucker

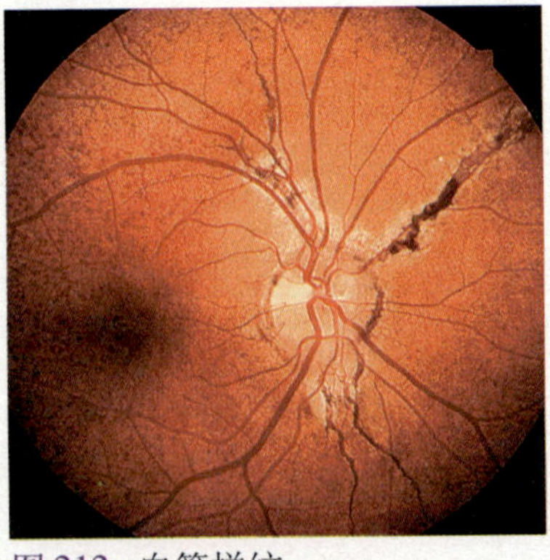

图 212　血管样纹
Angioid streaks

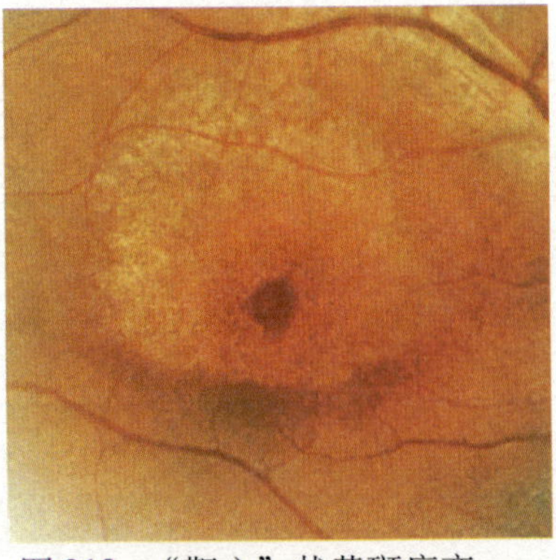

图 213　“靶心”状黄斑病变
Bull's eye maculopathy

色素性视网膜炎（视网膜色素变性）

少见，发病于10～20岁，伴夜盲。常染色体显性遗传、常染色体隐性遗传或X-连锁遗传。大多数遗传的异常导致临床表现，标志是赤道部－周边血管周围的"骨小体"状色素沉着，小动脉变细和视盘蜡黄(图214)。多伴黄斑水肿和白内障。许多是全身综合征表现之一。

Stargardt 病和黄点状眼底病

这两种病变是常染色体隐性遗传疾病的变异。表现为中心视力缺损：Stargardt病发病于少年，黄点状眼底病发病于青年。Stargardt病早期可见"青铜"样斑点，逐渐发展成萎缩区（图 215)。黄点状眼底病黄白色斑点分散在后极和赤道部－周边视网膜各处(图 216)，可发展为与 Stargardt 病相似的黄斑病。

Best 病（卵黄状黄斑营养不良）

罕见的常染色体显性基因遗传病，黄斑出现随着时间的进展从青少年的卵黄样（蛋黄形）病变（图217)至成人瘢痕形成和严重的视力下降。

脉络膜营养不良

无脉络膜症　极罕见的X-连锁遗传性疾病，10岁以内发病伴夜盲，具有特征性的视网膜赤道部扩大的脉络膜视网膜萎缩斑，在中心部进行性扩展但黄斑部受累极晚（图 218)。

脉络膜视网膜回旋形萎缩　极罕见的常染色体隐性遗传，先天性代谢异常，10 岁以内发病伴夜盲，具有特征的脉络膜视网膜萎缩形成的视网膜赤道部融合斑（图 219)。

37 Dystrophies of the fundus

Retinitis pigmentosa

Presentation of this uncommon condition is during the second decade of life with night blindness. Inheritance may be autosomal dominant, recessive or X-linked. A large number of genetic abnormalities have been found to cause the clinical picture, the hallmarks of which are mid-peripheral perivascular 'bone-spicule' pigmentation, arteriolar attenuation and waxy disc pallor (Fig. 214). Associated macular oedema and cataract are common. A number of systemic syndromes are associated.

Stargardt's disease and fundus flavimaculatus

These two uncommon conditions represent variants of the same underlying autosomal recessive disease. Presentation is with central visual impairment: in early adulthood in Stargardt's and early middle age in fundus flavimaculatus. In early Stargardt's disease a 'beaten-bronze' macular lesion is seen that slowly progresses to an atrophic lesion (Fig. 215). In fundus flavimaculatus yellow-white flecks are scattered throughout the posterior pole and mid-peripheral fundus (Fig. 216), and maculopathy similar to Stargardt's may develop.

Best's disease

In this rare dominantly inherited disorder the macular appearance evolves over time from a juvenile egg yolk (vitelliform) lesion (Fig. 217) to scarring and severe visual loss in adult life.

Choroidal dystrophies

Choroideremia Very rare X-linked disorder presenting during the first decade with night blindness characterized by enlarging midretinal patches of chorioretinal atrophy that progressively spread centrally but spare the macula till late on (Fig. 218).

Gyrate atrophy Very rare recessively inherited inborn error of metabolism presenting during the first decade with night blindness characterized by coalescing midretinal patches of chorioretinal atrophy (Fig. 219).

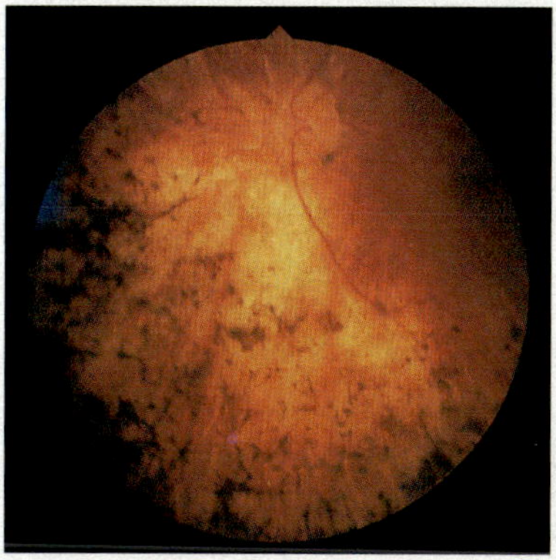

图 214 色素性视网膜炎
Retinitis pigmentosa

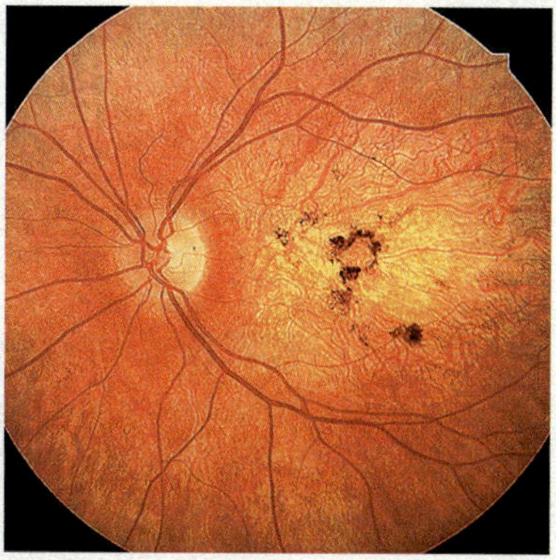

图 215 陈旧性 Stargardt 病
Advanced Stargardt's disease

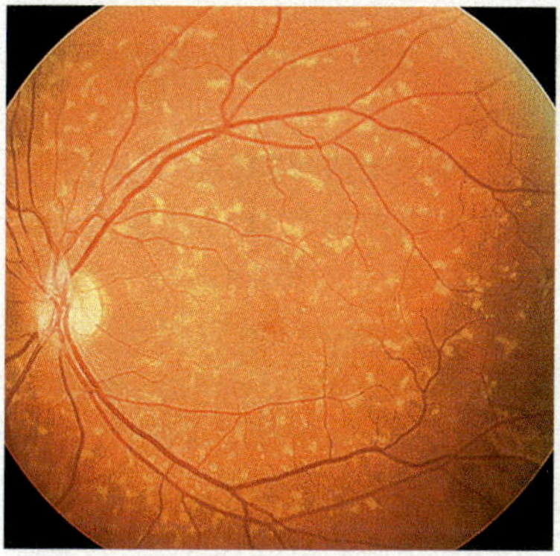

图 216 黄点状眼底病
Fundus flavimaculatus

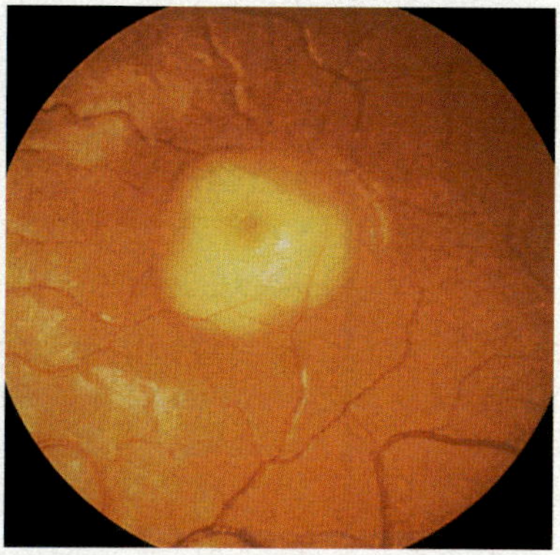

图 217 Best 病卵黄样病变
Vitelliform lesion in Best's disease

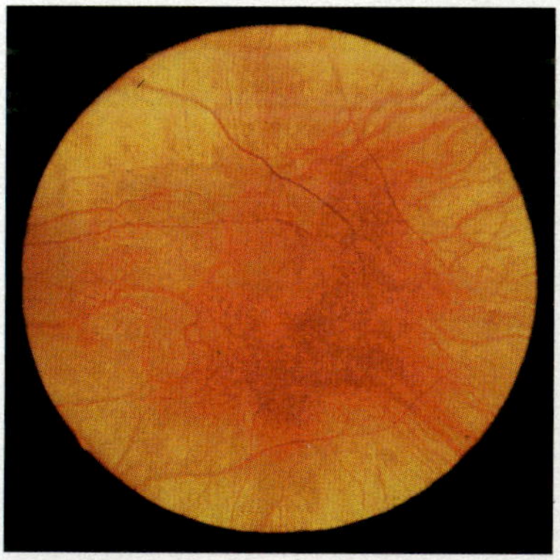

图 218 陈旧性无脉络膜症
Advanced choroideremia

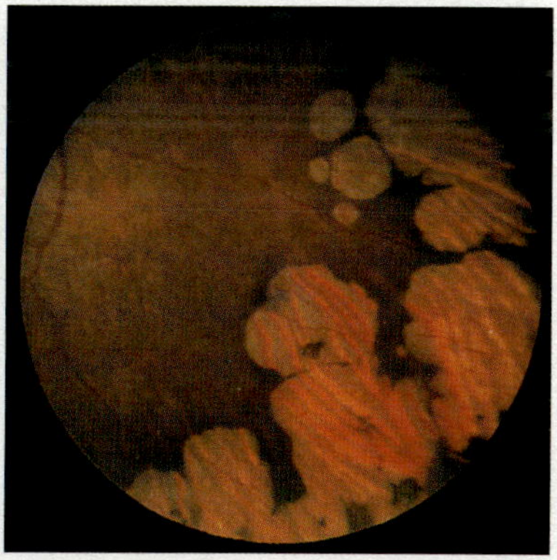

图 219 脉络膜视网膜回旋形萎缩
Gyrate atrophy

38 视网膜脱离

定义

视网膜神经上皮层被积聚的视网膜下积液（SRF）从下面的视网膜色素上皮层（RPE）分离。

孔源性视网膜脱离

病因学

由于玻璃体视网膜在周边视网膜的薄弱区域（如格子状变性，图221）牵引使视网膜撕裂（图220）而发展。

临床特征

- *急性*：活动性的隆起，半透明，波浪状的视网膜脱离（图 222）有裂孔。
- *长期*：视网膜变薄，叠峦状，有分界线（“高水位标志”），纤维化的固定的视网膜（增殖性玻璃体视网膜病变，PVR，图 223）。

治疗

- 巩膜扣带术可用于治疗不复杂的视网膜脱离。
- 玻璃体切割术结合玻璃体内注射气体或硅油用于治疗复杂的视网膜脱离。

牵引性视网膜脱离

纤维组织收缩引起无裂孔视网膜脱离，如由于增殖型糖尿病性视网膜病变；检查固定不动的视网膜凹面看到少量视网膜下液（图 224）。治疗是在睫状体平坦部行玻璃体切割术。

渗出性视网膜脱离

病因学

液体从脉络膜进入视网膜下间隙导致生理学的屏障破坏。原因包括眼内的肿瘤、炎症、严重的CNV、广泛的激光光凝和严重的高血压。

临床特征

球形脱离、视网膜活动度好、大量可移动液体、无裂孔（图 225）。积极寻找原发病。

Retinal detachment 38

Definition

A separation of the neuroretina from the underlying retinal pigment epithelium (RPE) by the accumulation of subretinal fluid (SRF).

Rhegmatogenous retinal detachment

Aetiology

A retinal tear (Fig. 220) develops as a result of vitreoretinal traction on a weak area in the peripheral retina (e.g. lattice degeneration - Fig. 221).

Clinical features

- *Acute*: mobile convex, slightly opaque, corrugated detached retina (Fig. 222) with break(s)
- *Long-standing*: retinal thinning, cysts, demarcation lines ('high water marks'), and fibrotic and immobile retina (proliferative vitreoretinopathy - PVR - Fig. 223).

Management

- Scleral buckling for uncomplicated cases
- Vitrectomy combined with intravitreal injection of gas or silicone oil for complicated cases.

Tractional retinal detachment

Contraction of fibrous tissue, e.g. associated with proliferative diabetic retinopathy, causes the retina to detach without a break; on examination concave immobile retina with shallow SRF is seen (Fig. 224). Treated by pars plana vitrectomy.

Exudative retinal detachment

Aetiology

The passage of fluid from the choroid into the subretinal space occurs following breakdown of physiological barriers. Causes include intraocular tumours, inflammation, severe CNV, extensive laser photocoagulation and severe hypertension.

Clinical features

Convex, very mobile retina with deep shifting fluid and absence of retinal breaks (Fig. 225). Treatment consists of addressing the cause.

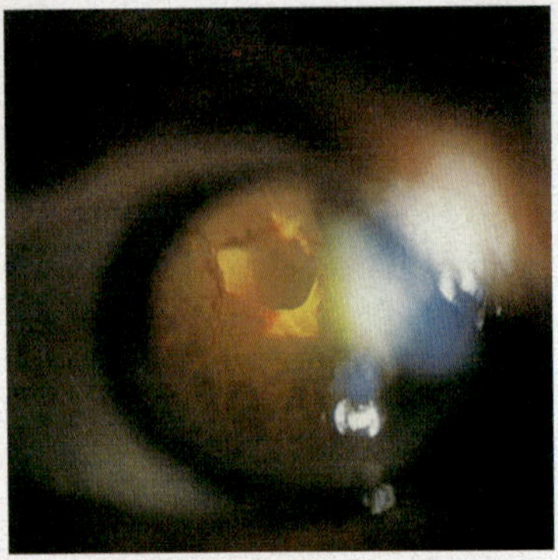

图 220　大的视网膜撕裂
Large retinal tear

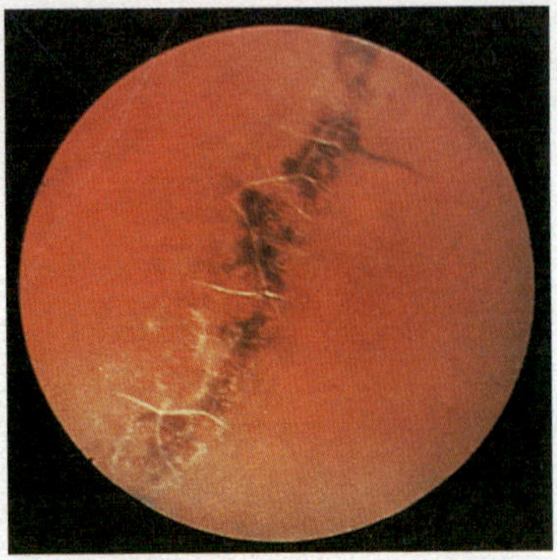

图 221　格子状变性
Lattice degeneration

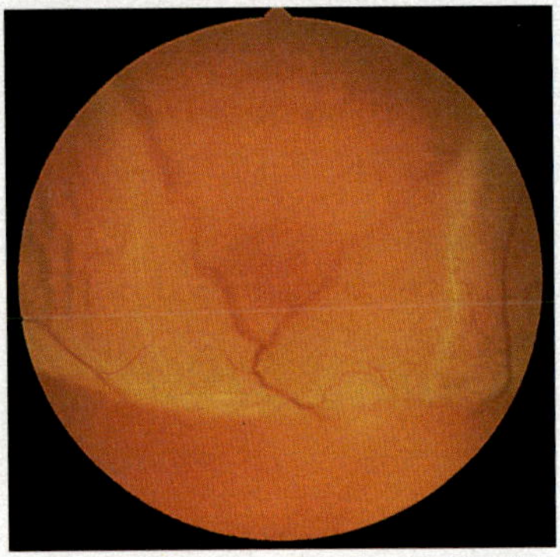

图 222　急性高度孔源性视网膜脱离
Acute superior rhegmatogenous retinal detachment

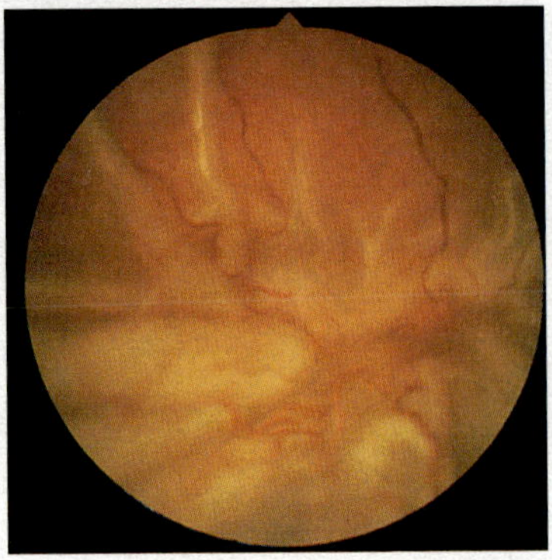

图 223　完全性孔源性视网膜脱离伴严重 PVR
Total rhegmatogenous detachment with severe PVR

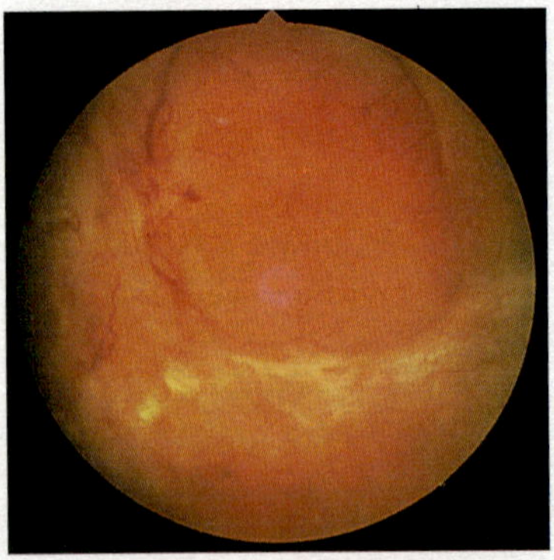

图 224　牵引性视网膜脱离
Tractional retinal detachment

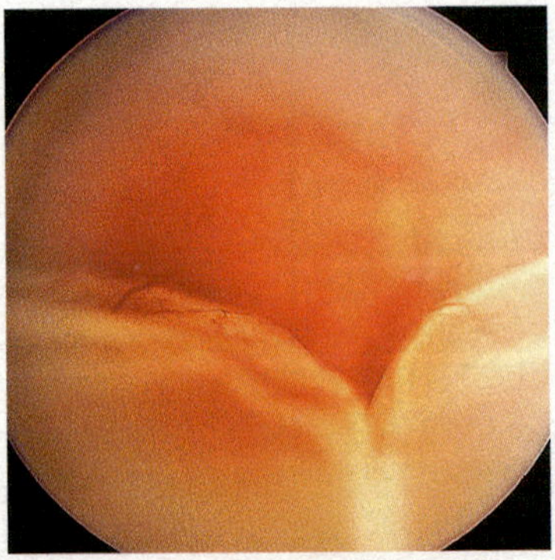

图 225　渗出性视网膜脱离
Exudative retinal detachment

脉络膜痣

临床特征 常见良性肿瘤，扁平的或轻度隆起、椭圆形或圆形、石灰色病变，直径通常小于3mm。痣表面常见玻璃疣（图226）。

脉络膜黑色素瘤

临床特征 成人最常见的原发性眼内恶性肿瘤。检查可见着色的或无色的视网膜下肿块伴渗出性视网膜脱离（图227）。

治疗 治疗包括眼球摘除术，点状或线状放射治疗，激光光凝或局部切除术。

虹膜黑色素瘤

临床特征 着色的或无色素的虹膜下结节（图 228）可伴瞳孔变形，色素层外翻和虹膜新生血管形成。

脉络膜血管瘤

临床特征 极罕见，圆顶状或鳞状、橙红色病变多位于后极（图229），多伴继发的囊样变性和色素斑。

（脉络膜）转移癌

临床特征 单个或多发，累及单眼或双眼，奶白色椭圆形病变，边界不清，多位于后极（图 230）。原发病灶多位于支气管或乳房。

脉络膜骨瘤

临床特征 极罕见的肿瘤，多发病于青年女性。轻度地隆起，橙黄色病变边界清楚，位于后极（图 231）。25% 的患者最后双眼发病。

39 Tumours of the uvea

Choroidal naevus

Clinical features

This common benign tumour is a flat or slightly elevated, oval or round, slate-grey lesion, usually less than 3mm in diameter. Overlying drusen are often present (Fig. 226).

Choroidal melanoma

Clinical features

This is the most common primary malignant intraocular tumour in adults. Examination shows a pigmented or amelanotic subretinal mass associated with exudative retinal detachment (Fig. 227)

Management

Options include enucleation, plaque or external beam irradiation, laser photocoagulation or local resection.

Iris melanoma

Clinical features

A pigmented or non-pigmented inferior iris nodule (Fig. 228) which may be associated with pupillary distortion, ectropion uveae and iris neovascularization.

Choroidal haemangioma

Clinical features

A very rare dome-shaped or placoid, orange-red lesion typically located at the posterior pole (Fig. 229) which may be associated with secondary cystoid degeneration and pigment mottling.

Metastatic carcinoma

Clinical features

Solitary or multiple, unilateral or bilateral, creamy-white, oval lesions with ill-defined borders, most commonly located at the posterior pole (Fig. 230). Common primary sites are the bronchus and breast.

Choroidal osteoma

Clinical features

This very rare tumour typically presents in a young female as a slightly elevated, orange-yellow lesion with well-demarcated borders, located at the posterior pole (Fig. 231). 25% are eventually bilateral.

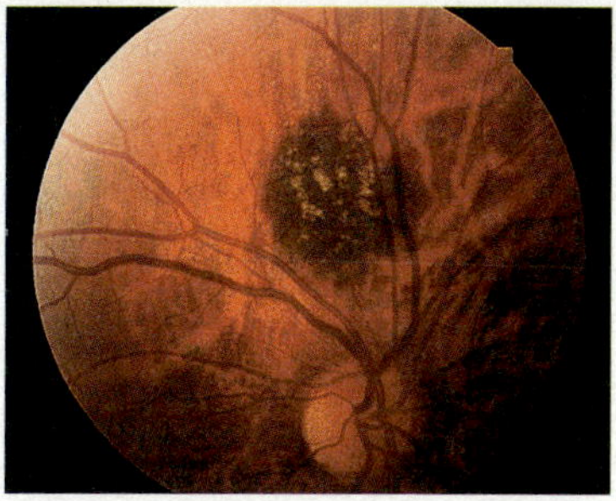

图 226 脉络膜痣伴表面玻璃疣
Choroidal naevus with overlying drusen

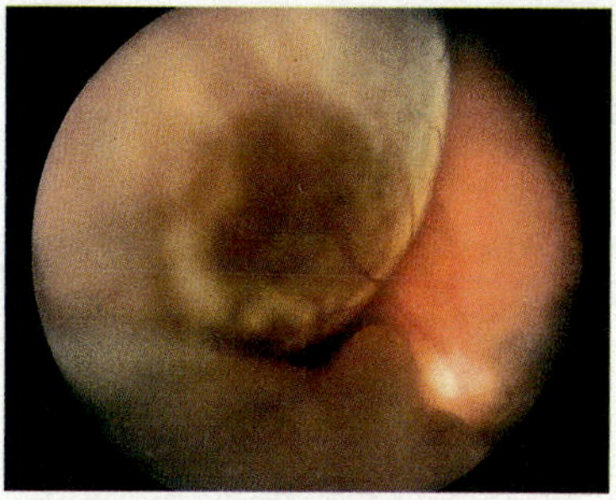

图 227 巨大脉络膜黑色素瘤伴渗出性视网膜脱离
Large choroidal melanoma with exudative retinal detachment

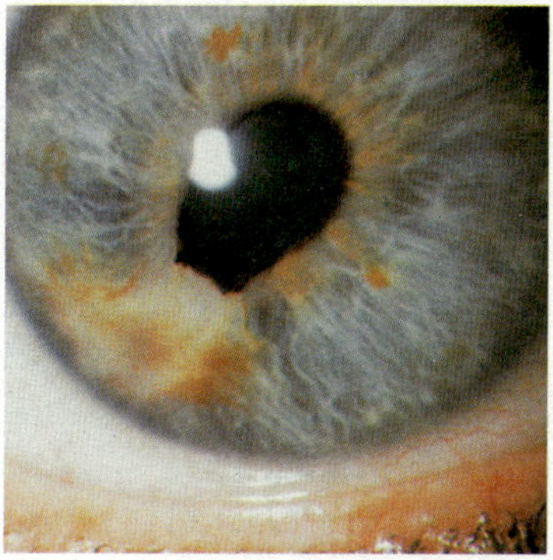

图 228 虹膜黑色素瘤
Iris melanoma

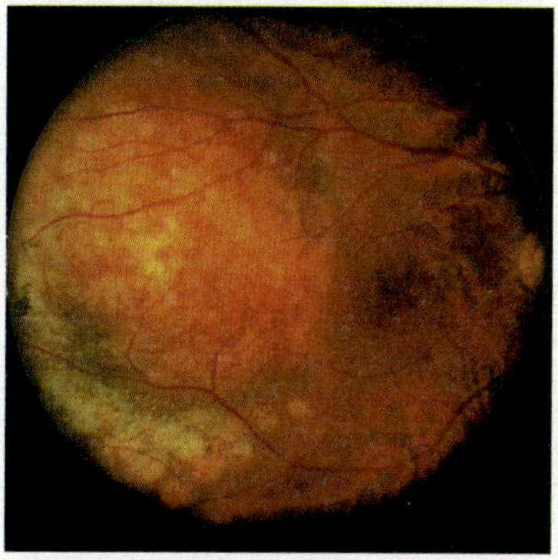

图 229 脉络膜血管瘤伴渗出性视网膜脱离
Choroidal haemangioma with exudative retinal detachment

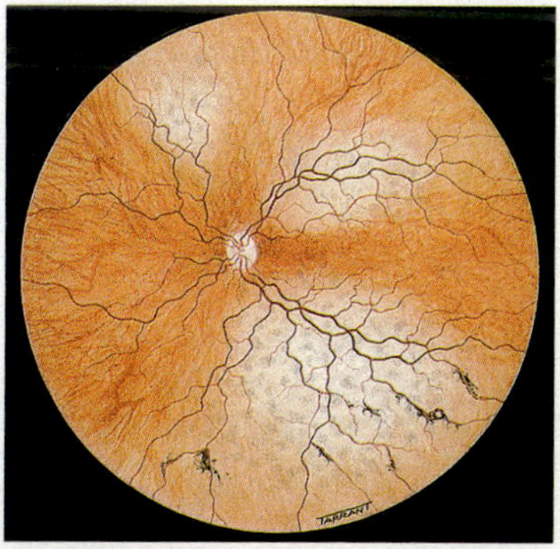

图 230 三个脉络膜转移癌
Three choroidal metastases

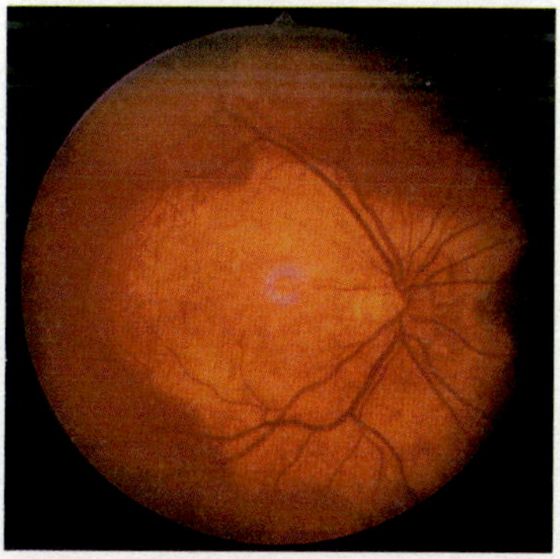

图 231 脉络膜骨瘤
Choroidal osteoma

视网膜和视盘肿瘤

视网膜母细胞瘤

临床特征 儿童最常见的眼内恶性肿瘤。30% 的患者双眼发病；6%患者有家族史。多在18个月左右发病，伴白瞳（瞳孔泛白，图 232）和肿瘤生长进入玻璃体腔（内生性）或视网膜下的空间（外生性）。

治疗 治疗包括点状或线状放射治疗、激光光凝、冷冻疗法、全身的化学治疗和剜出术。

视网膜的星形细胞瘤

临床特征 罕见，良性肿瘤，本病常伴有结节性硬化（Bourneville病）。白色，圆形肿块经常位于靠近视盘处（图 233）。多发，累及双眼。

视网膜毛细血管瘤

临床特征 罕见，良性肿瘤。圆形，橙红色病变伴随输入小动脉和输出小静脉的扩张（图 234）。常为多发的，50% 病例双眼受累。25% 患者有器官系统损害（von Hippel-Lindau综合征：即遗传性斑痣性错构瘤）。治疗包括激光光凝或冷冻疗法。

视网膜海绵状血管瘤

极罕见的先天性病变，特征是葡萄样的动脉瘤簇（图 235）。

视网膜蔓状血管瘤

极罕见的先天性动静脉畸形，包括显著扩张和扭曲的血管（图236）。部分患者有中枢神经系统疾病（Wyburn-Mason 综合征，即神经视网膜血管瘤综合征）。

视盘黑色素细胞瘤

罕见，良性黑色肿瘤伴羽毛状边缘（图 237），常见于皮肤色泽较深的患者。

Tumours of the retina and optic nerve head

Retinoblastoma

Clinical features

The most common malignant ocular tumour in children. Bilateral in 30% of cases; 6% of patients have a positive family history. Presents typically at about 18 months with a white pupil (leukocoria - Fig. 232) and grows either into the vitreous cavity (endophytic) or in the subretinal space (exophytic).

Management

Options include external beam or plaque irradiation, laser photocoagulation, cryotherapy, systemic chemotherapy, and enucleation.

Retinal astrocytoma

Clinical features

An uncommon, benign tumour that typically affects patients with tuberous sclerosis (Bourneville's disease). Whitish, round mass frequently situated near the optic nerve head (Fig. 233). May be multiple and bilateral.

Retinal capillary haemangioma

Clinical features

Uncommon benign tumour. Round, orange-red lesion associated with dilated supplying and draining vessels (Fig. 234). Frequently multiple, with both eyes affected in 50% of cases. 25% of patients have systemic lesions (von Hippel-Lindau syndrome). Treatment involves laser photocoagulation or cryotherapy.

Retinal cavernous haemangioma

Very rare congenital lesion characterized by grape-like aneurysmal clusters (Fig. 235).

Retinal racemose haemangioma

A very rare congenital arteriovenous malformation consisting of grossly dilated and tortuous vessels (Fig. 236). A proportion of patients will have central nervous system lesions (Wyburn-Mason syndrome).

Melanocytoma of the optic nerve head

Rare, benign black tumour with feathery edges (Fig. 237) which usually occurs in pigmented races.

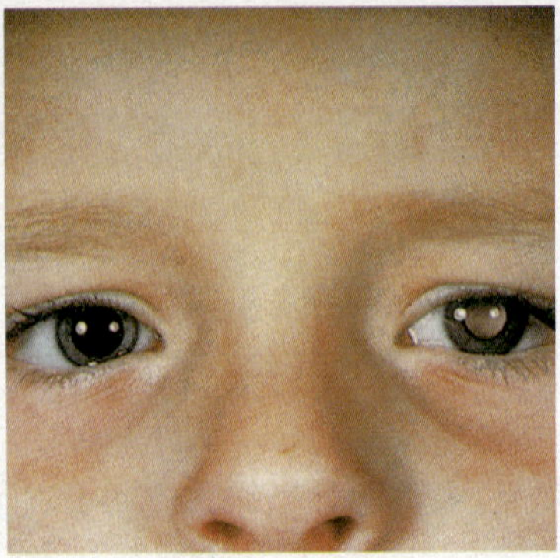

图 232 视网膜母细胞瘤引起左眼白瞳
Retinoblastoma causing left leukocoria

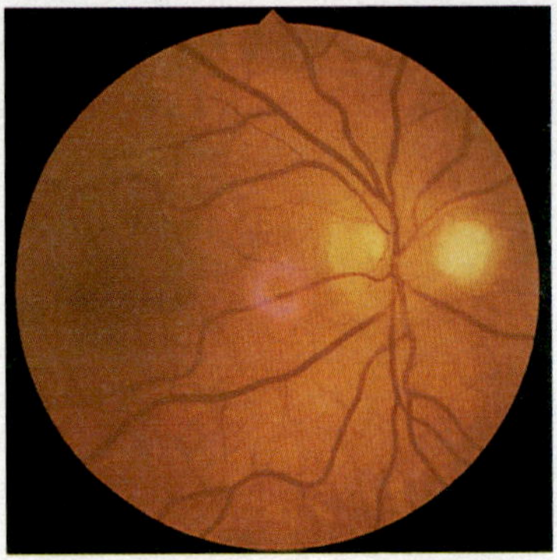

图 233 视网膜的星形细胞瘤
Retinal astrocytoma

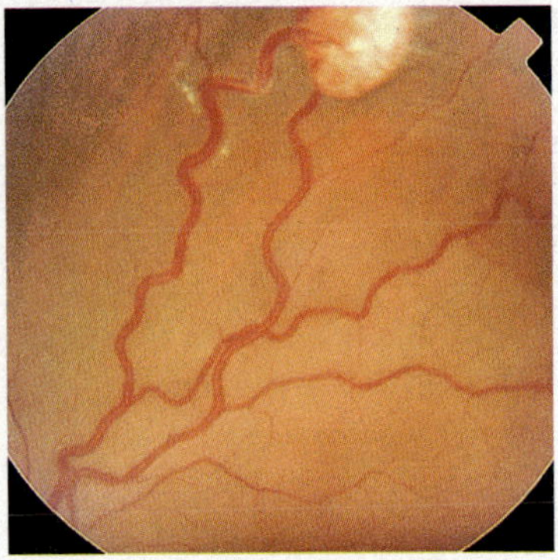

图 234 视网膜毛细血管瘤
Retinal capillary haemangioma

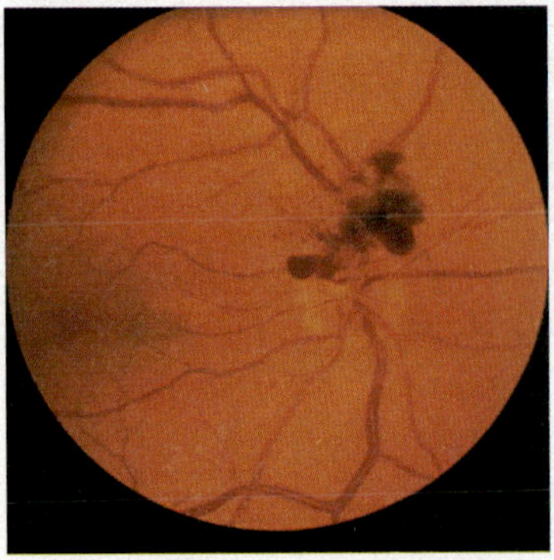

图 235 视网膜海绵状血管瘤
Retinal cavernous haemangioma

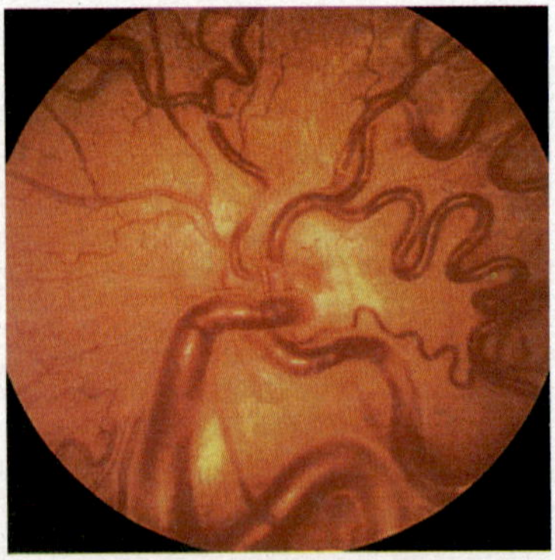

图 236 视网膜蔓状血管瘤
Retinal racemose haemangioma

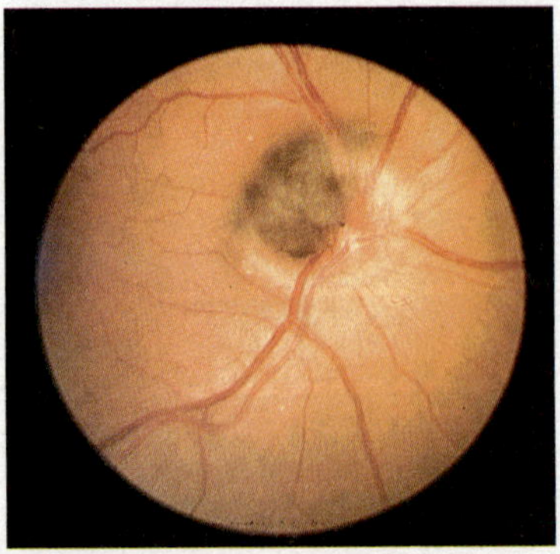

图 237 视盘黑色素细胞瘤
Melanocytoma of the optic nerve head

后天性视神经病变

视神经炎

定义 视神经的炎症，病因中最多的是多发性硬化症。

临床特征 亚急性发病，常累及单侧，中心视力下降伴随疼痛，尤其是眼球运动疼痛。视盘常正常（球后视神经炎），偶有水肿（视盘炎）。严重的或反复发作可导致视神经萎缩（图 238）。

前部缺血性视神经病变

定义 视盘的梗死。

分类

- *动脉炎*：伴随巨细胞性动脉炎，预后不良。
- *非动脉炎*：伴随高血压和动脉粥样硬化。

临床特征 严重的急性单眼视力丧失（动脉炎）或视力下降，伴随严重视野缺损（非动脉炎）。检查可见视盘苍白和水肿。视盘周围常有细小的出血（图 239）。

治疗 立即 ESR 是重要的。动脉炎型全身应用大剂量类固醇以保护另一眼。

视盘水肿

定义 颅内压升高导致视盘水肿。

临床特征 颅内压升高症状包括头痛和恶心。暂时的视物模糊，每次常持续几秒，但直到晚期视力常保持正常。

体征

- *早期*：视盘充血，边界模糊（图 240）。
- *发展完全期*：视盘显著隆起，周围出血（图241）和棉絮状斑。
- *长期静止期*：显著隆起“香槟酒软木塞”样表现（图 242）。

41 Acquired optic nerve disorders

Optic neuritis

Definition
Inflammation of the optic nerve, with a range of causes, the most important being multiple sclerosis.

Clinical features
Presents with subacute, usually unilateral, impairment of central vision that may be associated with pain, especially on eye movement. The optic disc is usually normal (retrobulbar neuritis) and occasionally swollen (papillitis). Severe or recurrent attacks may lead to optic atrophy (Fig. 238).

Anterior ischaemic optic neuropathy

Definition
Infarction of the optic nerve head.

Classification
- *Arteritic*: associated with giant cell arteritis and has a poor prognosis
- *Non-arteritic*: associated with hypertension and atherosclerosis.

Clinical features
Presents with severe acute unilateral visual loss (arteritic) or variable visual decrease associated with an altitudinal visual field defect (non-arteritic). On examination, the optic disc is pale and swollen. Splinter-shaped haemorrhages are common (Fig. 239).

Management
An immediate ESR is essential. The arteritic form is treated with high-dose systemic steroids to protect the other eye.

Papilloedema

Definition
Disc swelling caused by raised intracranial pressure.

Clinical features
Symptoms of raised intracranial pressure including headaches and nausea. Transient visual obscuration lasting a few seconds are common but visual acuity is normal until late.

Signs

- *Early*: hyperaemia with indistinct margins (Fig. 240)
- *Established*: obvious elevation, peripapillary haemorrhages (Fig. 241) and cotton wool spots
- *Long-standing*: markedly elevated 'champagne cork' appearance (Fig. 242).

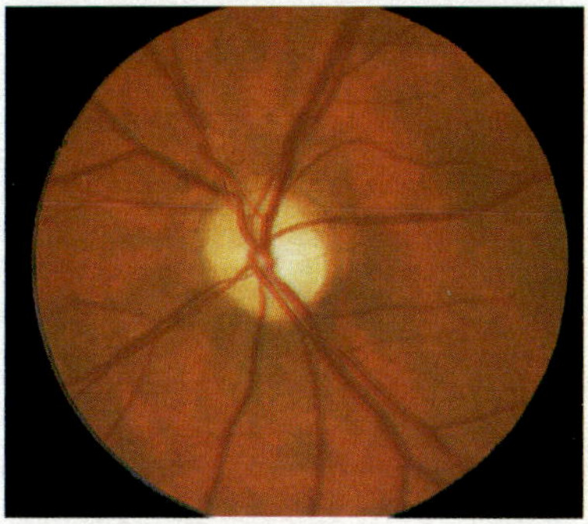

图 238 视神经萎缩
Optic atrophy

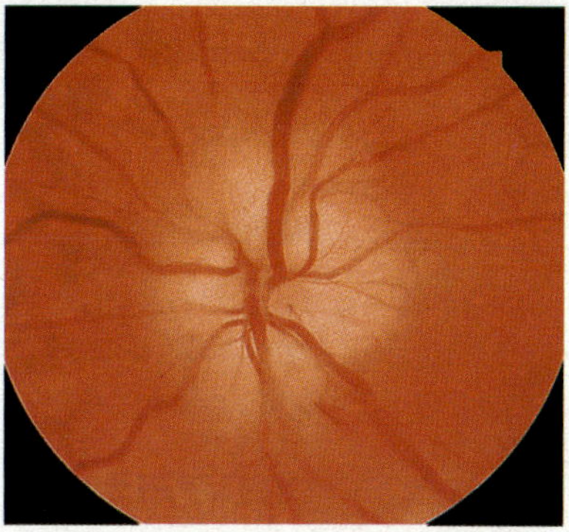

图 239 前部缺血性视神经病变
Anterior ischaemic optic neuropathy

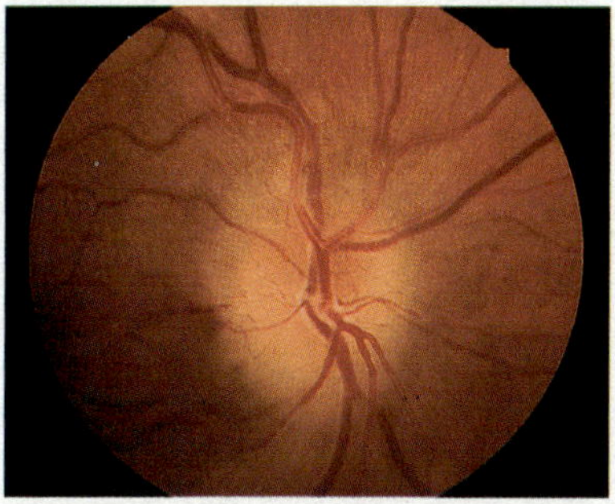

图 240 早期视盘水肿
Early papilloedema

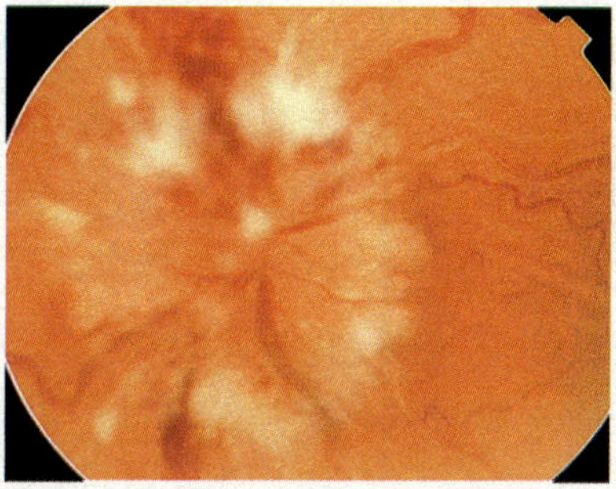

图 241 发展完全的视盘水肿
Established papilloedema

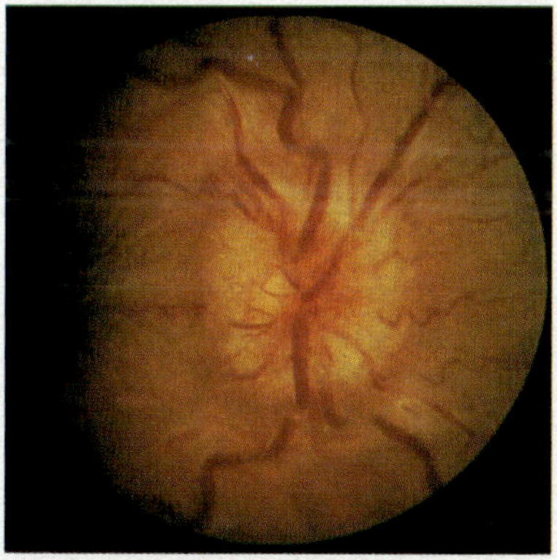

图 242 长期静止期的视盘水肿
Long-standing papilloedema

先天性视盘异常

倾斜的视盘

临床特征 椭圆形视盘由于它的垂直轴倾斜（图243），常伴发近视，多累及双眼。固定的颞上方视野缺损是因为病变未能超过垂直中线。

视盘玻璃疣

定义 视盘之内玻璃样沉着物，常累及双眼，多为家族性。

临床特征 类似视盘水肿外观（假性视盘水肿）。视盘呈多结节和隆起的外观，生理性视杯消失。新生血管分支不规则（图 244）。视野缺损或产生 CNV。

有髓神经纤维

临床特征 视网膜的神经纤维永存髓鞘形成。羽毛状白斑位于视盘周围可被误诊为“视盘水肿”（图 245）。

视盘小窝

临床特征 多为单侧发病，深色，圆形或椭圆形凹陷位于较大的视盘上（图 246）。大约 50% 病例发展为黄斑区浆液性脱离。

视盘缺损

临床特征 由于胚裂闭合异常所致。视盘包含下方的大凹陷（图 247）。典型的视力受损和上方视野缺损。可伴随许多先天性神经和全身的异常。

牵牛花综合征

临床特征 视盘扩大和凹陷，凹陷的底部有透明的残余物，放射状的新生血管（图 248）。视力可严重下降。可能伴有先天性中枢神经系统和其他的中线缺损。

Congenital optic disc anomalies

Tilted disc

Clinical features

Oval optic disc with its vertical axis directed obliquely (Fig. 243) often associated with myopia and usually bilateral. A stable upper temporal visual field defect that fails to respect the vertical midline is frequent.

Optic disc drusen

Definition

Deposits of hyaline-like material within the optic nerve head which are often bilateral and familial.

Clinical features

May mimic the appearance of optic disc swelling (pseudopapilloedema). The optic nerve head is lumpy and elevated, with no physiological cup. Emerging blood vessels branch anomalously (Fig. 244). Visual field defects or CNV may occur.

Myelinated nerve fibres

Clinical features

Persistent myelination of the retinal nerve fibres. Feathery white patches which may be mistaken for papilloedema when located around the optic disc (Fig. 245).

Optic disc pit

Clinical features

Usually unilateral dark, round or oval pit in a larger than normal disc (Fig. 246). About 50% of eyes develop a serous detachment of the macula.

Optic disc coloboma

Clinical features

Caused by defective closure of the fetal fissure. The optic nerve head contains a large inferior excavation (Fig. 247). Visual acuity is usually impaired and a superior visual field defect is typical. May be associated with a variety of congenital neurological and systemic anomalies.

Morning glory anomaly

Clinical features

The disc is enlarged and excavated with hyaloid remnants within its base and blood vessels emerging radially (Fig. 248). Vision may be severely impaired. Associated congenital central nervous system and other midline defects may be present.

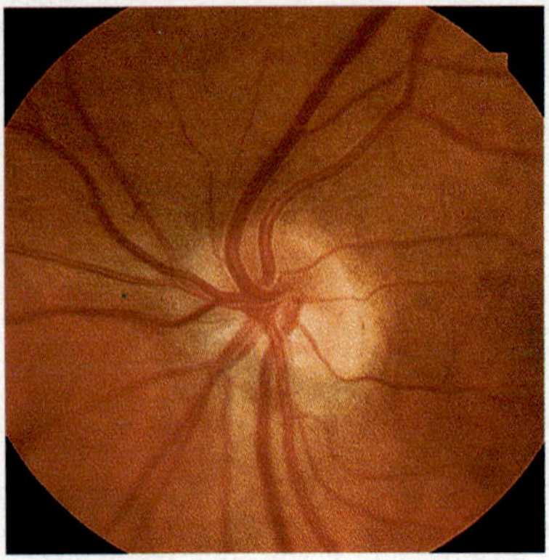

图 243 倾斜的视盘
Tilted disc

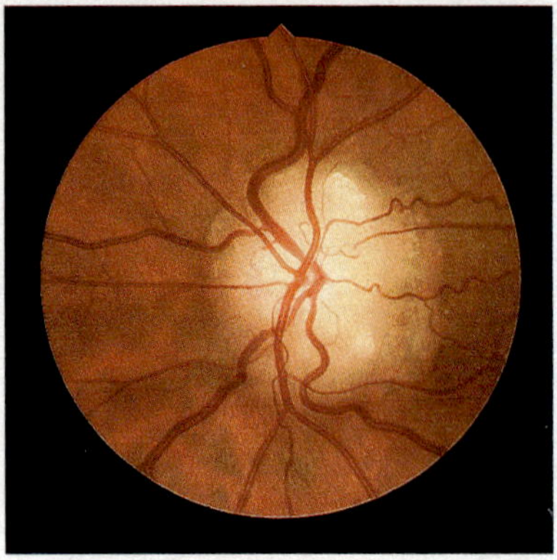

图 244 视盘玻璃疣
Optic disc drusen

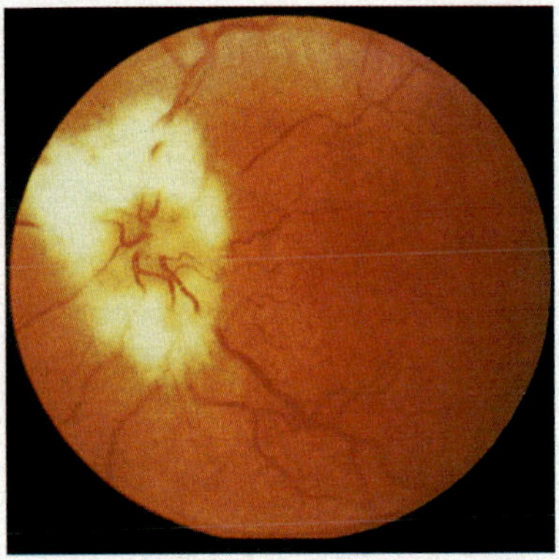

图 245 有髓神经纤维
Myelinated nerve fibres

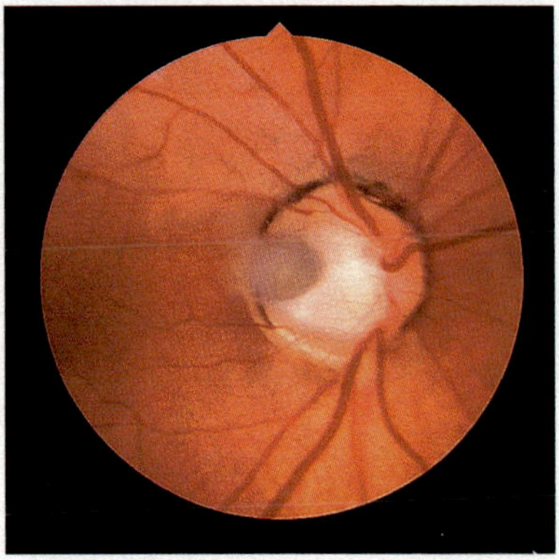

图 246 视盘小窝
Optic disc pit

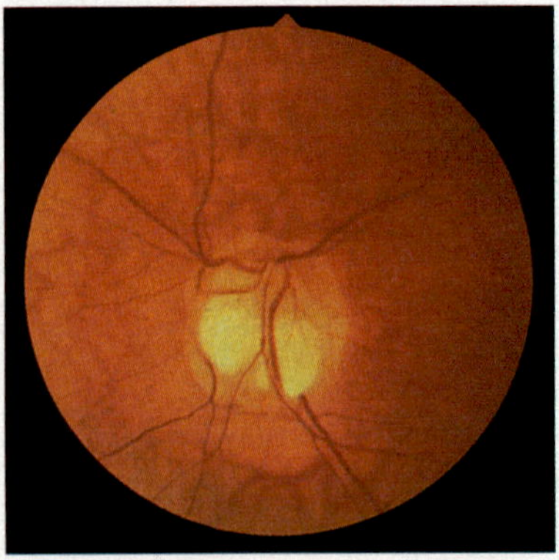

图 247 视盘缺损
Optic disc coloboma

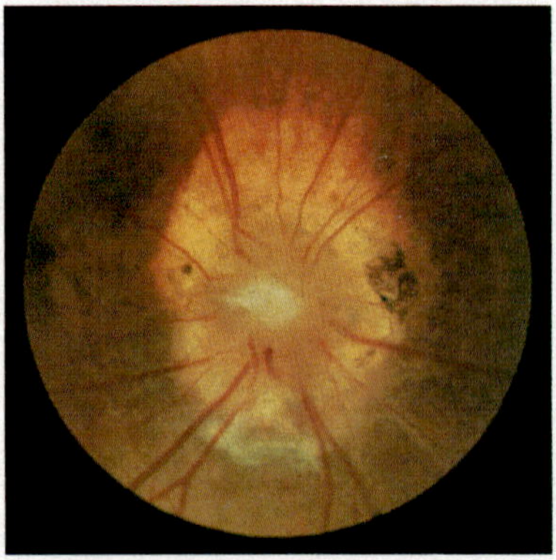

图 248 牵牛花综合征
Morning glory anomaly

斜视

定义

双眼视轴分离。

内斜视（会聚性斜视）

临床特征

婴儿型内斜视 生后 6 个月内发病；不会与假性内斜视混淆（图 249）。恒定的大斜视角度（图 250），偶尔伴下斜肌作用过度或眼球震颤。

调节性内斜视 内斜视集合过强，多在 2.5 岁出现。有一些远视的患者，可通过配戴眼镜将眼位矫正至正常。

非调节性内斜视 包含知觉性内斜视，使得在融合作用受损的一眼视力丧失，连续性内斜视于外斜视矫正手术后出现。

外斜视（散开性斜视，图 251）

分类

- *先天性*
- *间歇性*：婴儿和儿童。
- *继发性*：与内斜视相似。
- *连续性*：内斜视手术之后出现。

Duane 综合征

临床特征

少见的先天性病变，20%的患者双眼发病。第一眼位常为正位，但外展严重受限（图 252），伴眼球退缩和内转时睑裂狭窄（图 253）。

Brown 综合征

临床特征

罕见的先天性病变，10%的患者双眼发病。第一眼位为正位，但内转时向上运动受限（图 254）。

斜视的治疗

- 眼底检查除外屈光间质混浊或眼底病变。
- 矫正屈光不正。
- 治疗弱视（常用遮盖疗法）。
- 有适应证的患者可行眼外肌手术。

43 Childhood strabismus (squint)

Strabismus

Definition

A misalignment of the eyes.

Esotropia (convergent squint)

Clinical features

Infantile esotropia Presentation is in the first 6 months of life; should not be confused with pseudoesotropia (Fig. 249). Constant large angle (Fig. 250), occasionally inferior oblique overaction and nystagmus.

Accommodative esotropia Convergent squint linked with focussing, typically presenting at about 2.5 years. In some cases, the eyes can be straightened by spectacle correction of a hypermetropic refractive error.

Non-accommodative esotropia Includes sensory esotropia, caused by loss of vision in one eye impairing fusion, and consecutive esotropia, occurring after surgery to correct exotropia.

Exotropia (divergent squint- Fig. 251)

Classification

- *Congenital*
- *Intermittent*: in infants and older children
- *Secondary*: similar to esotropic counterpart
- *Consecutive*: following surgery for esotropia.

Duane's syndrome

Clinical features

Uncommon congenital condition, bilateral in 20% of cases. Eyes are usually straight in the primary position but abduction severely restricted (Fig. 252), with retraction of the globe and narrowing of the palpebral fissure on adduction (Fig. 253).

Brown's syndrome

Clinical features

Rare congenital condition, bilateral in 10% of cases. Eyes straight in the primary position, but there is limited elevation in adduction (Fig. 254).

Management of squint

- Ophthalmoscopy to exclude media opacity or fundus lesion
- Correction of significant refractive error
- Treatment of amblyopia (usually occlusion therapy)
- Extraocular muscle surgery, if appropriate.

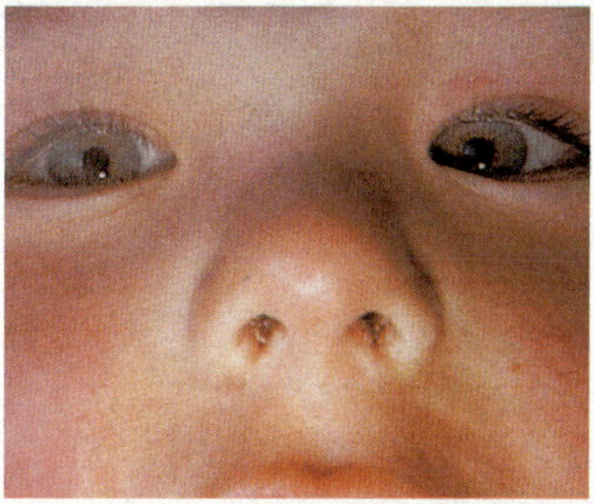

图 249 内眦赘皮的假性内斜视。注意对称性角膜反射
Pseudoesotropia due to epicanthic folds. Note symmetrical corneal reflexes

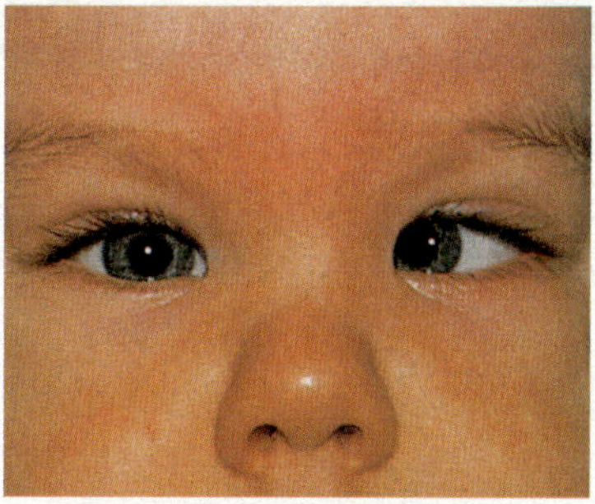

图 250 左眼婴儿型内斜视。注意不对称性角膜反射
Left infantile esotropia. Note asymmetrical corneal reflexes

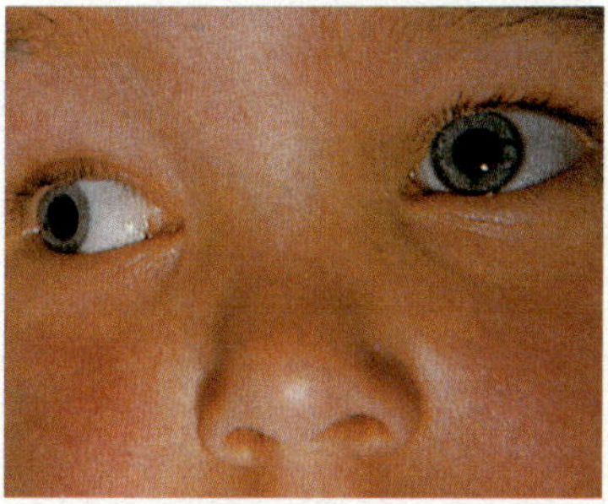

图 251 右眼外斜视
Right exotropia

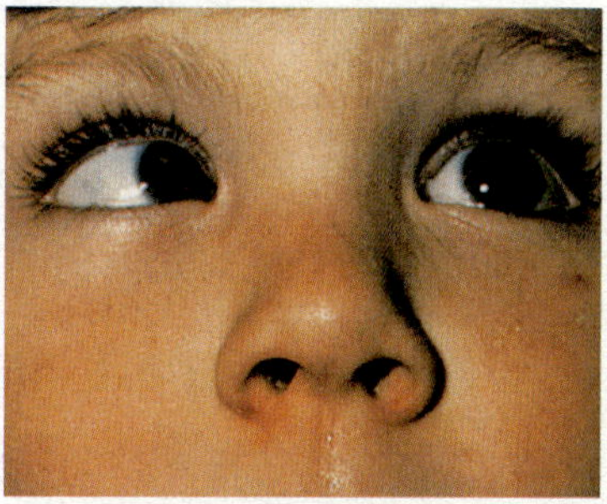

图 252 左眼Duane综合征，左眼企图外展
Left Duane's syndrome; attempted abduction of the left eye

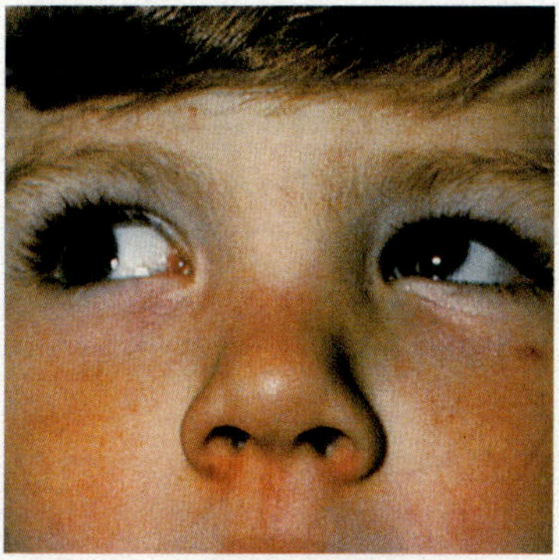

图 253 左眼 Duane 综合征，左眼内转时眼球退缩
Left Duane's syndrome; note retraction of the left eye on adduction

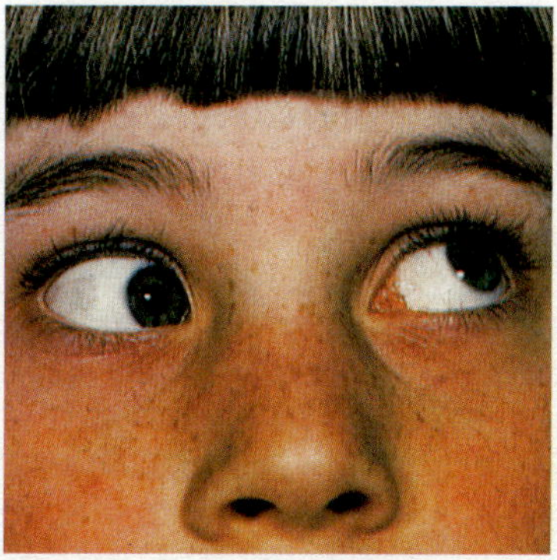

图 254 右眼 Brown 综合征
Right Brown's syndrome

44 第三、第四和第六脑神经麻痹

临床特征

第三脑神经（动眼神经）麻痹

- 上睑下垂是由于提上睑肌麻痹。
- 外斜视是由于外直肌活动不受限。
- 上转受限是由于上直肌和下斜肌麻痹（图 255）。
- 下转受限是由于下直肌麻痹（图 256）。
- 内转受限是由于内直肌麻痹（图 257）。
- 眼球向下转时有内旋转（上斜肌活动不受限）。
- 眼内肌麻痹－瞳孔散大，调节功能不足。

第四脑神经（滑车神经）麻痹

- 第一眼位呈上斜视（隐性或显性）；同侧的头部倾斜：Bielschowsky 试验阳性（图 258）。
- 内转受限（图 259）。
- 垂直复视，向下看时更明显。

第六脑神经（展神经）麻痹

- 外转运动时水平复视是最典型表现。
- 第一眼位呈内斜视是由于内直肌不受累。
- 外转受限（图 260）。

病因学

- *血管性疾病*（如动脉粥样硬化，高血压，糖尿病）：单纯眼科疾患或卒中的一个症状。
- *后交通动脉瘤*：考虑是第三脑神经麻痹，尤其是若伴有疼痛、瞳孔受累及缺乏血管危险因素时。
- *颅内压增高*：两侧的第六脑神经麻痹（假性定位征）。
- *外伤*：多为两侧的第四脑神经麻痹。
- *海绵窦病变*（如瘘管，血栓形成）：第四和第六脑神经麻痹。
- *肿瘤*（如听神经瘤，鼻咽癌）：第六脑神经麻痹。

Third, fourth and sixth nerve palsies

Clinical features

Third (oculomotor) nerve palsy

- Ptosis due to paralysis of the levator palpebrae superioris
- Divergence due to unopposed action of the lateral rectus
- Defective elevation due to paralysis of the superior rectus and inferior oblique muscles (Fig. 255)
- Defective depression due to paralysis of the inferior rectus (Fig. 256)
- Defective adduction due to paralysis of the medial rectus (Fig. 257)
- Intorsion on attempted downgaze (unopposed superior oblique)
- Internal ophthalmoplegia - dilated, poorly reactive pupil and defective accommodation.

Fourth (trochlear) nerve palsy

- Hyperdeviation (latent or manifest) in the primary position; accentuated by ipsilateral head tilt: positive Bielschowsky test (Fig. 258)
- Defective depression in adduction (Fig. 259)
- Vertical diplopia, worse in downgaze

Sixth (abducens) nerve palsy

- Horizontal diplopia most marked in abduction
- Convergence in the primary position due to unopposed medial rectus
- Limitation of abduction (Fig. 260).

Aetiology

- *Vascular disease* (e.g. atherosclerosis, hypertension, diabetes): isolated or as part of larger stroke
- *Posterior communicating artery aneurysm*: consider in 3rd nerve palsy especially if painful, pupil involved and absence of vascular risk factors
- *Raised intracranial pressure*: bilateral 6th nerve palsy (false localizing sign)
- *Trauma*: especially bilateral 4th nerve palsy
- *Cavernous sinus lesions* (e.g. fistula, thrombosis): 4th and 6th nerve palsy
- *Tumours* (e.g. acoustic neuroma, nasopharyngeal carcinoma): 6th nerve palsy.

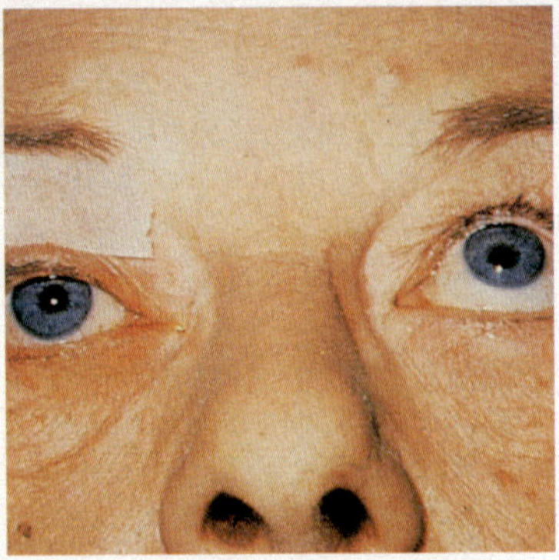
图 255　右眼第三脑神经麻痹，上转不能
Right third nerve palsy: failure of elevation

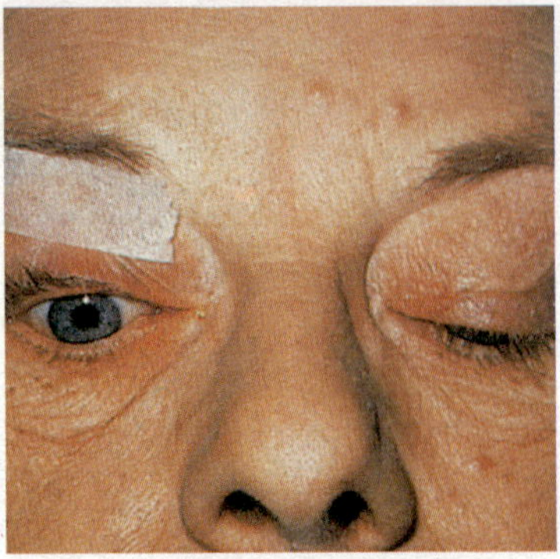
图256　右眼第三脑神经麻痹，下转不能
Right third nerve palsy: failure of depression

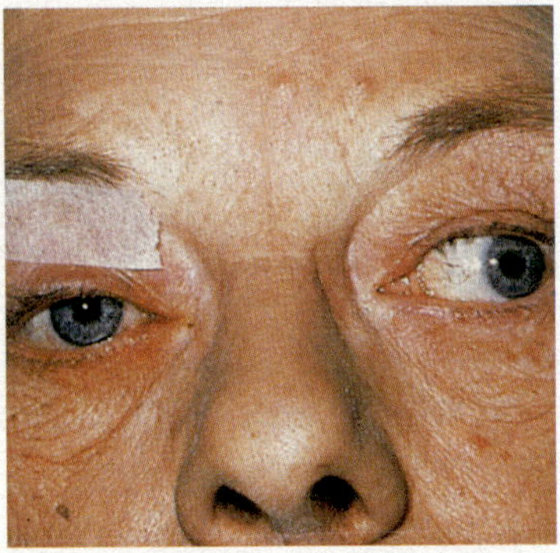
图 257　右眼第三脑神经麻痹，内转不能
Right third nerve palsy: failure of adduction

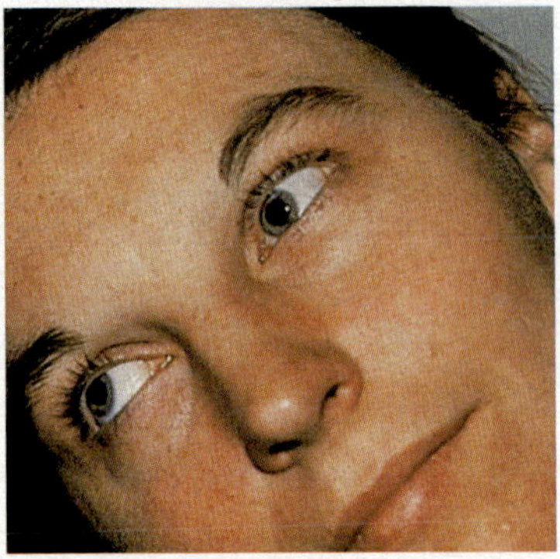
图 258　Bielschowsky 试验阳性，表现为右侧上斜视
Positive Bielschowsky test showing right hyperdeviation

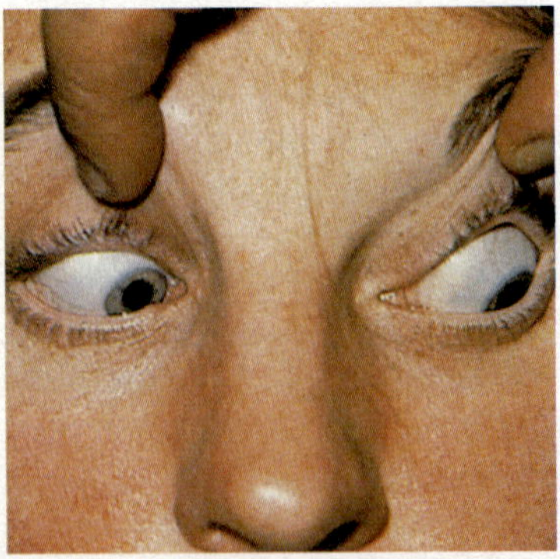
图 259　右眼第四脑神经麻痹：内转受限
Right fourth nerve palsy: failure of depression in adduction

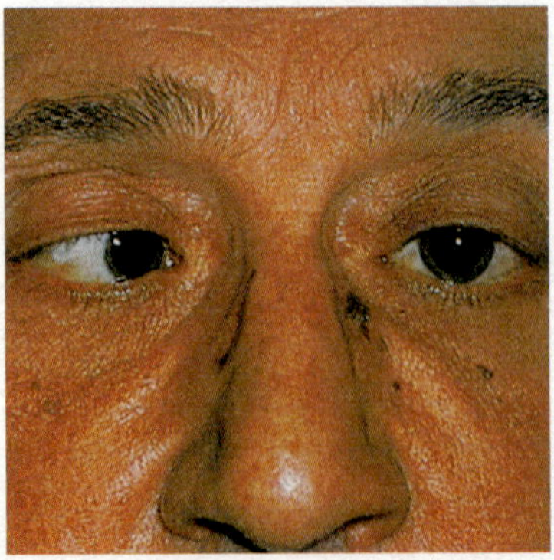
图 260　左侧第六脑神经麻痹：外转受限
Left sixth nerve palsy: failure of abduction

角膜上皮擦伤

临床特征

很常见，多由于指甲和植物造成。疼痛明显，伴有眼睑痉挛和流泪。角膜上皮缺损可被荧光素染色（图261），常于24小时内痊愈。一些患者可发展为复发性角膜糜烂。

治疗

抗生素油膏；大的角膜上皮缺损眼垫遮盖可改善症状，但不会加速愈合。

异物

- *睑板下沟异物*：常有角膜上方的划伤伴频繁瞬目。
- *角膜异物*：典型地有铁锈，可能伴周围的锈环（图262）。
- *穿透伤*：多由锤打金属碎片造成。合并症包括感染和白内障。

眼球前段钝挫伤

- *结膜下出血和眼周的淤血*。
- *前房积血*（图263）：再次出血可导致严重眼压升高，并有角膜血染的危险。
- *虹膜瞳孔括约肌损伤*。
- *虹膜根部离断*(图 264)。
- *前房角后退*（见图 154）：易患慢性青光眼。
- *晶状体损伤*：半脱位，脱位（见图181）和白内障形成。
- *巩膜破裂*：常由于严重的外伤。

眼球后段钝挫伤

- *玻璃体出血*：可掩盖原发病；超声检查可显示玻璃体出血。
- *视网膜震荡*（图 265）：外伤性水肿。
- *脉络膜破裂*（图 266）。
- *视网膜撕裂*：渗出，赤道或黄斑裂孔可导致视网膜脱离。
- *视神经撕脱*：见于严重外伤。

45 Trauma

Corneal abrasion

Clinical features

Very common and often caused by fingernails and plant stems. Pain is marked and associated with blepharospasm and lacrimation. The epithelial defect, which stains with fluorescein (Fig. 261), often heals within 24 hours. Some patients subsequently develop recurrent corneal erosions.

Management

Antibiotic ointment; padding may improve comfort in very large abrasions but does not enhance healing.

Foreign body

- *Subtarsal*: usually scratches the superior cornea with blinking
- *Corneal foreign body*: typically ferrous and may be associated with a surrounding rust ring (Fig. 262)
- *Penetrating*: commonly hammered metal fragments. Complications include infection and cataract.

Blunt anterior segment trauma

- *Subconjunctival haemorrhage and periocular ecchymosis*
- *Hyphaema* (Fig. 263): re-bleeding may result in a severe IOP rise with a risk of corneal blood staining
- *Iris sphincter damage*
- *Iridodialysis* (Fig. 264)
- *Angle recession* (see Fig. 154): risk of chronic glaucoma
- *Lens damage*: subluxation, dislocation (see Fig.181) and cataract formation
- *Scleral rupture*: usually caused by severe trauma.

Blunt posterior segment trauma

- *Vitreous haemorrhage*: may hide underlying damage; ultrasound indicated
- *Commotio retinae* (Fig. 265): traumatic oedema
- *Choroidal rupture* (Fig. 266)
- *Retinal tear*: dialysis, equatorial or macular holes may cause retinal detachment
- *Avulsion of the optic nerve*: in severe trauma.

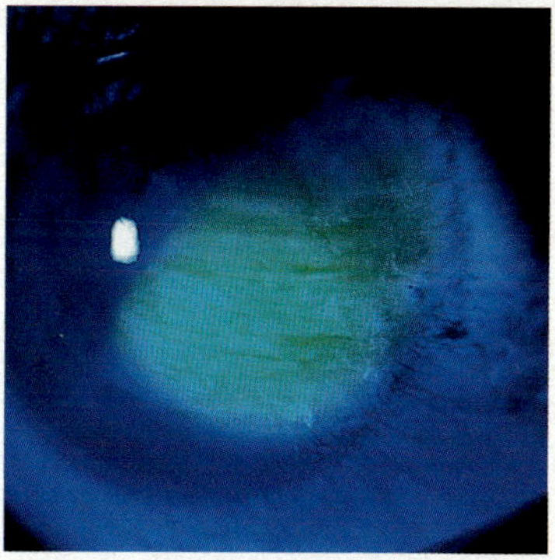

图261 角膜上皮擦伤荧光素染色
Corneal abrasion stained with fluorescein

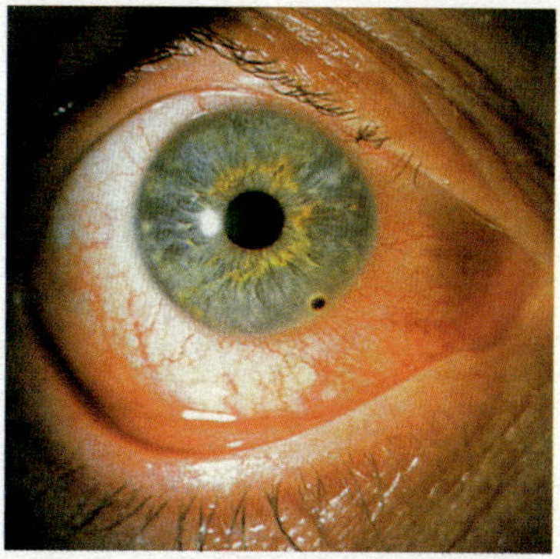

图 262 角膜异物伴锈环
Corneal foreign body with rust ring

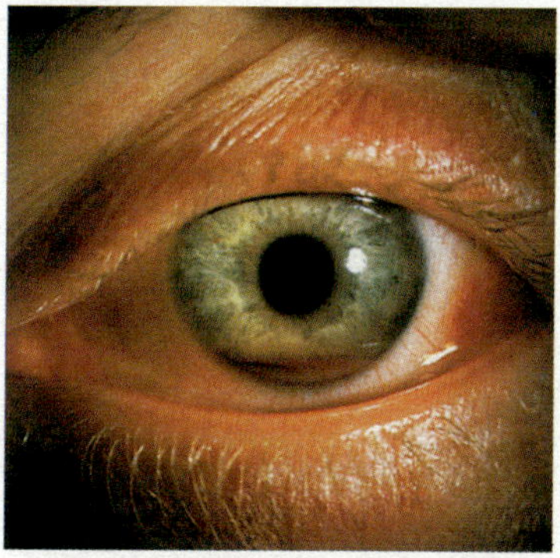

图 263 前房积血
Hyphaema

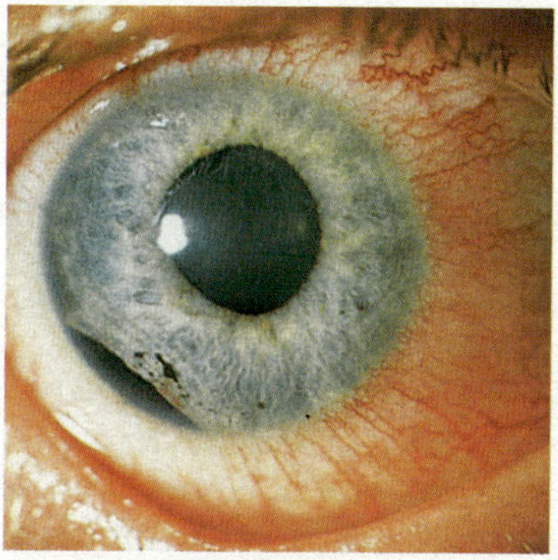

图 264 虹膜根部离断
Iridodialysis

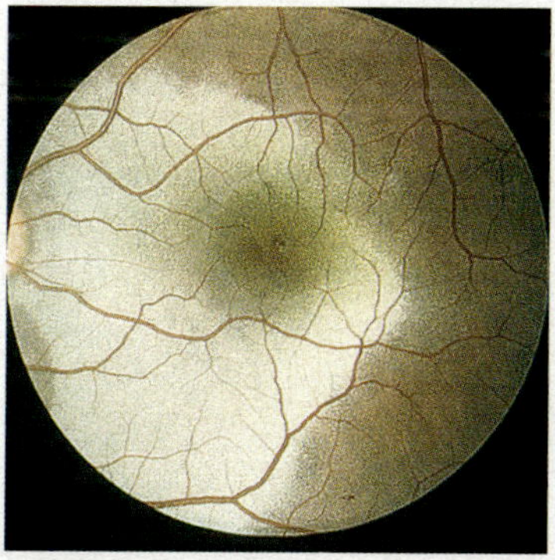

图 265 视网膜震荡
Commotio retinae

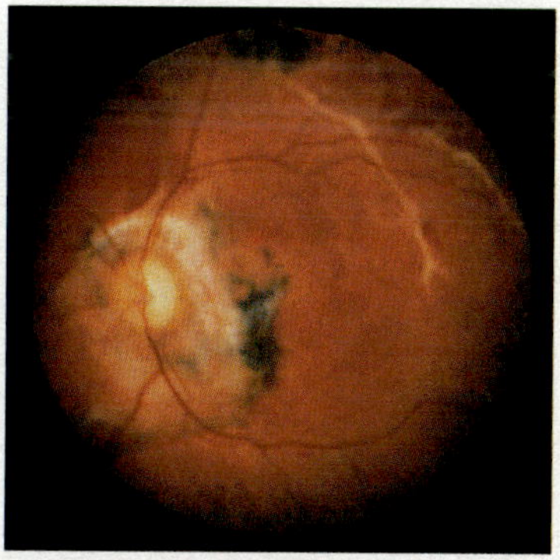

图 266 脉络膜破裂
Choroidal rupture

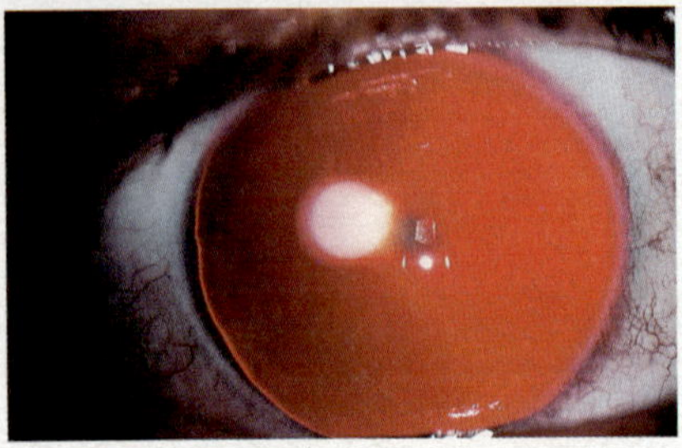

1. 15岁男孩生而具有双侧眼部异常。

a. 诊断是什么?

b. 哪里发生基因突变?

c. 一些人病变可发展成腹部的肿瘤。该患者兄弟、母亲和祖父全有眼部异常;该患者发展成肿瘤的可能性是多少?

d. 可出现什么其他的眼部特征?

This 15-year-old boy was born with the bilateral ocular abnormality shown.

a. What is the diagnosis?

b. Where is the genetic mutation?

c. Some individuals with this condition develop an abdominal tumour. This patient's brother, mother and grandfather all have the eye abnormality shown; what is the likelihood that the patient will develop the tumour?

d. What other ocular features may be present?

2. 患者76岁,病程至少1年,表面溃疡和结痂交替。

a. 可能的诊断是什么?

b. 不同的临床类型是什么?

c. 如何治疗?

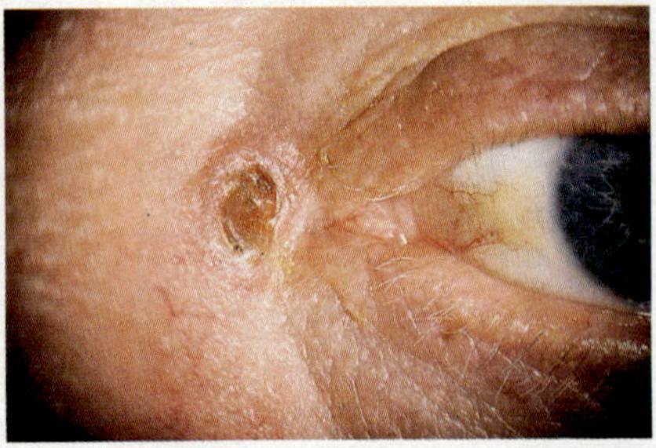

This patient is aged 76. The lesion shown has been present for at least a year, its surface intermittently breaks down and crusts.

a. What is the likely diagnosis?

b. What are the different clinical types?

c. What is the treatment?

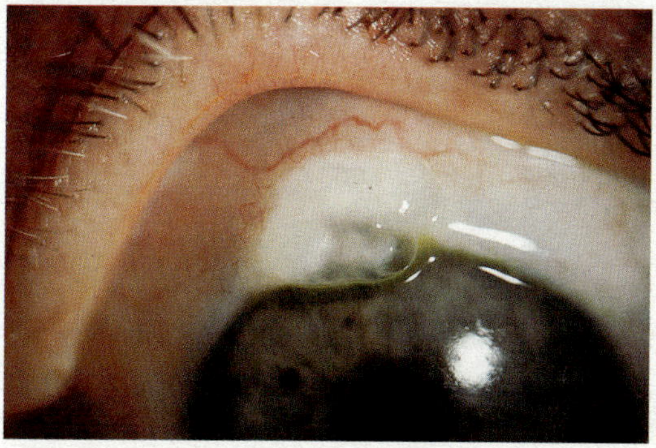

3. 64 岁女性最近做过眼睛手术。

a. 做过什么手术？

b. 该手术的主要适应证是什么？

c. 选择什么疗法有效？

d. 手术失败率高可使用什么附加药？

This 64-year-old woman recently underwent ocular surgery.

a. What was the surgical procedure?

b. What is the main indication for this operation?

c. What alternative therapy is available?

d. What adjunctive agents can be used if the risk of failure is high?

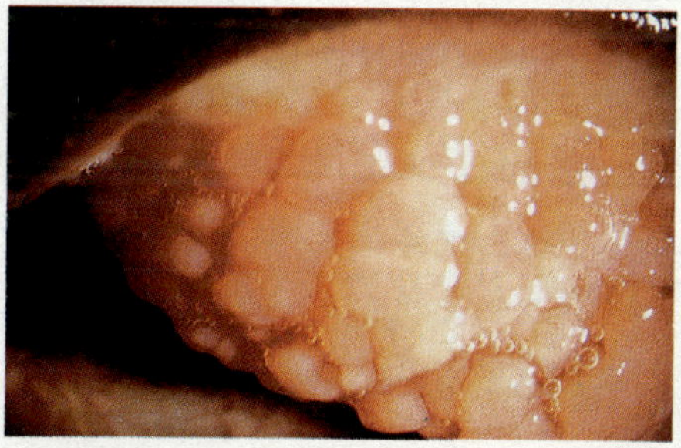

4. 患者戴硬性隐形眼镜 3 年。

a. 描述体征。

b. 有什么组织学表现？

c. 发病机理是什么？

d. 给出造成这种病变的其他两种原因。

This patient has worn rigid contact lenses for 3 years.

a. Describe the signs.

b. What is the histology?

c. What may be the pathogenesis?

d. Give two other causes of this condition.

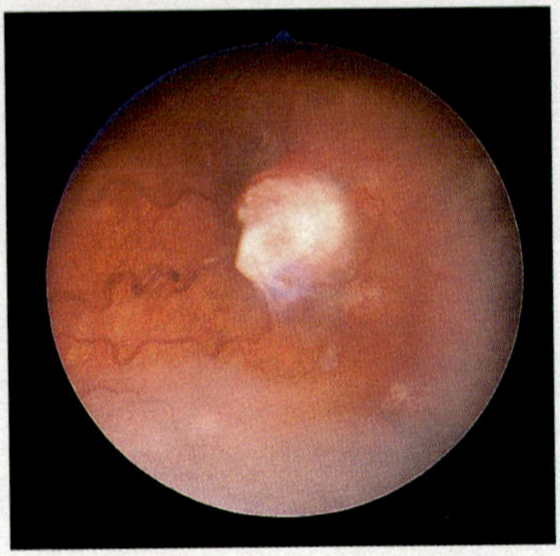

5. 这是一个视网膜毛细血管瘤。

a. 斑痣性错构瘤病伴随该病变的名称和遗传类型是什么？

b. 说出该斑痣性错构瘤病发生时的三种系统损害。

c. 单个视网膜毛细血管瘤的患者伴有全身病的比例是多少？

d. 视网膜病变是如何威胁视力的，怎样治疗？

This is a retinal capillary haemangioma.

a. What is the name and inheritance pattern of the phacomatosis associated with this lesion?

b. Name three systemic lesions occurring in this phacomatosis.

c. What proportion of patients with a solitary retinal capillary haemangioma have systemic involvement?

d. How do the retinal lesions threaten sight and how can they be treated?

6. 眼科医生发现 64 岁的男性患者单眼病变。

a. 疾病表现如何？

b. 这种眼部情况发展为青光眼的百分比大约是多少？

c. 常发生于什么地区？

d. 为什么白内障手术伴有高危并发症？

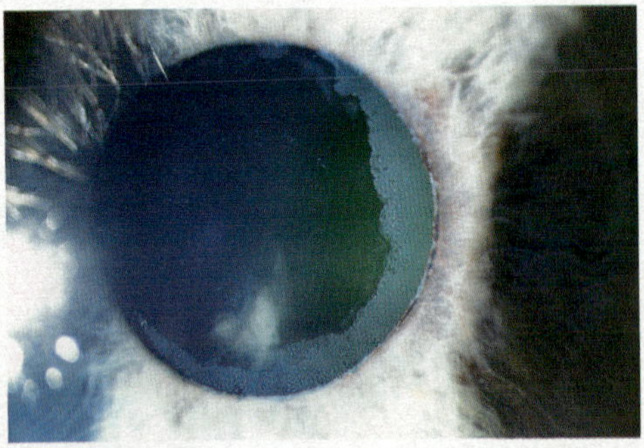

A 64-year-old man was found by his optometrist to have this condition in one eye.

a. What is the disorder shown?

b. Approximately what percentage of eyes with this condition develops glaucoma?

c. In which geographical region is it particularly common?

d. Why would cataract surgery be associated with a higher risk of complications?

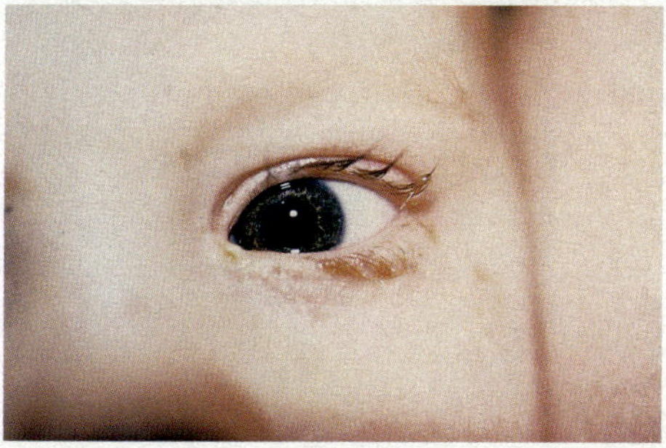

7. 父母发现6个月婴儿自出生起一眼持续流泪。
a. 可能的原因是什么?
b. 可采用什么保守治疗措施?
c. 在多大时考虑更有效的治疗，将采取什么治疗形式?
d. 婴儿眼流泪应该排除哪种最重要但少见的疾病?

The parents of this 6-month-old baby are concerned because the eye has watered persistently since birth.
a. What is the probable cause?
b. What conservative measures might be adopted?
c. At what age should more active intervention be considered, and what form should this take?
d. What is the most important, but much less common, condition that ought to be excluded in an infant with a watering eye?

8. 患者5天以前行小梁切除术。
a. 疾病表现是什么?
b. 该情况可能的原因是什么?
c. 临床上视网膜脱离的不同情况表现如何?

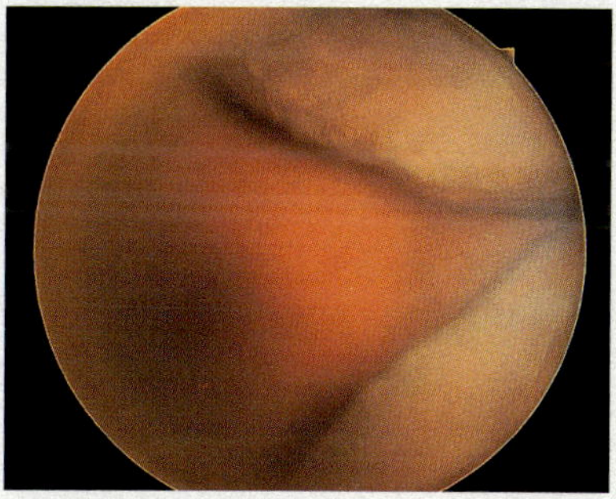

This patient underwent a trabeculectomy 5 days ago.
a. What is the condition shown?
b. What is the likely cause in this context?
c. Clinically, how does the appearance of this condition differ from that of retinal detachment?

9. 56岁白人男性6个月以前首先注意到缓慢扩大的褐色斑点。

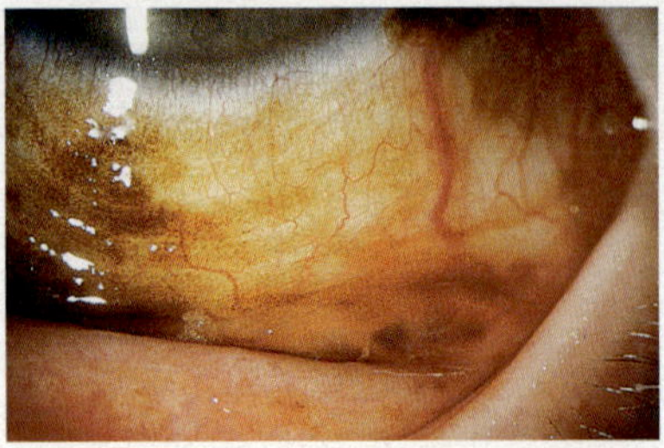

a. 诊断是什么?
b. 两个主要的组织学类型是什么?
c. 有恶变的可能吗?
d. 弥漫性结膜色素沉着的其他原因是什么?

This 56-year-old white man first noticed this slowly enlarging brown patch 6 months ago.

a. What is the diagnosis?
b. What are the two main histological types?
c. Is there any chance of malignant transformation?
d. What are the other causes of diffuse conjunctival pigmentation?

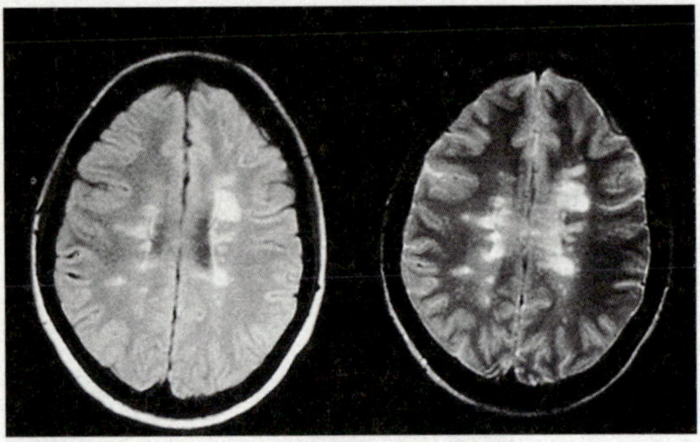

10. 这是一个33岁女性的MRI扫描，一周前发现左眼视力模糊。

a. 异常表现是什么?诊断是什么?
b. 眼底检查可见什么?
c. 她发作的时候其他的眼部症状是什么?
d. 该疾病的其他眼部并发症是什么?

This is the MRI scan of a 33-year-old woman who developed blurred vision in the left eye a week ago.

a. What abnormality is shown, and what is the diagnosis?
b. What might be seen on ophthalmoscopy?
c. What other ocular symptoms might she experience during the current episode?
d. What other ocular complications may be associated with this disease?

11. 这是6岁儿童眼眶蜂窝织炎。

a. 危及生命的合并症是什么?

b. 列出可能的诊断。

c. 如何治疗?

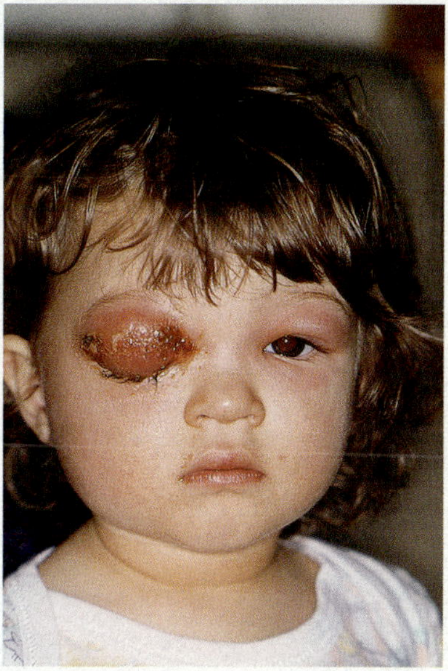

This is a 6-year-old child with orbital cellulitis.

a. What are the life-threatening complications?

b. List alternative diagnostic possibilities.

c. What is the management?

12. 这是36岁女性的视网膜,她患I型糖尿病20年。

a. 这是糖尿病性视网膜病变的什么阶段?

b. 糖尿病性视网膜病变其他阶段的体征是什么?

c. 糖尿病性视网膜病变最重要的危险因素是什么?

d. 列出糖尿病其他的眼部并发症。

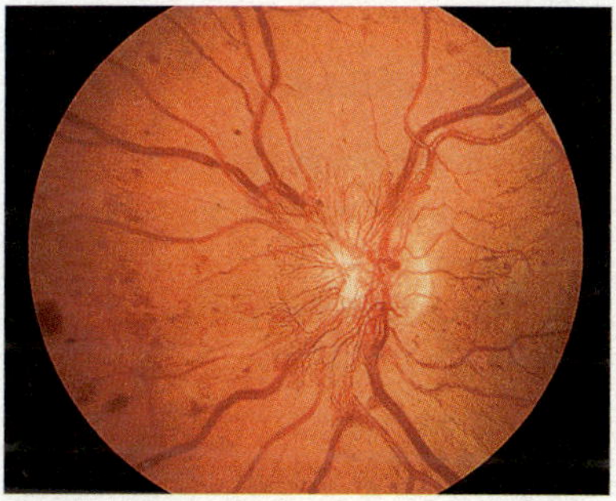

This is the fundus of a 36-year-old man who has had type 1 diabetes for 20 years.

a. What grade of diabetic retinopathy is shown?

b. What are the signs of the other grades of diabetic retinopathy?

c. What are the most important risk factors for diabetic retinopathy?

d. List the other ocular complications of diabetes.

13. 这是72岁女性的视网膜，她患II型糖尿病。

a. 视网膜可见什么？

b. 给三类临床意义显著的黄斑水肿(CSMO)下定义。

c. 怎样治疗CSMO。

d. 列出造成不良预后的因素。

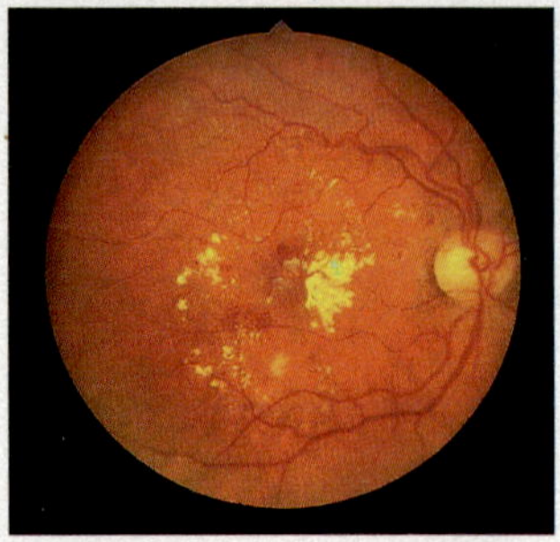

This is the fundus of a 72-year-old man with type 2 diabetes.

a. What does the fundus show?

b. Define the three categories of 'clinically significant macular oedema' (CSMO).

c. How is CSMO treated?

d. List factors conferring an adverse prognosis.

14. 这是脉络膜痣。

a. 什么临床特征可怀疑痣是小的黑色素瘤？

b. 对于黑色素瘤什么治疗形式是有效的？

c. 影响预后的因素是什么？

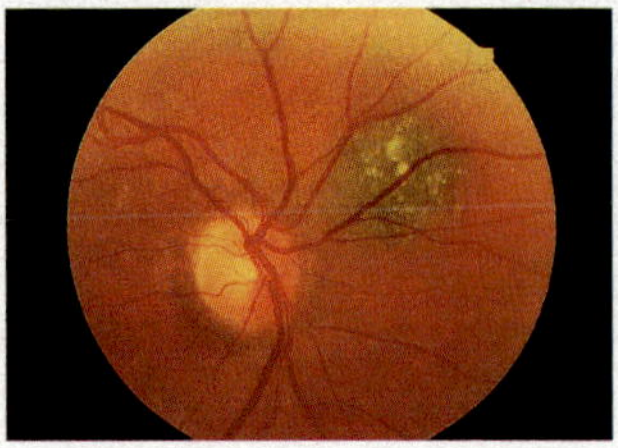

This is a choroidal naevus.

a. What clinical features might arouse suspicion that a naevus may be a small melanoma?

b. What treatment modalities are available for melanoma?

c. What factors influence prognosis?

15. 17岁有癫痫的男孩。

a. 脸部病变称为什么？

b. 可见的全身性表现是什么？遗传模式是什么？

c. 该疾病的眼部特点是什么？

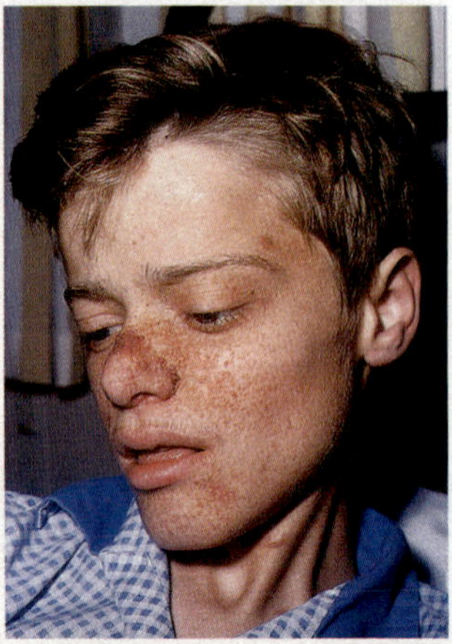

This is a 17-year-old boy with epilepsy.

a. What are the facial lesions called?

b. What is the systemic condition in which they are seen, and what is its inheritance pattern?

c. What are the ophthalmic features of the disease?

16. 70 岁女性高血压患者的眼底表现。

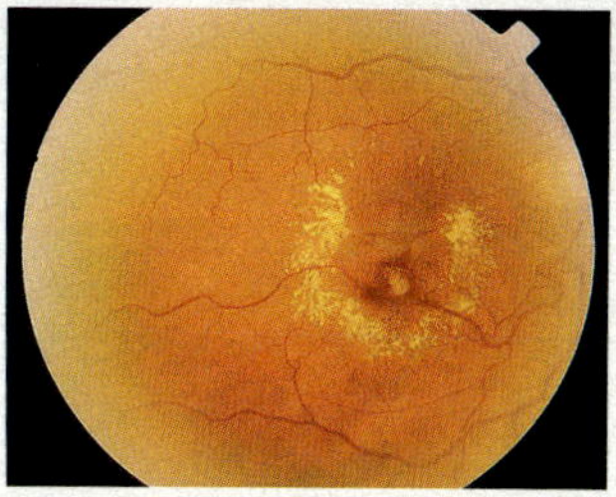

a. 损伤是什么?

b. 可发生什么并发症?

c. 如何治疗?

This is the fundal appearance of a 70-year-old hypertensive woman.

a. What is the lesion?

b. What complications may occur?

c. What is the management?

17. 这是青光眼引流方法。

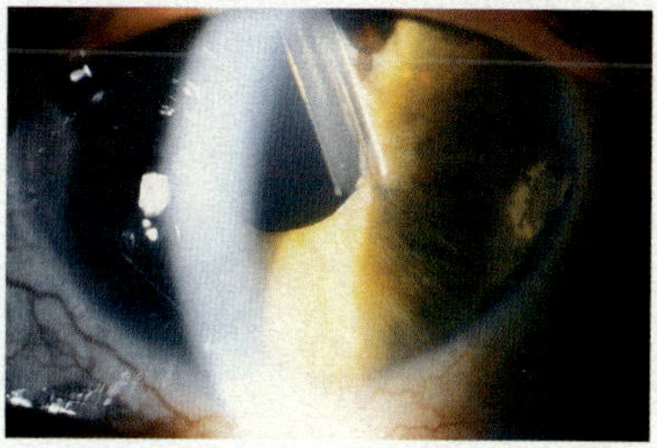

a. 该方法的适应证是什么?

b. 没有添加药物治疗情况下，植入后眼压控制理想的患者占多大比例?

c. 植入的并发症是什么?

This is a glaucoma drainage device.

a. What are the indications for such a device?

b. What proportion of patients undergoing implantation achieves adequate pressure control without additional medication?

c. What are the complications of implantation?

18. 25 岁女性双眼视网膜表现，右眼视力 6/36，左眼视力 6/18。

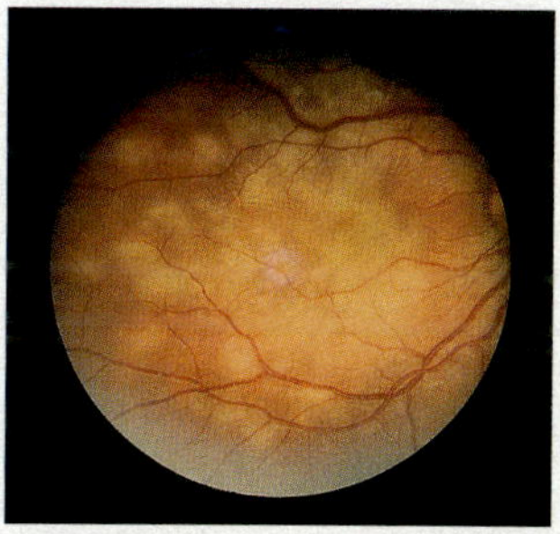

a. 荧光素眼底血管造影表明病变早期低荧光和晚期强荧光。最可能的诊断是什么?

b. 其他的眼部检查所见有哪些?

c. 可出现哪些全身性特征?

d. 预后如何?

This is the bilateral fundal appearance of a 25-year old man. Visual acuity in the right eye is 6/36 and in the left 6/18.

a. Fluorescein angiography shows early hypofluorescence and late hyperfluorescence of the lesions. What is the most likely diagnosis?

b. What other ocular findings may be evident?

c. What systemic features may be present?

d. What is the prognosis?

19. 19岁男性冠状位CT扫描。
a. 该异常表明什么?
b. 可能由于什么原因?
c. 可出现什么体征?
d. 如何治疗?

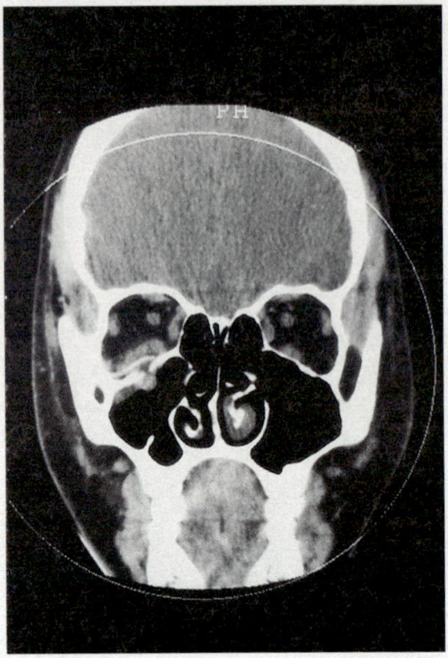

This is the coronal CT scan of a 19-year-old man.

a. What is the abnormality demonstrated?
b. What may be the cause?
c. What physical signs may be present?
d. What is the management?

20. 这是Grönblad-Strandberg综合征患者眼底的表现。
a. 异常表现是什么?
b. 该病的组织病理学是什么?
c. 在上下文中"橘皮"指什么?
d. 其他全身性伴随症状是什么?

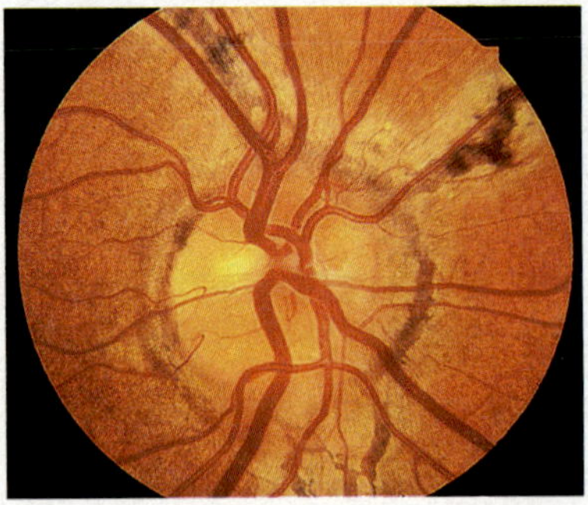

This is the fundal appearance in a patient with Grönblad-Strandberg syndrome.

a. What abnormality is shown?
b. What is the histopathology of the lesions?
c. What is *'peau d'orange'* in this context?
d. What are the other systemic associations?

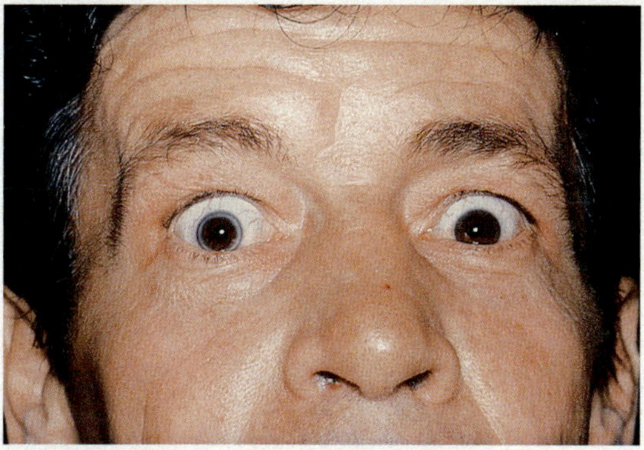

21. 72 岁患者 Parinaud(背侧中脑) ：合征，表现上转障碍。

a. Parinaud 综合征的其他临床体征是什么?

b. 这个年龄发病的可能原因是什么?

c. 在儿童期发病的重要原因是什么?

This is a 72-year-old patient with Parinaud's (dorsal midbrain) syndrome, showing failure of upgaze.

a. What are the other clinical signs of Parinaud's syndrome?

b. What are the likely causes in a patient of this age?

c. What are the important causes in children?

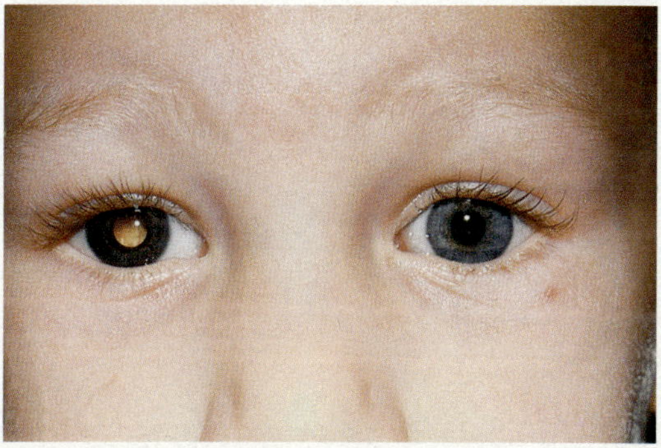

22. 父母注意到 18 个月婴儿的异常。

a. 这种阳性体征称作什么?

b. 该年龄的儿童应考虑的最重要原因是什么?

c. 列出其他的重要原因。

The parents of this 18-month-old baby noticed this abnormality.

a. What is this sign called?

b. What is the most important cause to be considered in a child of this age?

c. List the other important causes.

23. 这是眼带状疱疹。
a. 描述疱疹的演变。
b. Hutchinson 征是什么？有何意义？
c. 重要的眼部并发症是什么？

This shows herpes zoster ophthalmicus.
a. Describe the evolution of the rash.
b. What is Hutchinson's sign and what is its significance?
c. What are the important ocular complications?

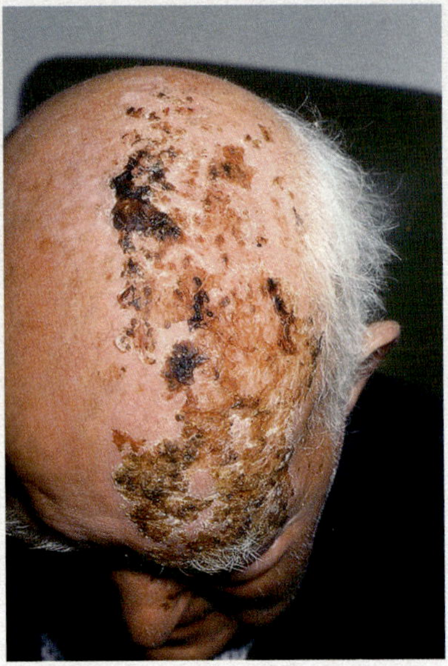

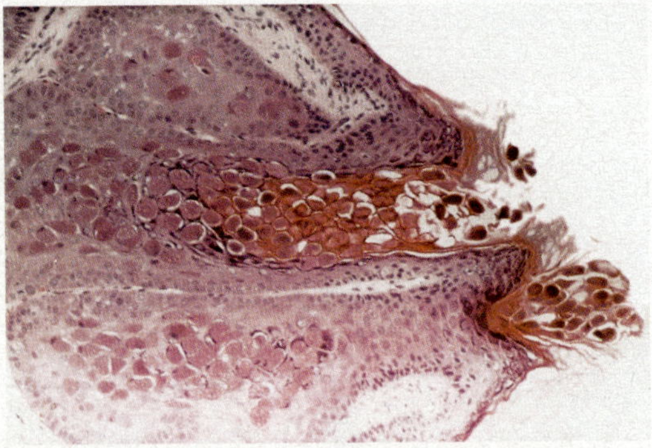

24. 病毒导致皮肤病损害的组织病理学表现。
a. 描述特点并确定诊断。
b. 病变的眼部表现特征是什么？
c. 患者有哪种全身性疾病可特征性地发展为这种类型的多发损害？

This shows the histopathology of a skin lesion caused by a virus.
a. Describe the features and give the diagnosis.
b. What is the characteristic mode of ocular presentation of this condition?
c. Patients with what systemic disease characteristically develop multiple lesions of this type?

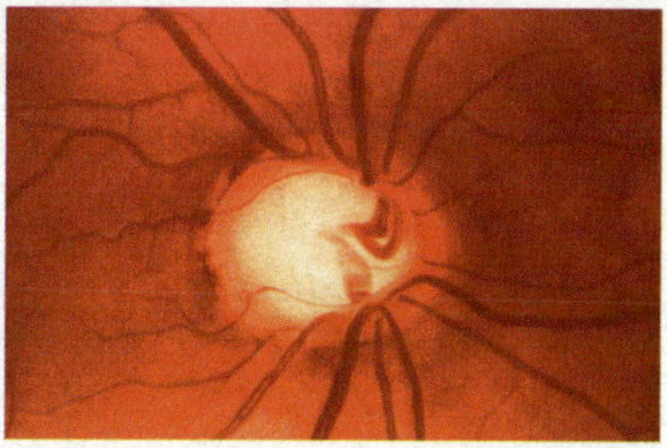

25. 81 岁男性的视盘，眼压是 12。
a.最可能的诊断是什么？
b.可出现哪些全身性特点？
c.该病特征性的视野缺损是什么？

This is the optic disc of an 81-year-old man whose intraocular pressure is 12.
a. What is the most likely diagnosis?
b. What systemic features may be present?
c. What are the characteristic visual field defects in this condition?

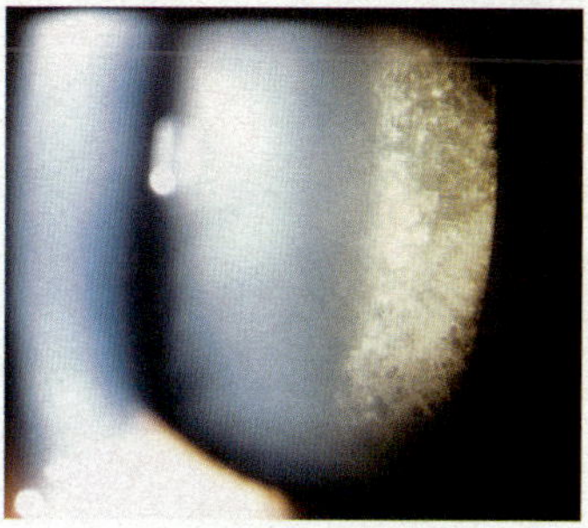

26. ：将进行白内障手术的患者。
a. 晶状体混浊的类型是什么？
b. 虽然矫正视力是 6/9，：状仍存在。可能出现哪些症状？
c. 该患者 46 岁患有哮喘，这和白内障有什么关系？

This patient is about to undergo cataract surgery.
a. What is the morphological type of this lens opacity?
b. Although corrected visual acuity is 6/9, symptoms are substantial. What form are these likely to take?
c. The patient, who is aged only 46, has asthma. What connection might this have with the cataract?

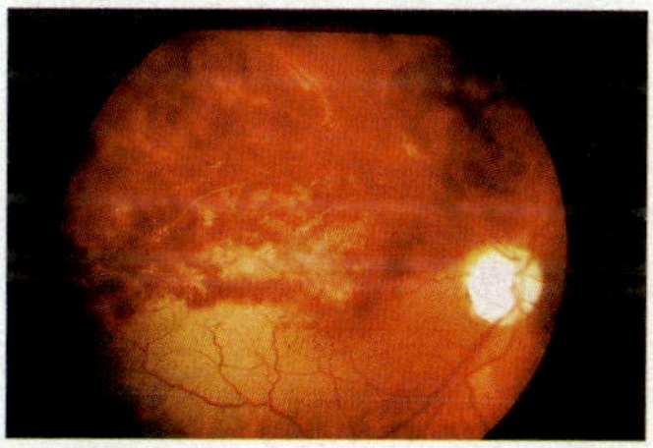

27. 37 岁土耳其人的眼底表现，他患有复发性口腔溃疡和下肢关节痛。
a. 眼部的诊断是什么？
b. 可能的系统性诊断是什么？
c. 他曾经治疗伴前房积脓的前葡萄膜炎，有效吗？
d. 可能的 HLA 分型是什么？

This is the fundal appearance of a 37-year-old Turk, who has experienced recurrent mouth ulcers and lower limb arthralgia.
a. What is the ocular diagnosis?
b. What is the probable systemic diagnosis?
c. He has been treated previously for anterior uveitis with hypopyon. Is this significant?
d. What is the likely HLA association?

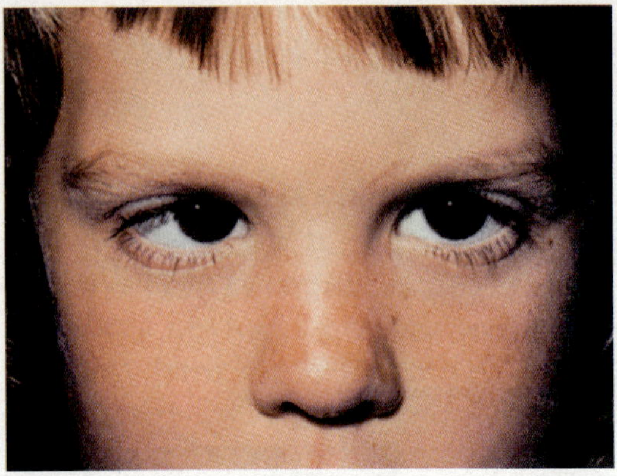

28. 数月以前，该 4 岁儿童的父母注意到孩子的一只眼向鼻子方向转。

a. 在病史中应注意什么?

b. 开始应该进行什么检查?

c. 这个年龄的内斜视怎么治疗?

A few months ago, the parents of this 4-year-old child noticed that one eye turns in towards the nose.

a. What points should be covered in the history?

b. How should the child be assessed initially?

c. What is the management of convergent squint presenting at this age?

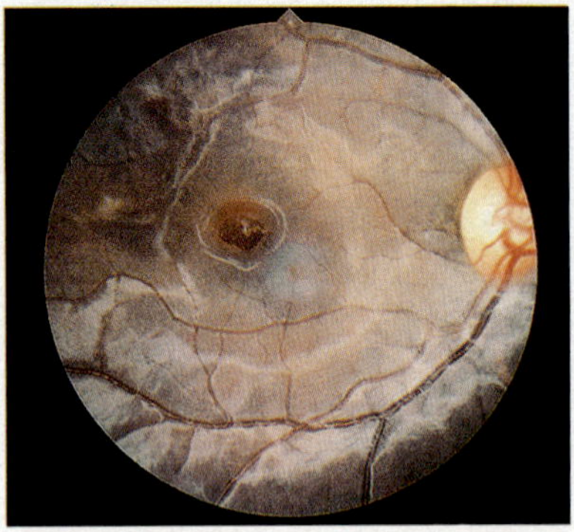

29. 63 岁女性的眼底表现，最近她注意到一只眼的视野中心有小的缺损区。

a. 诊断是什么?

b. 视力可能会有什么变化?

c. 什么可以改善她的视力?

d. 影响另一眼的几率是多少?

This is the fundal appearance of a 63-year-old woman who recently became aware of a small missing patch in the centre of the vision in one eye.

a. What is the diagnosis?

b. What is the visual acuity likely to be?

c. Can anything be done to improve her vision?

d. What is the chance of the condition affecting the other eye?

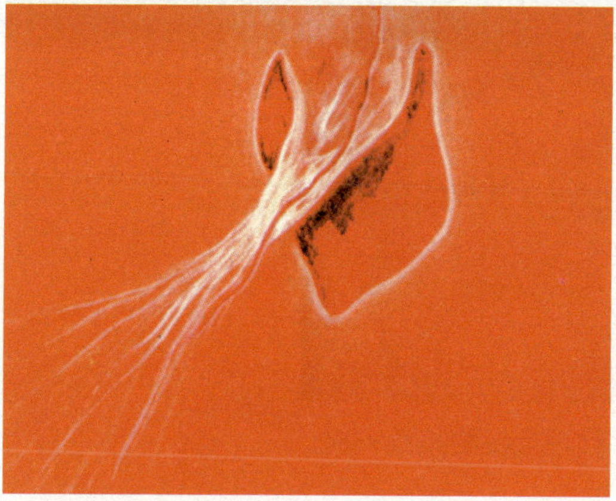

30. 该患者突然发现眼前悬浮物。
a. 表现出什么异常?
b. 应该怎样治疗?
c. 什么情况诱发视网膜脱离?

This patient experienced the sudden onset of floaters.
a. What abnormality is shown?
b. How should it be treated?
c. What conditions predispose to the development of retinal detachment?

31. 该患者畏光、充血和异物感2天。
a. 诊断是什么?
b. 测量眼压前应该检查什么关键体征?
c. 鉴别诊断是什么?
d. 怎么治疗?

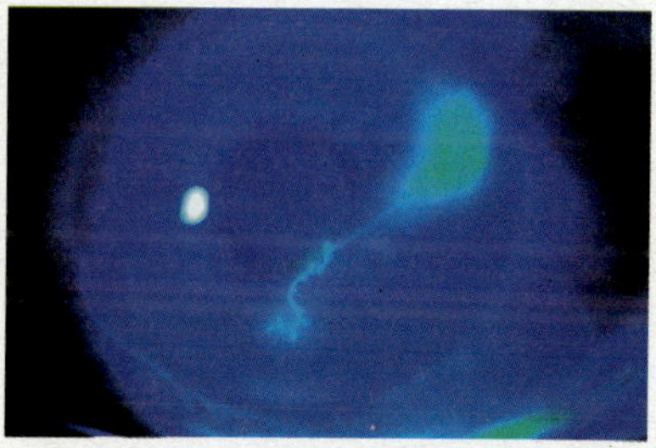

This patient has had a photophobic, red and gritty eye for 2 days.
a. What is the diagnosis?
b. What key physical sign should be checked prior to measuring the intraocular pressure?
c. What is the differential diagnosis?
d. What is the treatment?

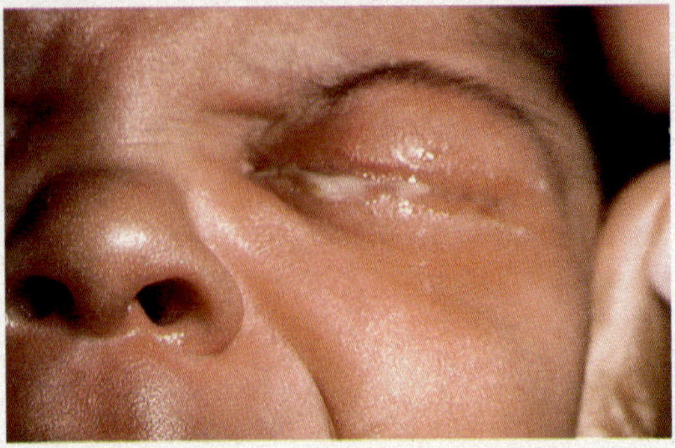

32. 2 周大婴儿，眼部粘性分泌物持续一周。

a. 按定义是什么诊断？

b. 病因是什么，从何时有明显症状？

c. 新生儿衣原体感染的全身表现是什么？

The eyes of this 2-week-old baby have been very sticky for the last week.

a. By definition, what is the diagnosis?

b. What are the causes, and when does each typically present?

c. What are the systemic manifestations of chlamydial infection in neonates?

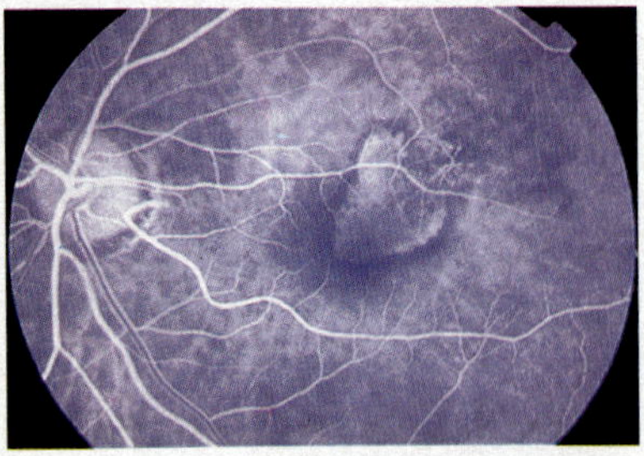

33. 70 岁女性荧光眼底血管造影照片。

a. 照片显示的病变是什么？

b. 已知患者的年龄，可能的原因是什么？

c. 其他潜在的病理是什么？

This is the fluorescein angiogram of a 70-year-old woman.

a. What lesion is demonstrated?

b. Given the patient's age, what is the likely cause?

c. What other underlying pathology might be responsible?

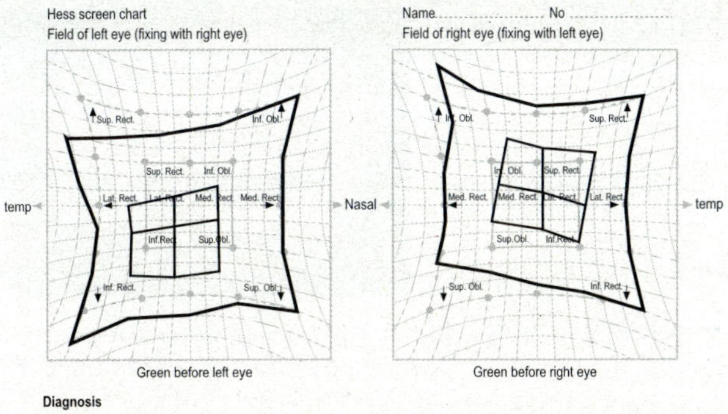

34. 48 岁复视患者 Hess 图。
a. 诊断是什么？
b. 详细描述图上显示的变化。

This is a Hess chart of a 48-year-old patient with double vision.
a. What is the diagnosis?
b. Describe in detail the changes shown on the chart.

35. 这是失明患者在白天的视网膜表现。
a. 描述体征。
b. 诊断是什么？
c. 需要做什么检查？为什么？
d. 突然单侧视力丧失其他的常见原因是什么？

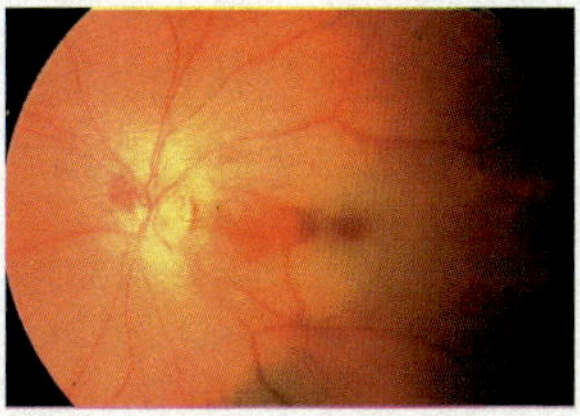

This is the fundal appearance of a patient who lost vision in the eye earlier in the day.
a. Describe the signs.
b. What is the diagnosis?
c. What imaging investigations might be appropriate and why?
d. What are the other common causes of sudden, profound, unilateral loss of vision?

36. 眼科医生认为该患者可能是黑色素瘤。
a. 诊断是什么？
b. 支持本诊断的特征是什么？
c. 关心全身性合并症吗？

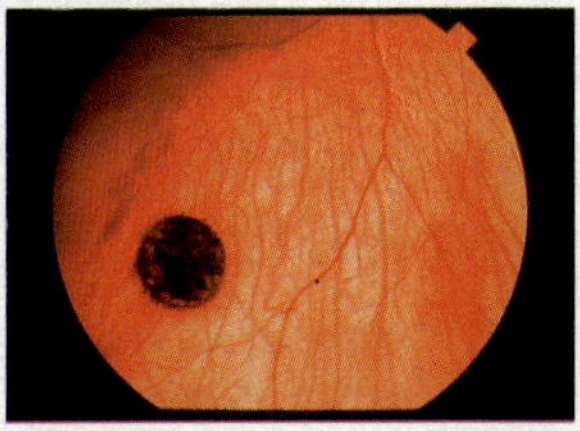

This patient's optometrist was concerned that this might be a melanoma.
a. What is the diagnosis?
b. What are the characteristics that support this?
c. Are you concerned regarding systemic implications?

37. 该患者在近几年有渐增的夜间视物困难（夜盲症）

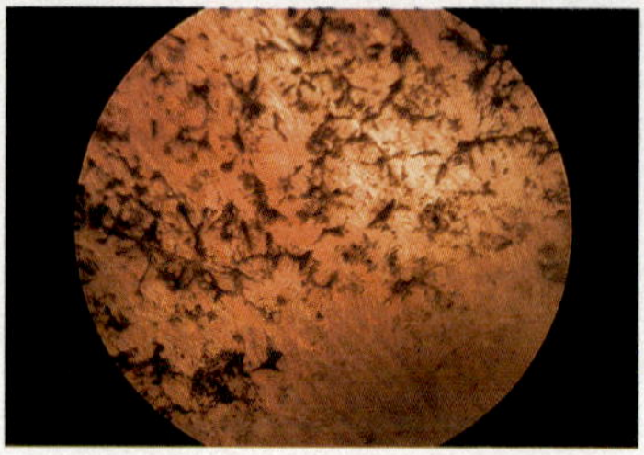

a. 体征是什么？诊断是什么？
b. 可出现哪些其他眼部特点？
c. 电生理检查可见什么？
d. 哪些全身病可以出现这种症状？

This patient has had increasing difficulty with night vision (nyctalopia) over the last few years.

a. What are the signs and what is the diagnosis?
b. What other ocular features may be present?
c. What are the electrodiagnostic findings?
d. What systemic disorders may be associated with this condition?

38. 该患者注意到她一侧脸汗多。

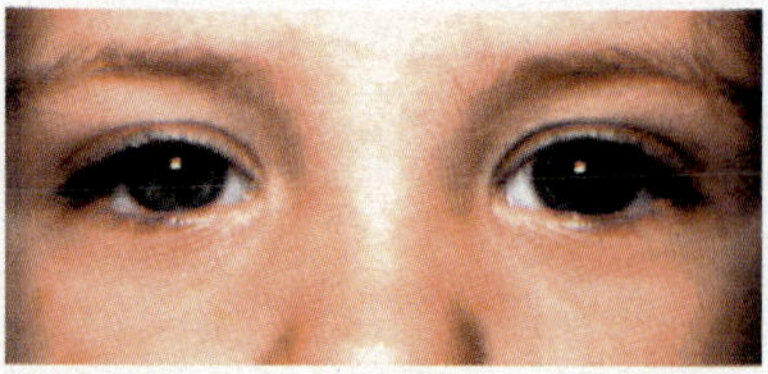

a. 描述体征，做出诊断。
b. 可出现哪些其他的眼部特点？
c. 哪些药理学试验有用？

This patient has noticed that she sweats much more on one side of her face.

a. Describe the signs and give the diagnosis.
b. What other ocular features may be present?
c. What pharmacological tests might be useful?

39. 这是先天性梅毒的老年患者的角膜。

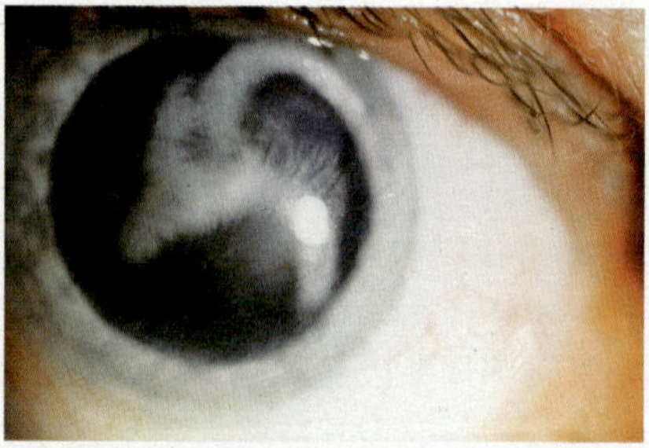

a. 这是什么病？
b. 罕见的角膜基质内出血。其机理是什么？
c. 列出先天性梅毒的晚期全身性体征。

This is the cornea of an elderly patient with congenital syphilis.

a. What is the condition?
b. Rarely, an intrastromal corneal haemorrhage may occur. What is the mechanism?
c. List the late systemic signs of congenital syphilis.

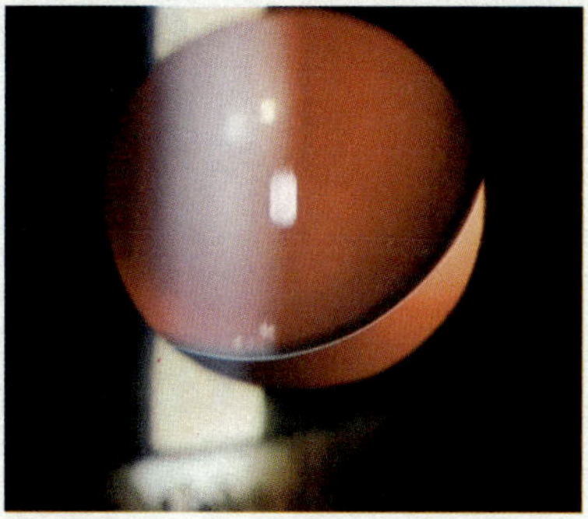

40. 该患者个高，有细长的手指（蜘蛛足样指／趾）和高腭穹。
a. 眼部的表现是什么？
b. 诊断是什么？遗传基础是什么？
c. 其他的全身性特征是什么？
d. 该眼部表现还合并什么其他的全身症状？

This patient has long, spindly fingers (arachnodactyly) and a high-arched palate.
a. What is the ocular sign?
b. What is the systemic diagnosis, and what is its genetic basis?
c. What other systemic features may be present?
d. What other systemic conditions are associated with this ocular finding?

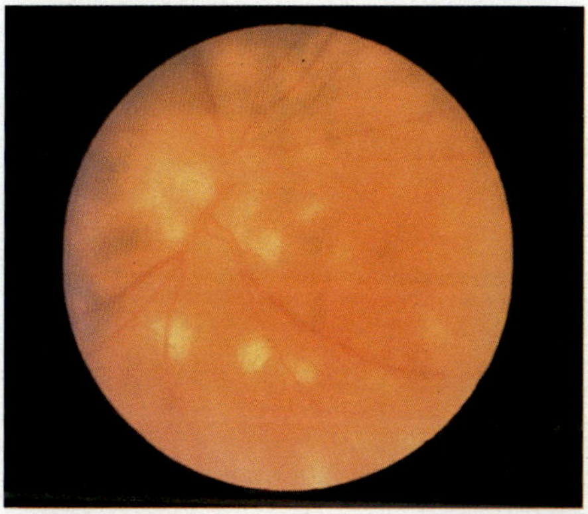

41. 56岁女性视网膜的表现，鸟枪弹视网膜脉络膜病变。
a. 与HLA有什么关联？
b. 玻璃体炎在这个疾病中常见吗？
c. 当决定开始治疗时什么特殊的检查是有用的？
d. 视力丧失最常见的原因是什么？

This is the retinal appearance in a 56-year-old woman with birdshot retinochoroidopathy.
a. What is the HLA association?
b. Is vitreitis common in this condition?
c. What special investigation is useful when deciding to start treatment?
d. What are the most common causes of visual loss?

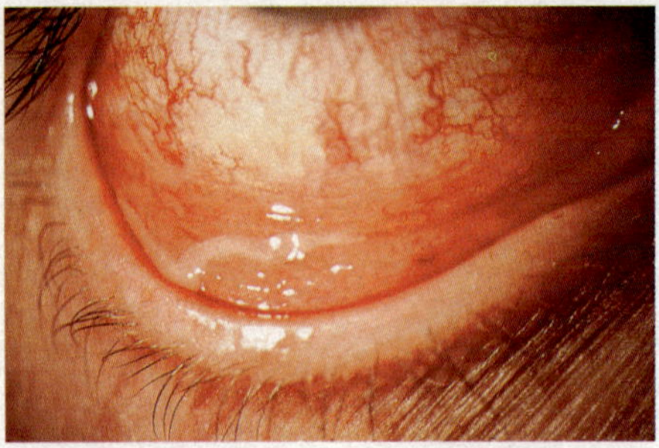

42. 这是20多岁男性眼部表现，他最近感染尿道炎。怀疑是Reiter综合征。

a. 他可能有什么其他的全身性表现？

b. 眼部的特征性表现是什么？

c. 什么血液化验有助于确诊？

d. 可出现什么心脏并发症？

This is the eye of a man in his twenties who recently contracted urethritis. Reiter's syndrome is suspected.

a. What other systemic features might he have?

b. What other ocular feature is characteristic?

c. What blood test will help to confirm the diagnosis?

d. What cardiac complication can occur?

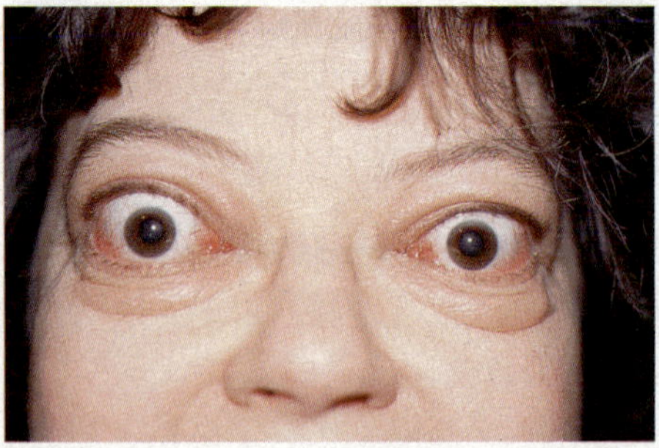

43. 40岁女性患甲状腺眼病。

a. 病变的症状是什么？

b. 甲状腺眼病多由于甲状腺功能低下还是甲状腺功能亢进造成？

c. 最少见的眼球运动障碍是什么？

d. 眼眶软组织肿胀常导致视神经病变。哪些治疗是有效的？

This woman aged 40 has thyroid eye disease.

a. What are the symptoms of this condition?

b. Is thyroid eye disease more commonly associated with primary hypo- or hyperthyroidism?

c. What is the least common ocular motility defect?

d. Orbital soft tissue swelling can sometimes lead to optic neuropathy. What treatments are available?

44. 该中年女性眼部的瘢痕性类天疱疮。

a. 特有的皮肤损害是什么？

b. 并发症是什么？

c. 活动性疾病怎样治疗？

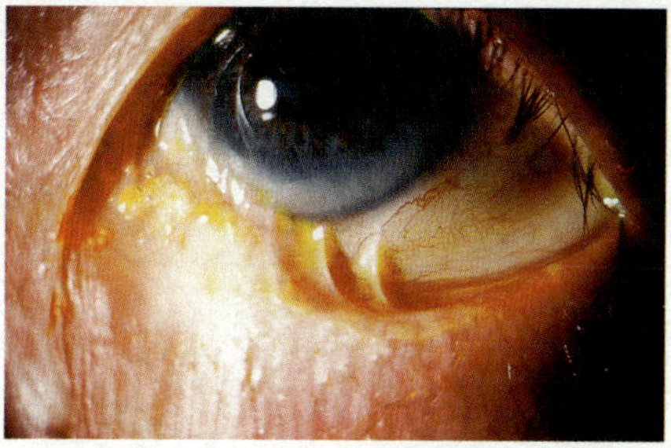

This middle-aged woman has ocular cicatricial pemphigoid.

a. What are the typical cutaneous lesions?

b. What are the complications?

c. How is the active disease treated?

45. 这是30岁女性双侧视盘表现，她主诉头痛、恶心和暂时的视物模糊。

a. 可能的诊断是什么？

b. 最主要的并发症是什么？

c. 治疗包括什么？

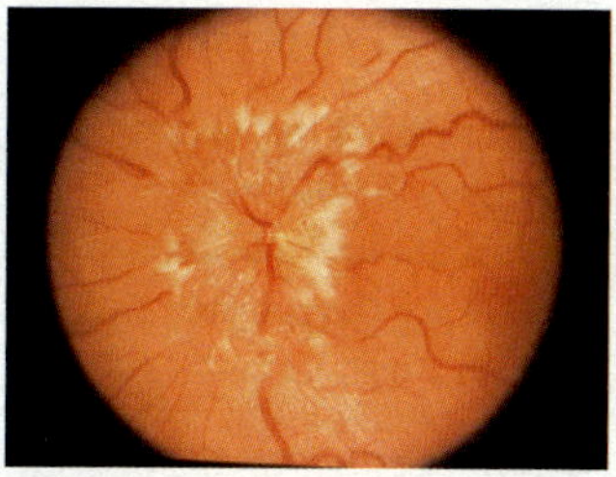

This is the bilateral optic disc appearance of an obese 30-year-old woman complaining of headache, nausea and transient visual obscurations.

a. What is the likely diagnosis?

b. What is the most important complication?

c. What are the treatment options?

46. 该患者一年前行全层角膜移植术。从上个月起该眼由于移植失败视物模糊。

a. 临床上，移植失败与排斥反应有何不同？

b. 排斥反应怎样治疗？

c. 列出角膜移植术预后不良的影响因素。

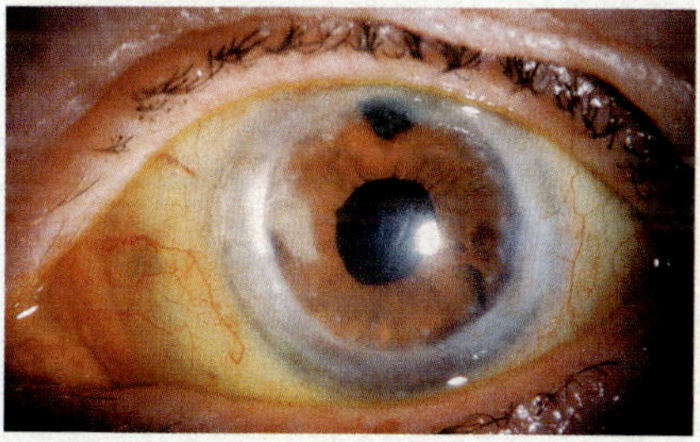

This patient underwent penetrating keratoplasty a year ago. For the past month vision in the eye has been blurred as a result of graft failure.

a. Clinically, how does graft failure differ from rejection?

b. How is rejection treated?

c. List factors conferring a poor prognosis for corneal grafting.

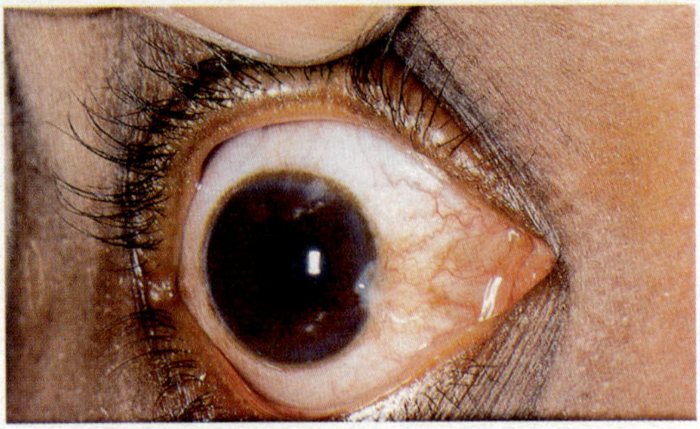

47. 该患者在中东工作多年。

a. 病变是什么?

b. 切除的适应证是什么?

c. 适当的手术操作是什么?

This patient has been working in the Middle East for several years.

a. What is the lesion?

b. What are the indications for its removal?

c. What are the possible surgical techniques?

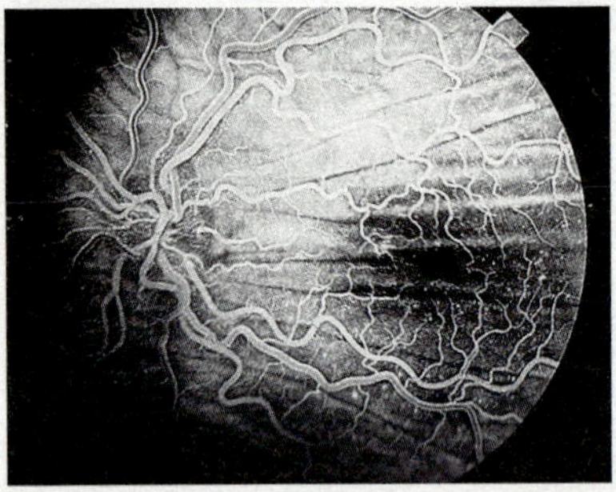

48. 在常规检查中，医生在双眼无症状的远视患者发现该情况(荧光素眼底血管造影照片显示)。

a. 诊断是什么?

b. 原因是什么?

c. 列出其他的原因。

At a routine sight test, an optometrist discovered this condition (a fluorescein angiogram is shown) in both eyes of an asymptomatic hypermetropic patient.

a. What is the diagnosis?

b. What is the cause?

c. List other causes.

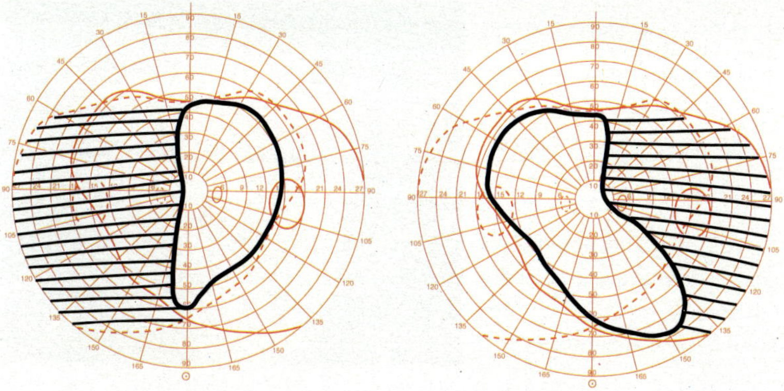

49. 50 岁女性的视野，有青光眼家族史但眼压正常。

a. 这是典型的青光眼视野吗？

b. 怀疑的病理改变是什么？

c. 有助于诊断的其他检查是什么？

These are the visual fields of a 50-year-old woman with a family history of glaucoma but normal intraocular pressures.

a. Are the visual fields typically glaucomatous?

b. What other pathology might be suspected?

c. What other investigation is indicated?

50. 女性患有慢性关节炎，主诉持续的眼部沙砾感。

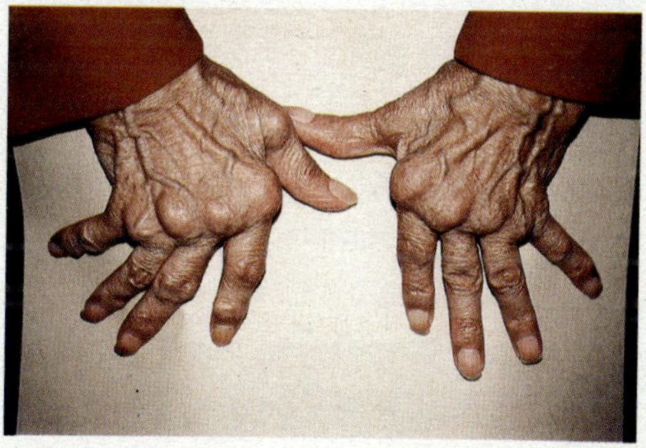

a. 全身性疾病的诊断是什么？

b. 她的沙砾感是什么？

c. 有助于确定诊断的简单检查是什么？

d. 可以出现什么其他眼部并发症？

This woman has chronic arthritis and complains of persistently gritty eyes.

a. What is the systemic diagnosis?

b. Why are her eyes gritty?

c. What simple tests can help to confirm the diagnosis?

d. What other ocular complications may occur?

51. 该病人2周前行听神经瘤切除术。
a. 异常表现是什么？
b. 可出现什么眼部问题？
c. 如何治疗？

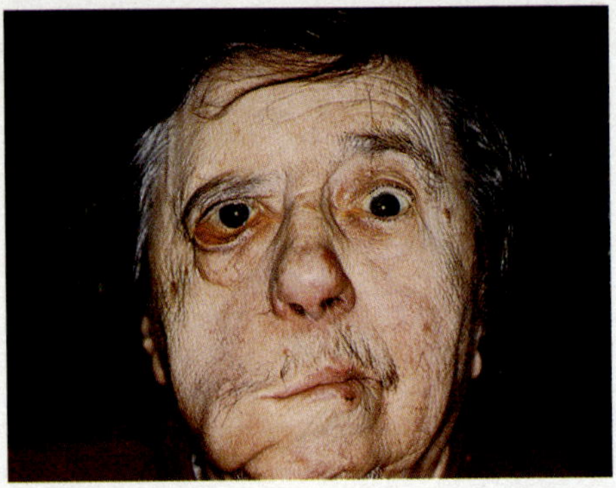

This patient underwent removal of an acoustic neuroma 2 weeks ago.
a. What is the abnormality shown?
b. What ocular problems may develop?
c. What is the management?

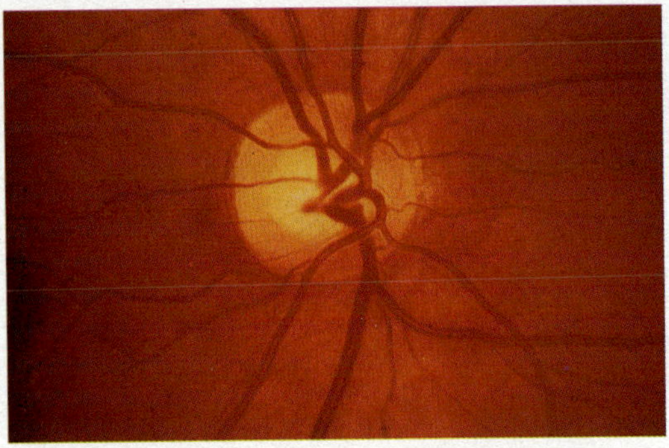

52. 57岁男性双眼眼压26 mmHg。
a. 他有青光眼吗？
b. 这种眼压的患者发展为青光眼的比例是多少？
c. 如果视神经正常，怎样测量视盘直径将有助于确定诊断？
d. 其他有用的检查是什么？

This 57-year-old man has intraocular pressures of 26mmHg in both eyes.
a. Does he have glaucoma?
b. What percentage of patients with this intraocular pressure develop glaucoma?
c. How will measuring the optic disc diameter help to determine if the nerve is normal?
d. What other investigations may be useful?

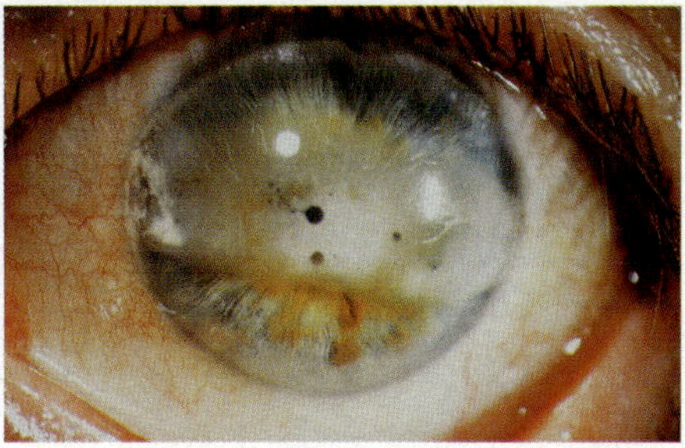

53. 9岁女孩患青少年原发性关节炎(JIA)。
a. 体征是什么?
b. JIA的眼部表现是什么?
c. 列出伴随眼部病变高发的三个JIA特征。

This 9-year-old girl suffers from juvenile idiopathic arthritis (JIA).
a. What are the signs shown?
b. What are the ocular manifestations of JIA?
c. List three characteristics in JIA which are associated with a high risk of eye problems.

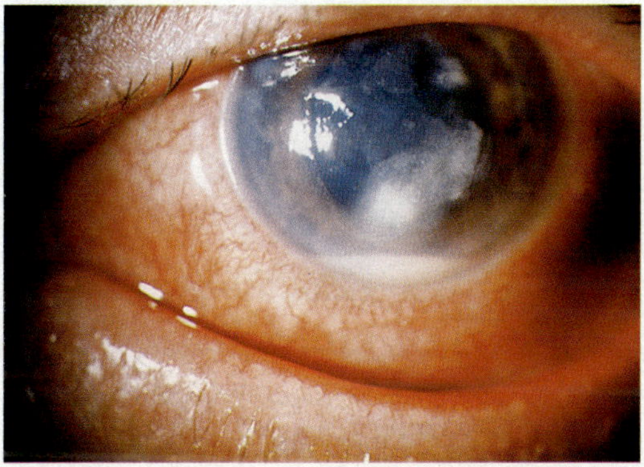

54. 戴软性隐形眼镜患者的角膜。眼红，非常不舒服24小时。
a. 诊断是什么?
b. 如何处理?
c. 列出微生物在普通培养基不生长的原因，但如果不处理会对视力构成严重威胁。

This is the cornea of a patient who wears soft contact lenses. The eye has been red and very uncomfortable for 24 hours.
a. What is the diagnosis?
b. What is the management?
c. List the causative microorganisms that do not grow on common culture media but may constitute a serious threat to vision if untreated.

55. (a) 该患者正在尝试向左看；左眼可见微小眼球震颤。(b) 向右注视无异常。(c) 集合正常。
a. 诊断是什么？
b. 病变位于哪里？
c. 指出该患者最有可能的原因。
d. 列出其他的原因。

(a) The patient is attempting to look to the left; a fine nystagmus can be seen in the left eye. (b) No abnormality is seen on right gaze. (c) Convergence is normal.
a. What is the diagnosis?
b. Where is the lesion located?
c. Give the most likely cause in this patient.
d. List other causes.

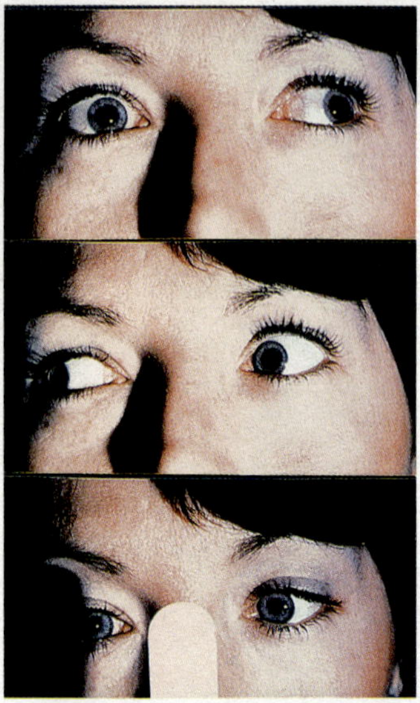
(a) (b) (c)

56. 37 岁男性患肉芽肿性虹膜炎。检眼镜检查可见中度玻璃体炎和视网膜炎。
a. 他没有感染 HIV。可能的诊断是什么？
b. 有助于确诊的检查是什么？
c. 如何治疗？

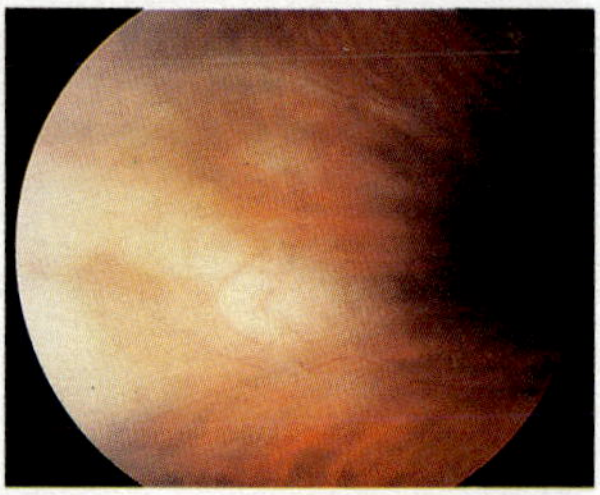

This 37-year-old man has granulomatous iritis. Ophthalmoscopy shows moderate vitreitis and retinitis, as shown.
a. He has no risk factors for HIV infection. What is the probable diagnosis?
b. What investigations might help to confirm the diagnosis?
c. What is the management?

57. 该患者持续缺血型视网膜中央静脉阻塞 3 个月。
a. 出现什么并发症？可能出现什么后遗症？
b. 列出出现这种情况的其他常见原因。
c. 该患者将怎样处理？

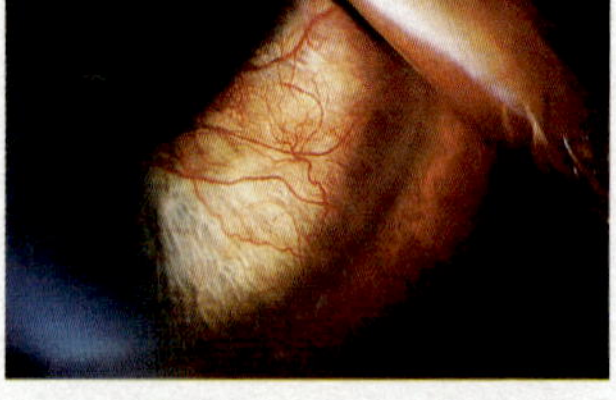

This patient sustained an ischaemic central retinal vein occlusion 3 months ago.
a. What complication has occurred, and what is the likely sequel?
b. List other common causes of the condition shown.
c. How should this patient be managed?

58. 老年女性出现全身性症状，由于腹痛和恶心来急诊科。急诊室工作人员注意到她眼睛红。
a. 诊断是什么？
b. 如何治疗？
c. 剧痛和眼红的其他常见的原因是什么？

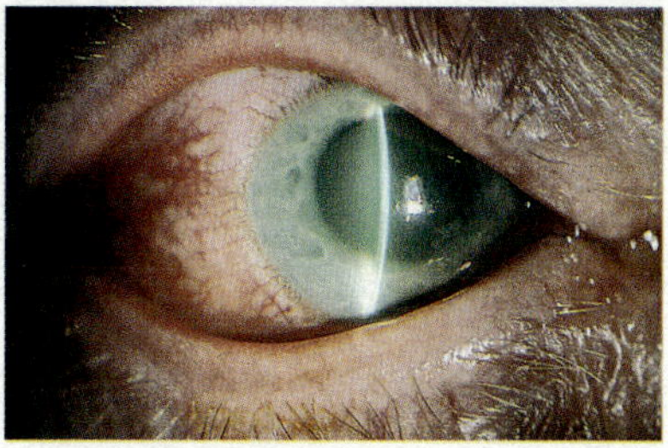

This elderly woman presented to the general accident and emergency department with abdominal pain and nausea. The casualty officer noticed that she had a red eye.
a. What is the diagnosis?
b. What is the management?
c. What are the other common causes of a very painful and red eye?

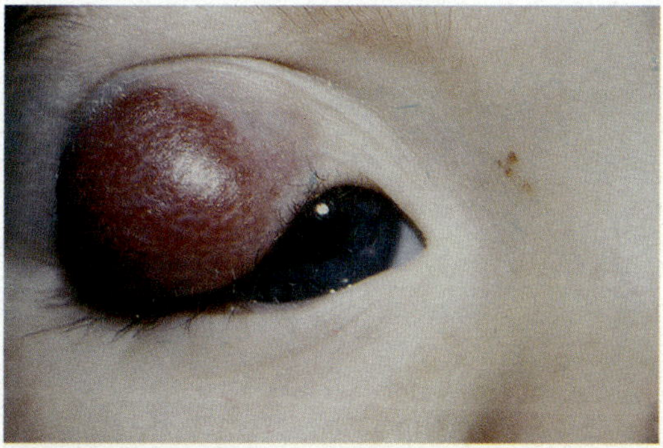

59. 婴儿的父母担心这个快速生长的病变会损害孩子的视力，并且以后会影响外观。
a. 诊断是什么？
b. 父母的担心对吗？
c. 最常用的治疗方式是什么？
d. 与全身性疾病有关系吗？

This baby's parents are concerned that this rapidly growing lesion may damage the child's eyesight, and also about its long-term cosmetic effect.
a. What is the diagnosis?
b. Is the parents' concern justified?
c. What is the most common form of treatment?
d. Are there any systemic implications?

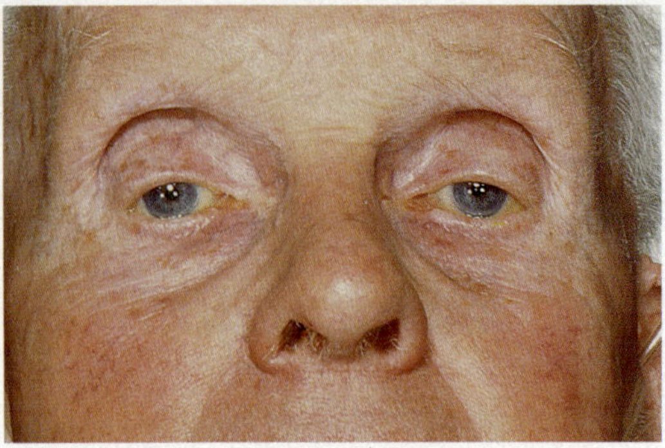

60. 双侧上睑下垂。

a. 什么肌肉负责上眼睑的升降，它们由什么神经支配?

b. 上睑下垂的原因是什么?

c. 假性上睑下垂的原因是什么?

Bilateral ptosis is shown.

a. What are the muscles responsible for elevating the upper lid, and what is their innervation?

b. What are the causes of ptosis?

c. What are the causes of pseudoptosis?

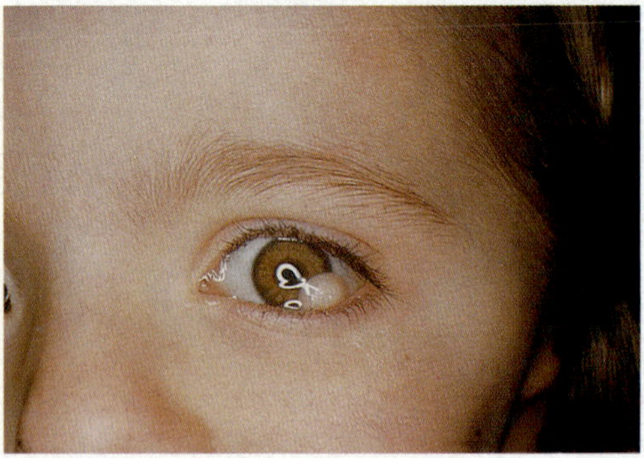

61. 婴儿的父母非常担心该疾病。

a. 诊断是什么?

b. 病理分类是什么?

c. 什么时候治疗?

d. 有全身并发症吗?

This infant's parents are extremely worried by this lesion.

a. What is the diagnosis?

b. What is its pathological categorization?

c. When might treatment be indicated?

d. Are there any systemic implications?

62. 该儿童正试图向上看和向右看。

a. 描述这种异常运动，给出诊断，假定在其他眼位眼运动正常。

b. 如何治疗？

c. 这类疾病最多见的原因是先天性的，但这类疾病后天性的原因是什么？

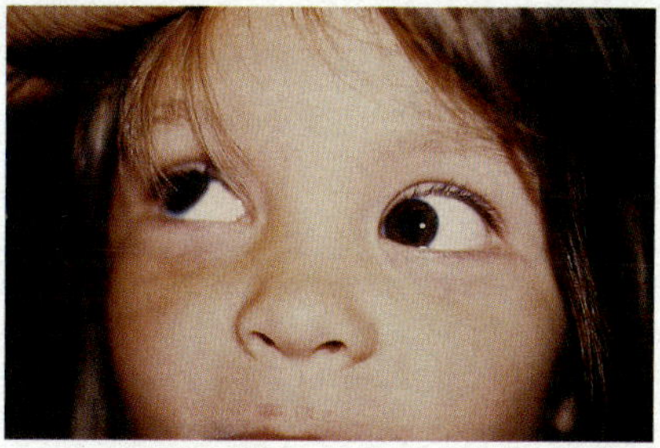

This child is attempting to look up and to the right.

a. Describe the motility abnormality and give the diagnosis, assuming eye movements are normal in other positions of gaze.

b. What is the management?

c. Most cases are congenital but what are the causes of an acquired lesion of this type?

63. 老年患者突然一眼视力丧失。眼底检查显示苍白肿胀的视盘。

a. 患者突然出现视力丧失和这样的视盘表现，最基本的问题是什么？

b. 急检什么血液项目可以确诊？

c. 需要做什么其他的检查？

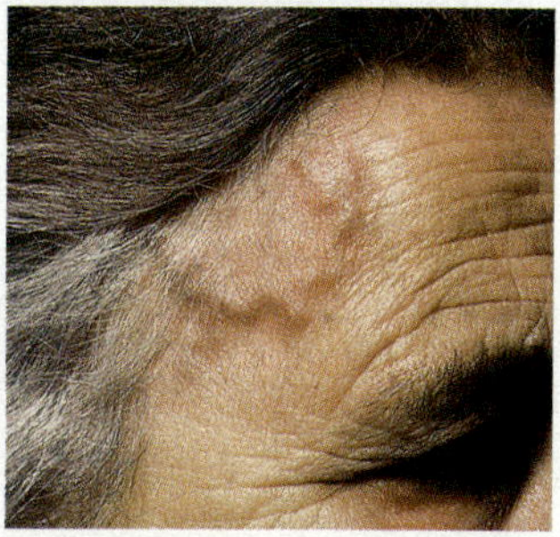

This elderly patient suddenly lost vision in one eye. Ophthalmoscopy revealed a pale, swollen optic disc.

a. What questions are essential in a patient presenting with sudden loss of vision and this disc appearance?

b. What urgent blood tests are indicated?

c. What further investigation is necessary?

64. 这个孩子上睑下垂和进展性两侧眼外肌无力。

a. 诊断是什么？

b. 根本的遗传异常是什么？

c. 除遗传分析之外，什么检查对确诊可能有帮助？

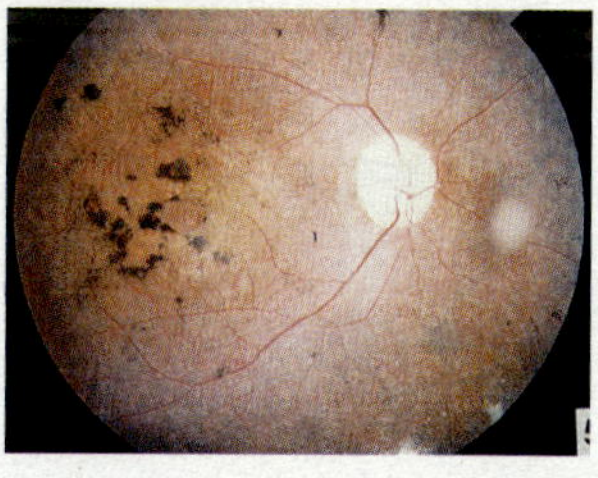

This child also has ptosis and progressive bilateral extraocular muscle weakness.

a. What is the diagnosis?

b. What is the underlying genetic abnormality?

c. In addition to genetic analysis, what investigations might be helpful in confirmation of the diagnosis?

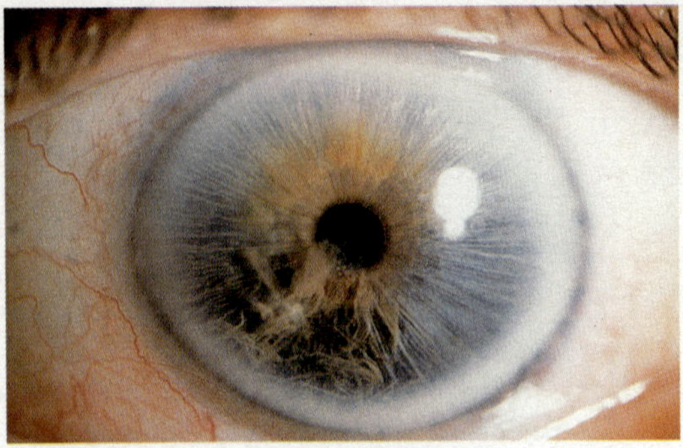

65. 78 岁老年男性双眼出现这种情况。

a. 诊断是什么?

b. 是如何威胁视力的?

c. 如何治疗?

This 78-year-old man has this condition in both eyes.

a. What is the diagnosis?

b. How is sight threatened?

c. What is the treatment?

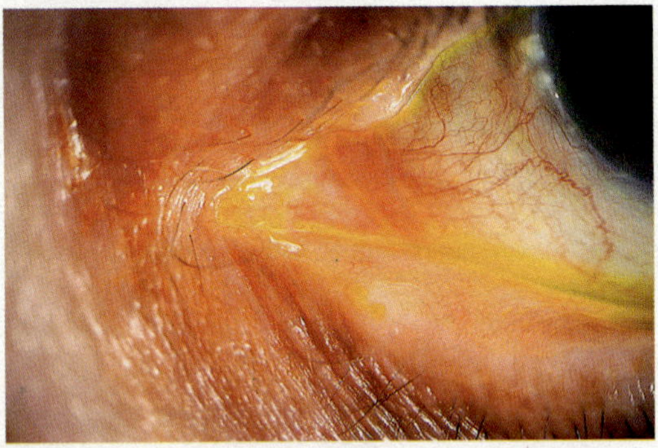

66. 60 岁老年女性主诉近 6 个月该眼流泪。

a. 异常表现是什么?

b. 进一步进行哪些检查可以排除流泪的其他原因?

c. 假如上述的异常造成流泪，如何选择治疗?

This 60-year-old woman complains of watering of the eye for the last 6 months.

a. What abnormality is shown?

b. What further investigations should be performed to exclude other causes of the watering?

c. Assuming the abnormality above is responsible for the symptoms, what are the treatment options?

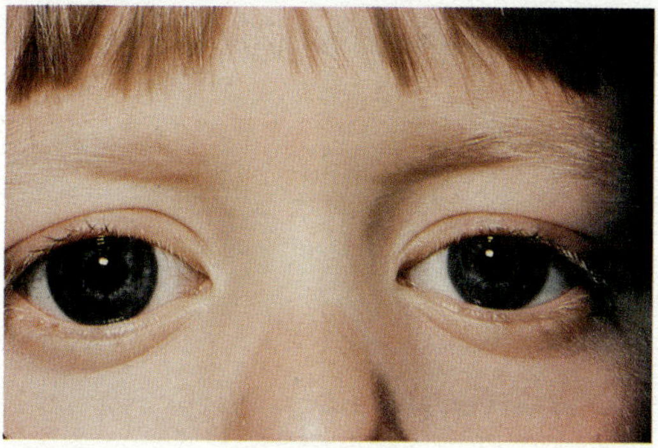

67. 这个孩子天生这种情况。

a. 描述体征；可能的诊断是什么？

b. 在这种情况可能出现什么其他的体征？

c. 怎样确定诊断？

This child was born with the condition shown.

a. Describe the signs; what is the likely diagnosis?

b. What other signs might be present in this condition?

c. How can the diagnosis be confirmed?

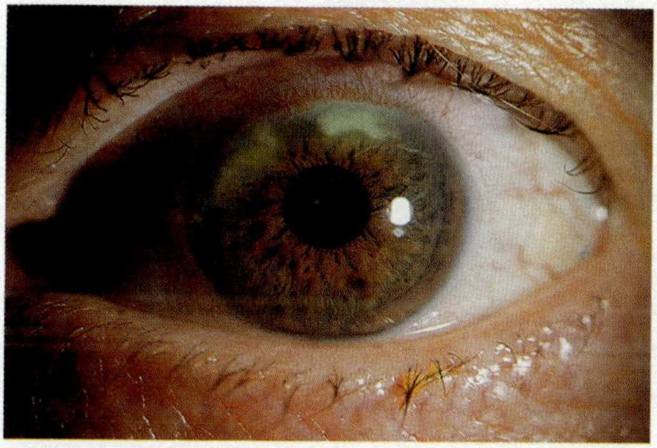

68. 33 岁女性主诉轻度眼部刺激持续 3 天。

a. 诊断是什么？

b. 什么特征提示这不是细菌性角膜炎？

c. 如何治疗？

This 33-year-old man complains of mild ocular irritation for the last 3 days.

a. What is the diagnosis?

b. What features suggest that this is not a bacterial keratitis?

c. What is the treatment?

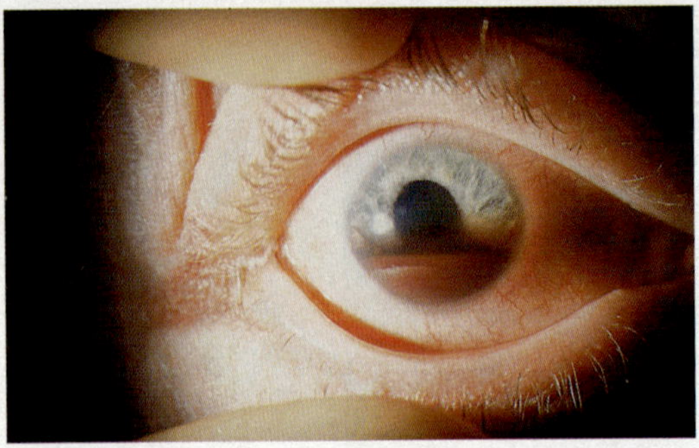

69. 15岁男孩一眼被网球击中。

a. 阳性表现是什么?

b. 该病严重的并发症是什么?

c. 将制定什么处理方案?

This 15-year-old boy was struck in the eye by a tennis ball.

a. What is the sign shown?

b. What is the most important complication of this condition?

c. What management should be instituted?

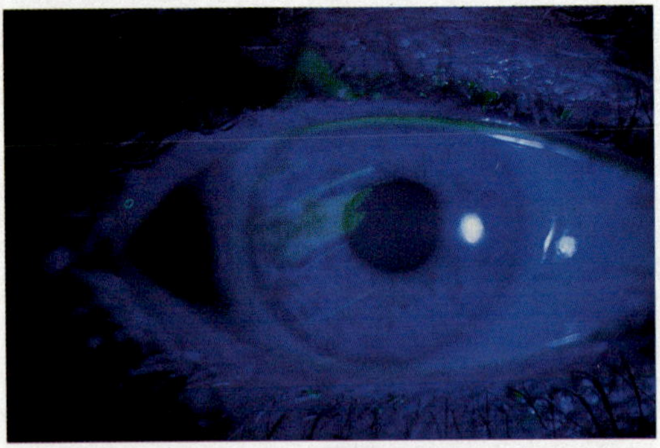

70. 早晨该患者一眼被孩子戳伤。

a. 损伤是什么?

b. 症状是什么?

c. 怎样治疗?

This patient was poked in the eye by a baby earlier in the day.

a. What is this lesion?

b. What are the symptoms?

c. What is the management?

71. 50岁患者突然出现上睑下垂和复视伴随同侧的额痛。
a. 诊断是什么?
b. 必须尽快排除什么潜在的病变?
c. 寻找病因时重要的临床特征是什么?

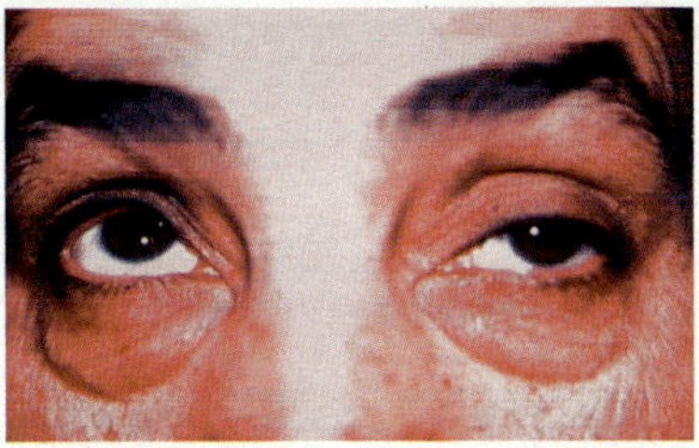

This 50-year-old suddenly developed a droopy eyelid and double vision associated with ipsilateral frontal headache.
a. What is the diagnosis?
b. What underlying condition must be urgently excluded?
c. What clinical features are important when considering the cause?

72. 该患者最近做过视网膜脱离手术。
a. 视网膜脱离并发症是手术复位失败的最常见原因。并发症是什么?
b. 列出这种疾病的体征。
c. 什么术式可能使视网膜复位?

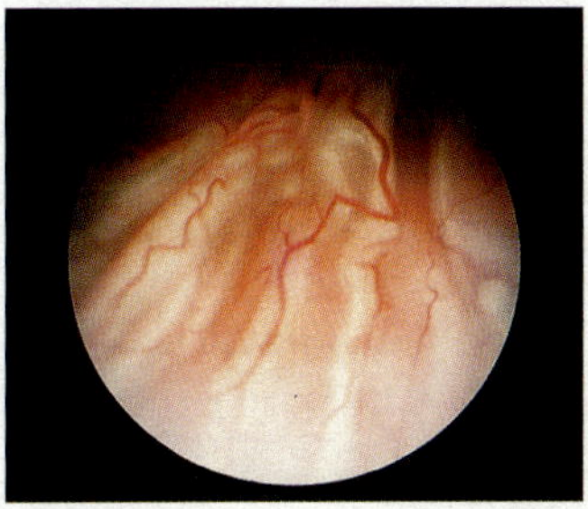

This patient recently underwent retinal detachment surgery.
a. The complication of retinal detachment shown is the most common cause of failure of surgical repair. What is it?
b. List the signs of the condition.
c. What form of surgery is likely to be used to attempt re-attachment?

73. 35岁女性突然出现眼前漂浮物。
a. 这是什么表现?
b. 看不到眼底，需进行什么检查?
c. 列出出现这种情况的原因。

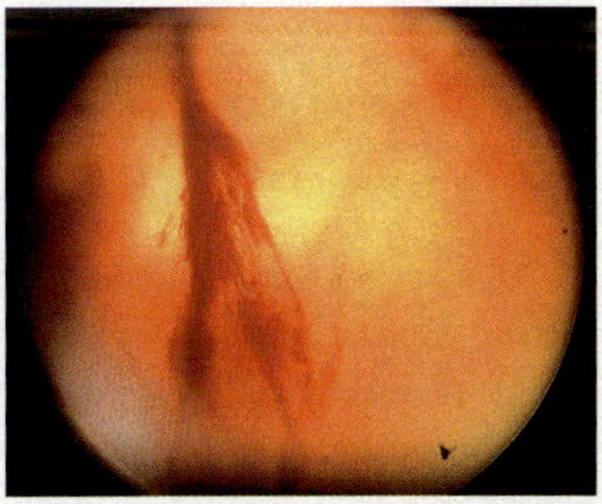

This healthy 35-year-old woman presented with the sudden onset of floaters.
a. What is shown?
b. As there is no useful view of the fundus, what investigation should be performed?
c. List the causes of the condition shown.

74. 中年患者主诉视物变形渐进性恶化。
a. 表现是什么异常？
b. 组织病理学基础是什么？
c. 病因是什么？

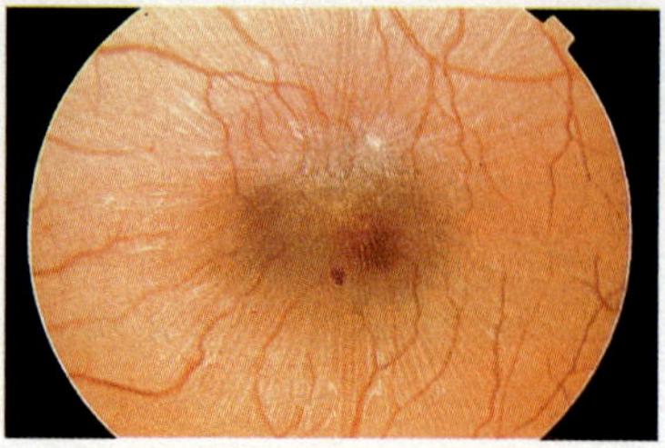

This middle-aged patient complains of gradually worsening distortion of vision.
a. What abnormality is shown?
b. What is its histopathological basis?
c. What are the causes?

75. 这是睫状体平坦部玻璃体切割术（PPV）的操作。
a. 器械的名称。
b. 列出 PPV 的主要适应证。

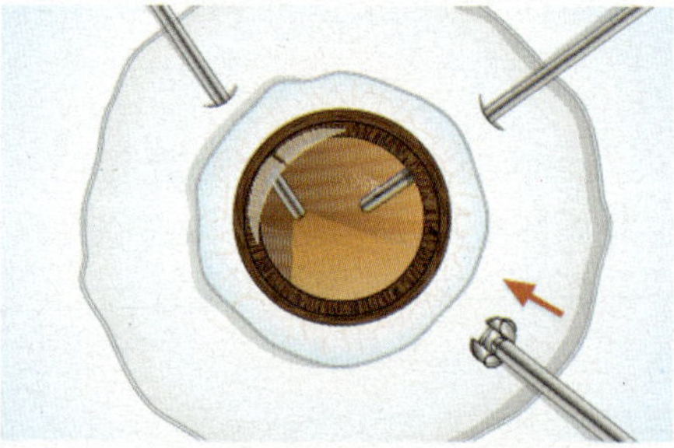

These are instrumentation used to perform pars plana vitrectomy (PPV).
a. Name the instruments.
b. List the important indications for PPV.

76. 灰白色圆形和多角形混浊点位于角膜浅层，中心高密度，蜂窝状外形；诊断是 Thiel-Behnke 角膜营养不良（Bowman 层 2 型营养不良）。
a. 这个疾病典型的临床表现是什么？
b. 描述组织学所见。
c. 遗传方式和基因是什么？
d. 影响 Bowman 层的其他营养不良是什么？临床上怎样区分两者？

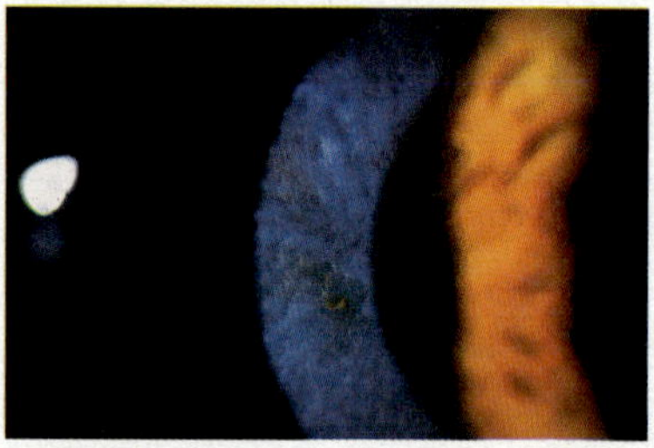

This patient has grey-white round and polygonal opacities in the superficial cornea, densest centrally and forming a honeycomb pattern in places; the diagnosis is Thiel-Behnke corneal dystrophy (Bowman layer dystrophy type 2).
a. What is the typical clinical presentation of this condition?
b. Describe the histology.
c. What is the inheritance pattern and where is the gene?
d. What is the other dystrophy affecting the Bowman layer and how do the two differ clinically?

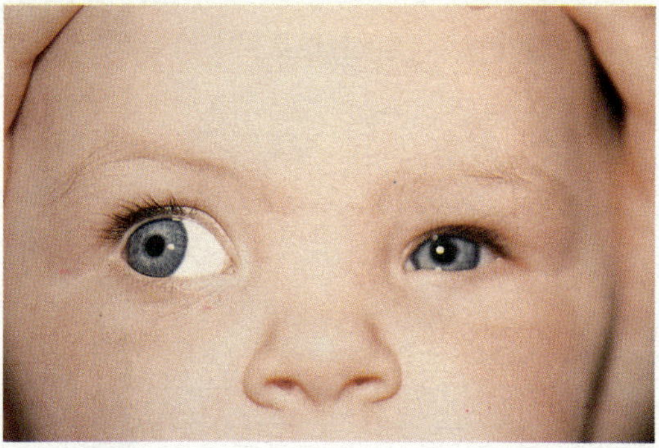

77. 该男孩先天性眼球运动性疾病，正试图向右看。

a. 描述体征，给出诊断。

b. 在这类疾病中按 Huber 标准怎样分类?

c. 除外其他的运动性体征，眼部的伴随症状是什么?

This boy with a congenital ocular motility disorder is attempting right gaze.

a. Describe the signs and give the diagnosis.

b. How would he be categorized in the Huber classification of this disorder?

c. Excluding other motility signs, what are the ocular associations of this condition?

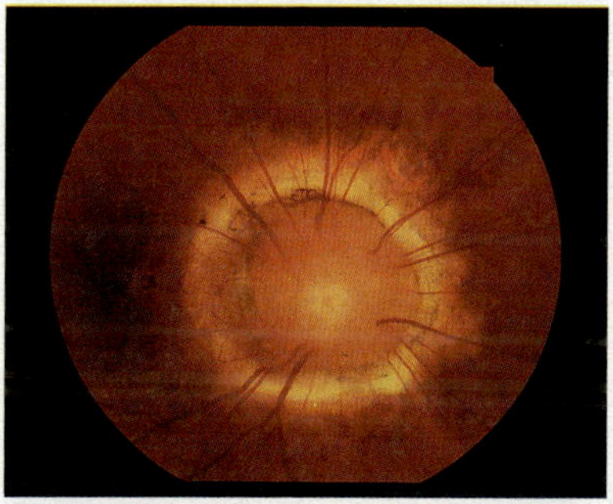

78. 该眼视力很差；对侧眼正常。

a. 描述体征，给出诊断。

b. 继发浆液性视网膜脱离的发病率是多少?

c. 全身性的先天异常有什么?

Vision is very poor in this eye; the fellow eye is normal.

a. Describe the signs and give the diagnosis.

b. What is the incidence of subsequent serous retinal detachment?

c. What are the systemic implications?

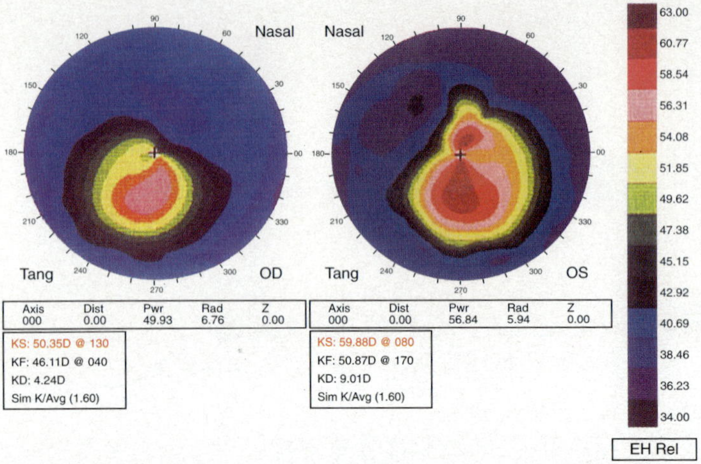

79. 23 岁女性渐增性散光角膜评估的检查所见。

a. 这是什么检查？

b. 彩色编码表示什么？

c. 角膜扫描正常吗？

This investigation was used to assess the cornea of a 23-year-old woman with increasing astigmatism.

a. What was the investigation employed?

b. What is represented by the colour coding used?

c. Is the cornea normal according to the scan?

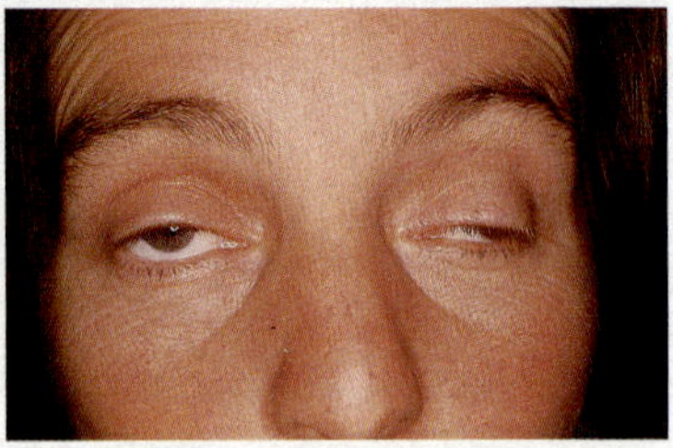

80. 患者主诉傍晚上睑下垂加重，间歇性复视。

a. 可出现这个症状的全身性疾病是什么？

b. 支持假定诊断的其他眼部体征是什么？

c. 有助于确定诊断的血液检验是什么？

d. 应进行的药理学检验是什么？

This patient complains of drooping eyelids worse towards the end of the day and intermittent double vision.

a. What underlying systemic disease may be present?

b. What other eye signs would reinforce the putative diagnosis?

c. What blood test can be useful in helping to confirm the diagnosis?

d. What pharmacological test might be indicated?

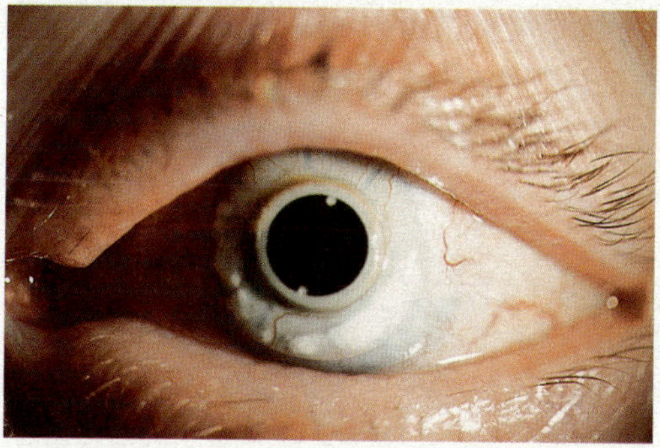

81. 3年前该患者双眼严重化学损伤。

a. 显示的方法是什么?

b. 这类手术的适应证是什么?

c. 并发症是什么?

This patient sustained a severe bilateral chemical injury 3 years ago.

a. What is the device shown?

b. What are the indications for surgery of this type?

c. What are the complications?

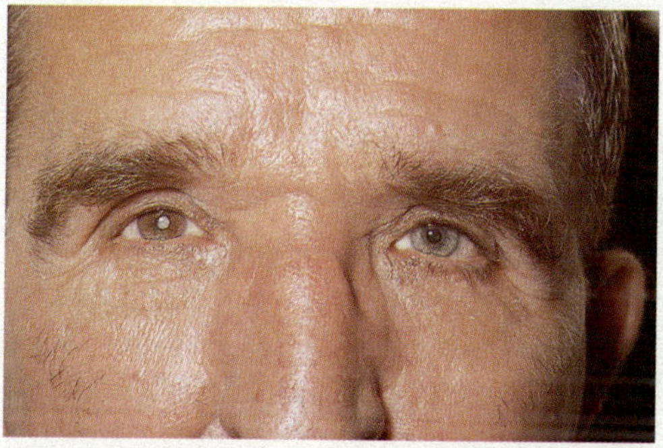

82. 该男性注意到几个月前左眼视力下降。裂隙灯检查发现弥漫的星状角膜后沉着物。

a. 描述体征，给出诊断。

b. 可能发生哪些其他威胁视力的并发症?

c. 怎样处理?

This man has noticed worsening vision in the left eye over the past few months. Diffuse stellate keratic precipitates are present on slit lamp examination.

a. Describe the signs and give the diagnosis.

b. Besides that shown, what other sight-threatening complication might occur?

c. How is the condition treated?

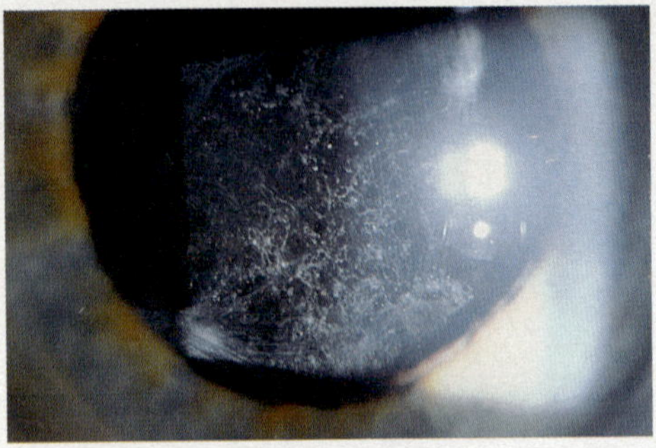

83. 人工晶状体眼视力渐进性下降几个月。

a. 叙述白内障术后并发症。

b. 该患者可能出现的其他症状是什么?

c. 怎样治疗?

d. 治疗的并发症是什么?

The vision in this pseudophakic eye has gradually been getting worse for several months.

a. Describe the complication of cataract surgery shown.

b. What other symptoms is the patient likely to be experiencing?

c. What is the treatment?

d. What are the complications of the treatment?

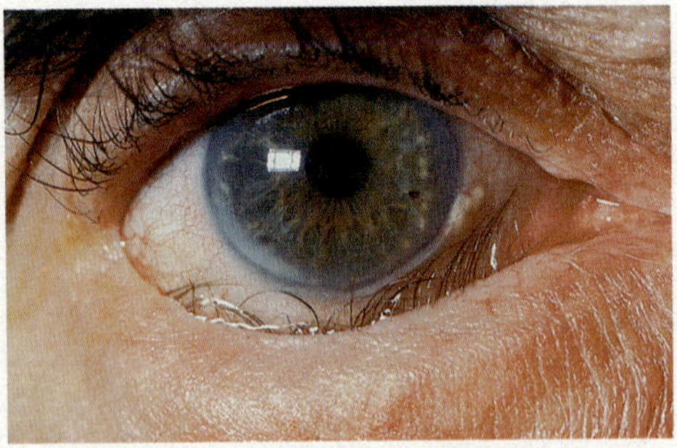

84. 该患者眼部异物感和充血持续几周。

a. 出现此症状的原因是什么?

b. 退行性改变的发病机理是什么?

c. 怎样治疗?

This patient's eye has been gritty and red for several weeks.

a. What is the cause of the symptoms?

b. What is the pathogenesis of the involutional form of this condition?

c. What is the treatment?

85. 这位81岁女性患者有严重的“湿性”年龄相关性黄斑变性。她的医生注意到该眼最近视力下降。
a. 这个疾病的表现是什么？
b. 如果临床上怀疑脉络膜新生血管形成(CNV)，可行什么检查？
c. 什么措施可使这只眼减少CNV的风险？

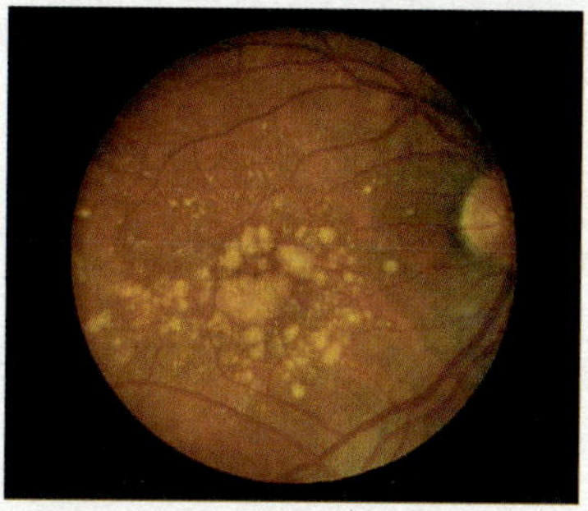

This 81-year-old woman has severe 'wet' age-related macular degeneration in her other eye. Her optometrist was concerned about a recent fall in the vision of the eye shown above.
a. What is the condition shown?
b. If there is clinical suspicion of choroidal neovascularization (CNV), what investigation should be performed?
c. Is there anything that can be done to reduce the risk of CNV in this eye?

86. 上述这位老年患者有圆顶状黄斑部隆起的异常表现。
a. 这项检查是什么？
b. 这种病变是什么？
c. 发病机理是什么？
d. 可采用什么治疗？

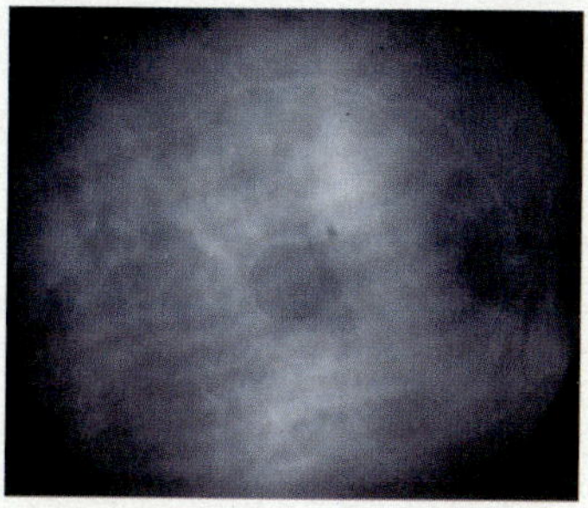

This elderly patient has a dome-shaped macular elevation corresponding to the abnormality shown above.
a. What is the investigation shown?
b. What is the lesion?
c. What is the pathogenesis?
d. How might it be treated?

87. 16岁女孩不舒服持续几周。医生检查眼底所见。
a. 描述病变，它们被称为什么？
b. 白血病可能是首要诊断。列出其他病因。
c. 该眼可能出现哪些其他的白血病表现？

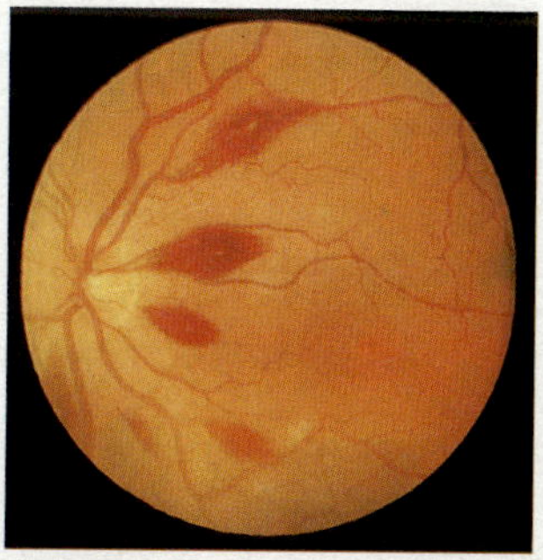

This 16-year-old girl has been unwell for several weeks. A physician identified this fundal appearance.
a. Describe the lesions. What are they called?
b. Leukaemia is a possible underlying diagnosis. List others.
c. How else might leukaemia manifest in the eyes?

88. 患者患有眼皮肤白化病，伴白发和极苍白的皮肤。
a. 他可能是酪氨酸酶阴性或阳性吗?
b. 视觉诱发电位检查对患者的诊断有帮助吗?
c. 说出与该病变有关的两个全身性综合征的名称。
d. 该患者患有这两个综合征之一吗?

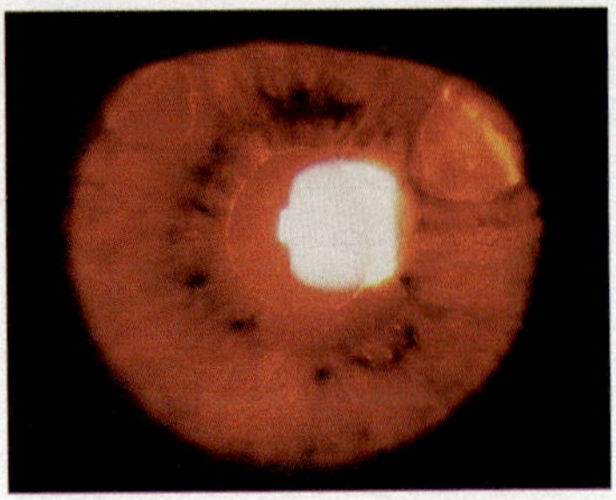

This patient has oculocutaneous albinism with white hair and very pale skin.
a. Is he likely to be tyrosinase-negative or -positive?
b. How would visual-evoked potential analysis help in the assessment of this patient?
c. Name two systemic syndromes associated with this condition.
d. Could this patient have either of these syndromes?

89. 30岁男性眼部检查偶然所见。
a. 描述该病变，其最可能的原因是什么?
b. 有免疫能力的人在什么年龄可复发这种病变?
c. 可用什么诊断试验?

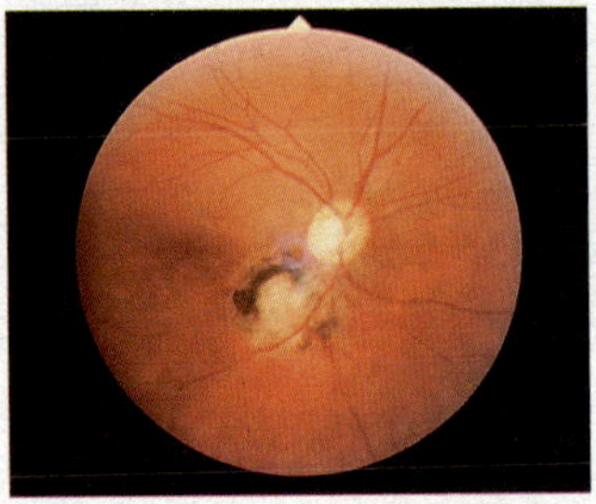

This was an incidental finding in a 30-year-old man.
a. Describe the lesion. What is the most likely cause?
b. At what age do such lesions tend to reactivate in immunocompetent individuals?
c. What diagnostic tests are available?

90. 该患者最近行白内障手术并出现玻璃体丢失。
a. 显示出什么?
b. 什么导致玻璃体丢失?
c. 玻璃体丢失的术后并发症是什么?

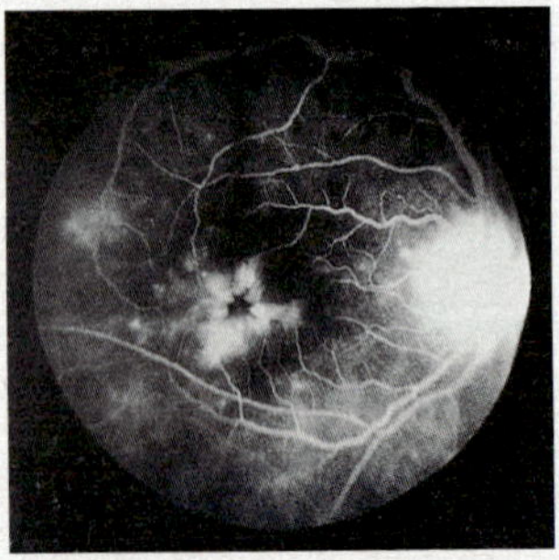

This patient recently underwent cataract surgery complicated by vitreous loss.
a. What is shown?
b. What is meant by 'vitreous loss'?
c. What are the postoperative complications of vitreous loss?

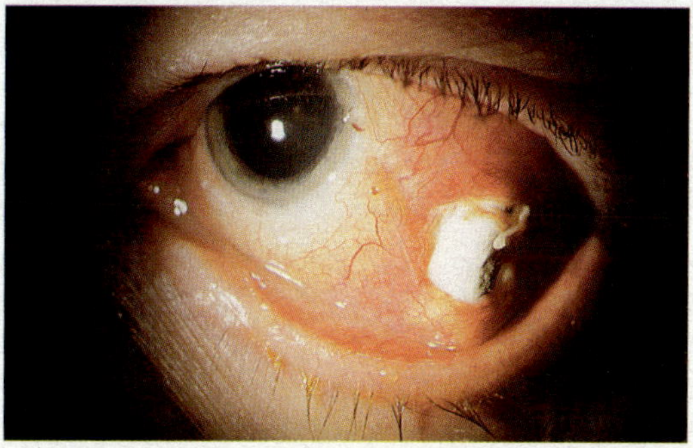

91. 1年前患者行视网膜脱离手术，放置外植块。

a. 发生的并发症是什么？

b. 除去外植块是否会发生再次脱离？

c. 怎样将外植块取出？

Retinal detachment surgery involving placement of an explant was carried out on this patient's eye 1 year ago.

a. What complication has occurred?

b. Could removal of the explant precipitate re-detachment?

c. How should the explant be removed?

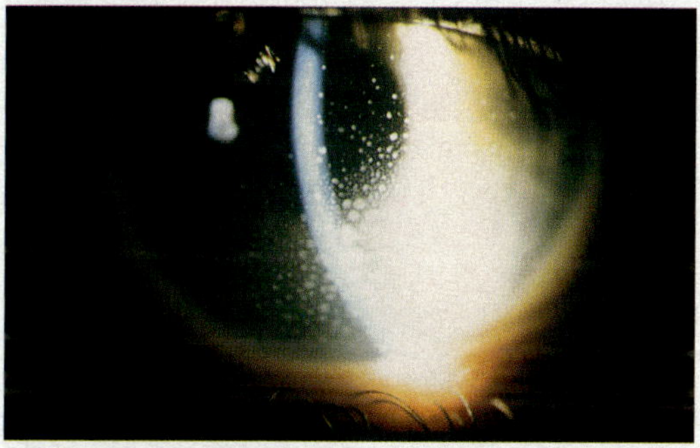

92. 该患者出现眼部发红、疼痛。

a. 出现的体征是什么？

b. 该患者以前没有眼病，其他方面也健康。是否需要全身检查？

c. 可进行的筛选检查是什么？

This patient presented with a sore red eye.

a. What sign is present?

b. The patient has had no previous eye problems and is otherwise healthy. Is systemic investigation indicated?

c. What screening investigations might be carried out?

93. 该患者患有全身性疾病，伴有多发性骨折和耳聋。
a. 全身性疾病是什么？
b. 异常表现的病理学基础是什么？
c. 哪些其他全身性疾病伴随该体征？

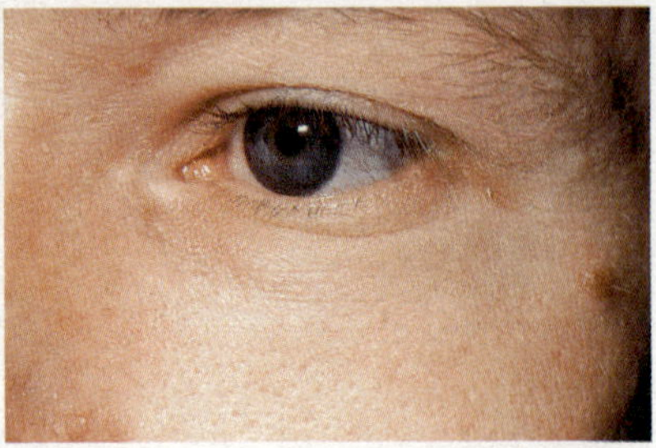

This patient has a systemic disorder associated with multiple fractures and deafness.
a. What is the systemic disorder?
b. What is the pathological basis of the abnormality shown?
c. What other systemic diseases are associated with this sign?

94. 该患者大约 10D 近视。
a. 病理过程是什么？
b. 列出高度近视的其他眼部表现。
c. 这个患者眼轴长度可能接近 20 mm 还是 30 mm？

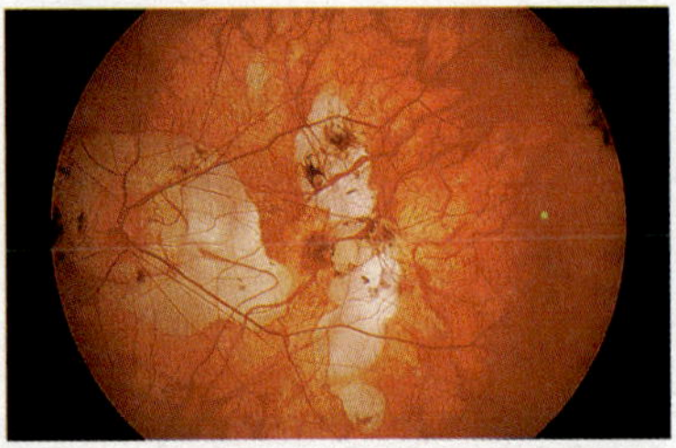

This patient has approximately 10 dioptres of myopia.
a. What is the pathological process shown?
b. List other ocular associations of high myopia.
c. Is this patient's ocular axial length likely to be nearer 20mm or 30mm?

95. 该近视患者正在进行屈光手术。
a. 该操作是什么？
b. 该操作可用于矫正远视或散光吗？
c. 可发生什么并发症？

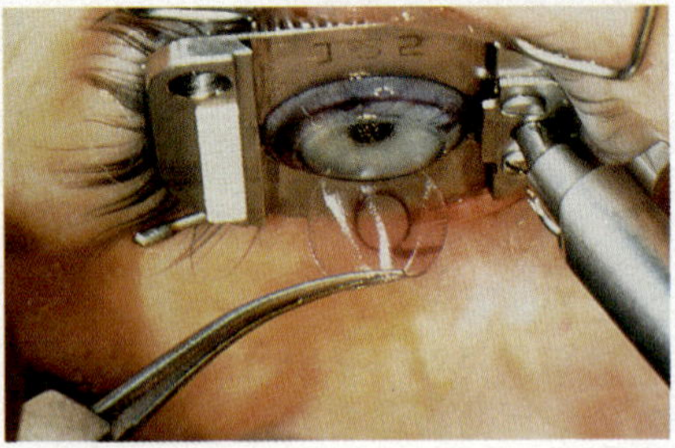

This myopic patient is undergoing refractive surgery.
a. What is the procedure?
b. Can this procedure also be used to correct hypermetropia or astigmatism?
c. What complications may occur?

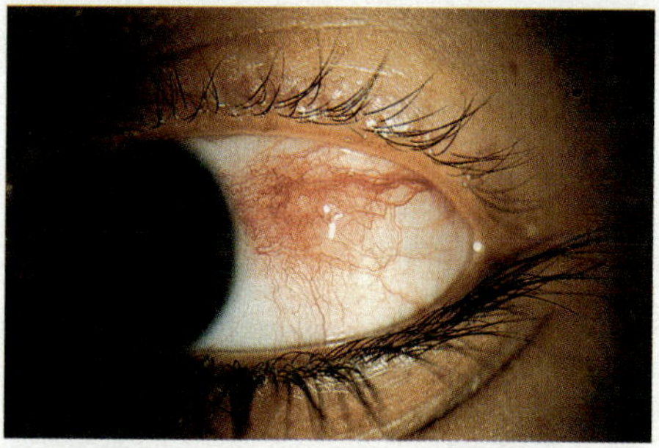

96. 30 岁女性的这只眼出现三角形红色区域并且轻度疼痛持续 3 天。

a. 诊断是什么?

b. 该疾病的分类。

c. 应该进行全身性检查吗?

d. 怎样治疗?

This 30-year-old woman has been aware of this triangular red patch and mild aching in the eye for 3 days.

a. What is the diagnosis?

b. Classify this condition.

c. Should systemic investigations be performed?

d. What is the treatment?

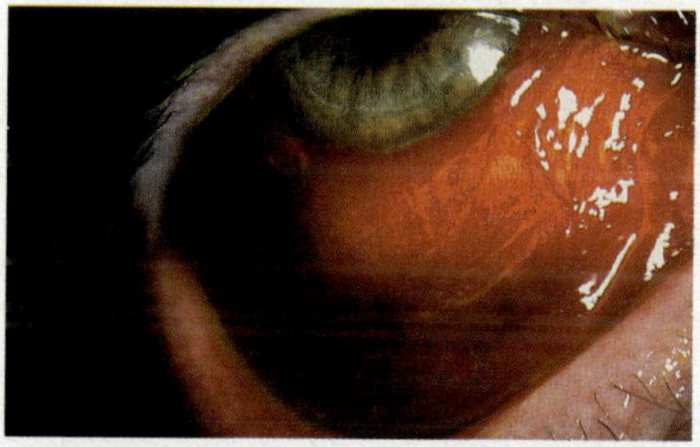

97. 刮胡须的时候，该患者注意到这个情况。

a. 诊断是什么?

b. 可能出现什么症状?

c. 需要做什么检查?

While shaving, this patient noticed the appearance shown.

a. What is the diagnosis?

b. What symptoms may be present?

c. What investigations are required?

98. 30岁男性近日右眼视力下降。
a. 可能的诊断是什么？
b. 视力可能是多少？
c. 如果对该诊断怀疑，应做什么检查？

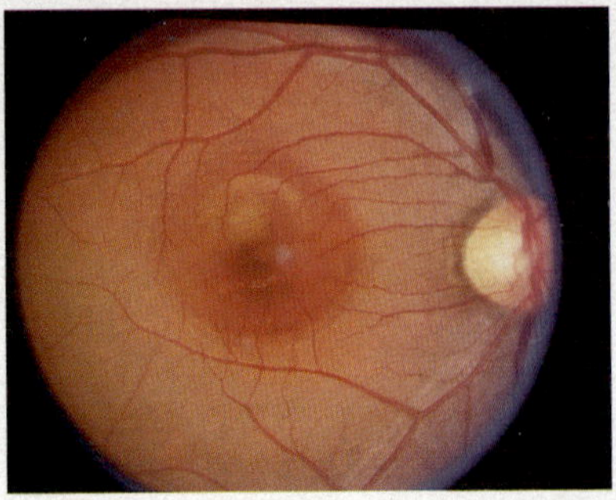

The visual acuity in this 30-year-old man's right eye has deteriorated over the last couple of days.
a. What is the likely diagnosis?
b. What is the visual acuity likely to be?
c. If there is any doubt regarding the diagnosis, what investigation is appropriate?

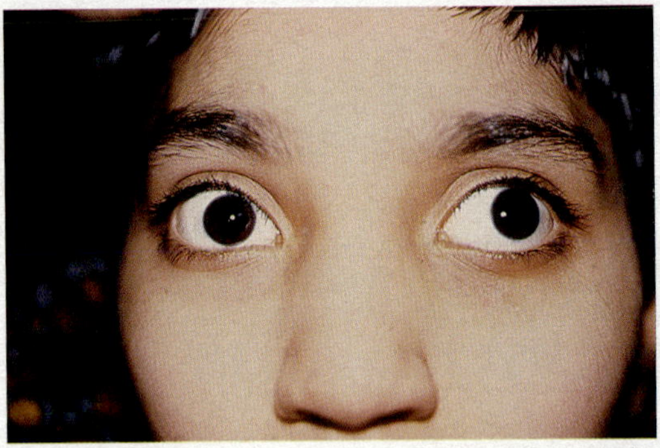

99. 当该儿童疲倦、注意力不集中或强光的时候，左眼外转。
a. 诊断是什么？
b. 这种类型斜视的临床分类是什么？
c. 怎样处理？

This child's left eye turns outward when he is tired, day-dreaming or exposed to bright light.
a. What is the diagnosis?
b. What are the clinical categories of this form of strabismus?
c. How is it managed?

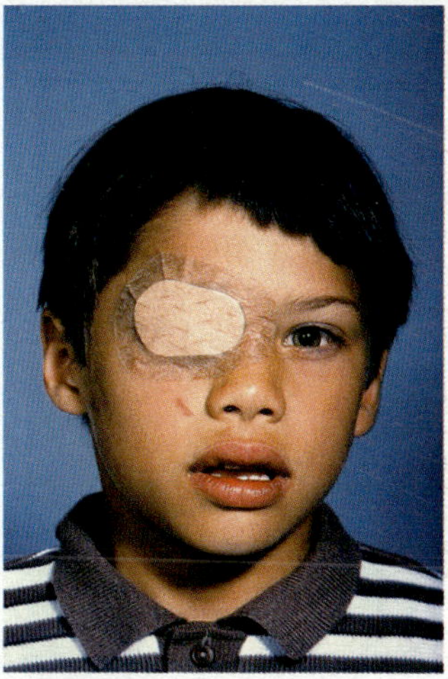

100. 该儿童正在行弱视的遮盖疗法。
a. 弱视是什么?
b. 原因是什么?
c. 弱视治疗有效的年龄限度是多少?

This child is undergoing occlusion therapy for amblyopia.
a. What is amblyopia?
b. What are the causes?
c. What is the usual age limit for useful treatment of amblyopia?

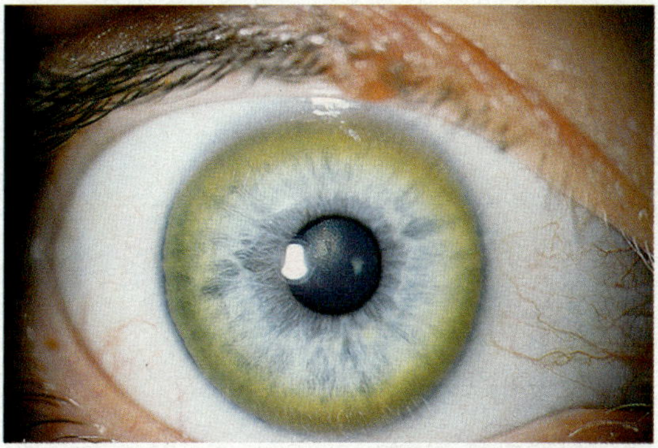

101. 年轻女性在做精神病的检查时;医生注意到她的眼部体征。
a. 该体征是什么?
b. 组织学改变是什么?
c. 原发病的诊断是什么?
d. 其他常见的眼部体征是什么?
e. 其他主要的全身异常是什么?

This young woman has been undergoing psychiatric investigation; one of her doctors noticed this ocular sign.
a. What is the sign called?
b. What is the histology?
c. What is the underlying diagnosis?
d. What is the other common ocular sign?
e. What are the other major systemic abnormalities?

102. 老年患者服用抗心律失常药。

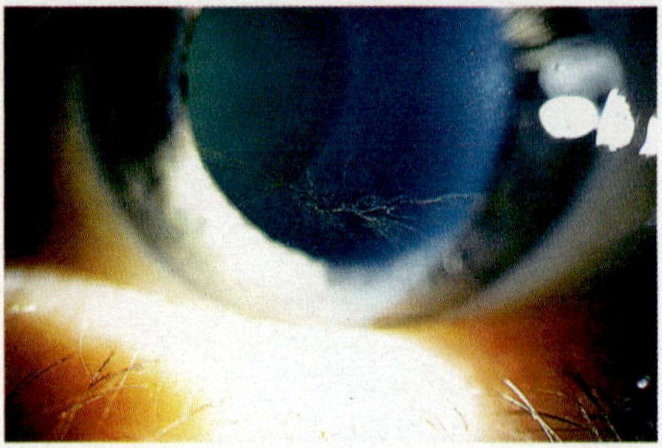

a. 描述该角膜外观，说出它的名称。
b. 该患者服用的药可能是什么？
c. 服用心脏药物的患者出现这种情况的比例是多少？
d. 其他还有哪些药和哪些疾病可出现类似的表现？

This elderly patient takes a drug for cardiac arrhythmia.

a. Describe and name the corneal appearance.
b. What drug is the patient likely to be taking?
c. What proportion of patients on the cardiac drug develop this?
d. What other drugs, and what disease, can give a similar appearance?

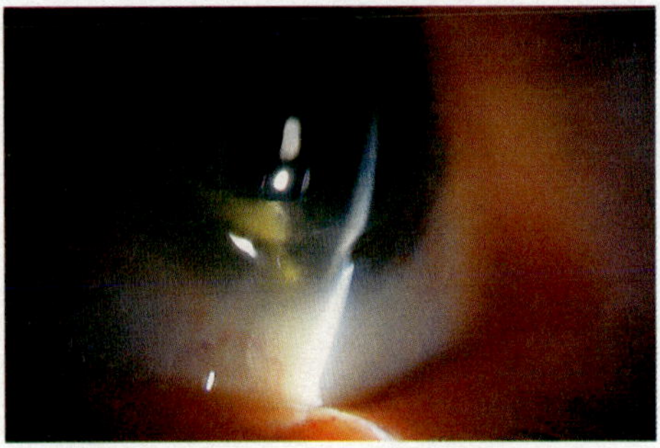

103. 其他方面健康的 55 岁男性，双眼发生渐增的散光几个月。在上网查询后他怀疑是否患圆锥角膜。

a. 不考虑角膜形态，你认为该患者的诊断正确吗？
b. 对所示病变精确定位的重要性是什么？
c. 可能的诊断是什么？

This otherwise healthy 55-year-old man has developed increasing astigmatism over several months in both eyes. After an Internet search he wonders whether he has keratoconus.

a. Regardless of the corneal appearance, do you think the patient's diagnosis is correct?
b. What is the significance of the precise location of the changes shown?
c. What is the likely diagnosis?

104. 40 岁女性主诉左眼渐进性变大；眼眶 CT 显示肌圆锥内边界清楚的椭圆形病变。

a. CT 显示的病变及体征是什么？

b. 该病变是成人最常见的眼眶良性肿瘤，诊断是什么？

c. 可能出现哪些其他眼部体征？

d. 怎样治疗？

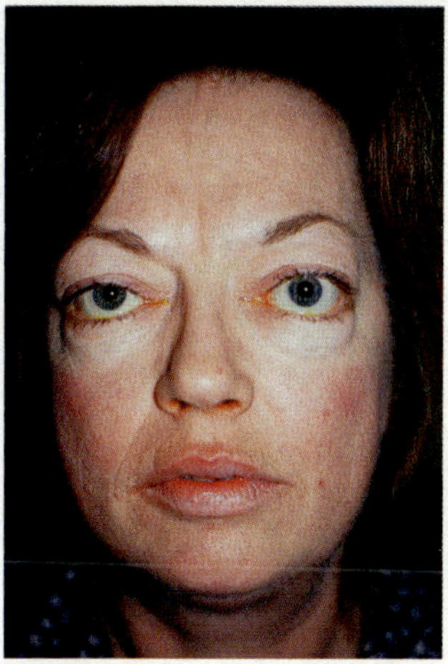

This 40-year-old woman complains that her left eye is gradually getting larger. CT of the orbit showed a well-circumscribed oval lesion within the muscle cone.

a. Bearing in mind the CT finding, what is the sign shown?

b. This lesion is the most common benign orbital tumour in adults; what is the diagnosis?

c. What other ocular signs might be present?

d. What is the treatment?

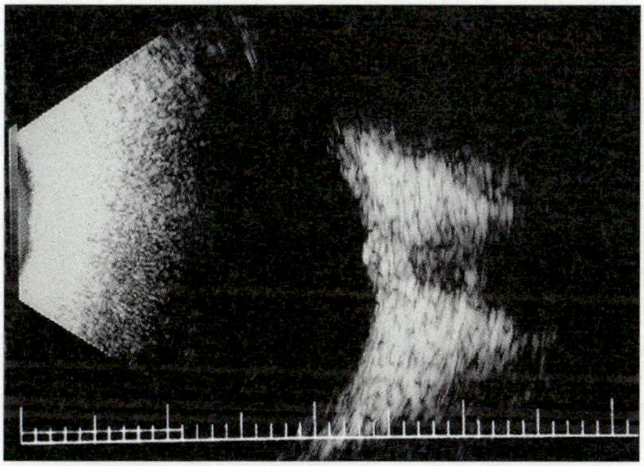

105. 内科医生不能确定该青年的视盘水肿，要求眼科检查。

a. 这是什么检查？

b. 异常表现是什么？

c. 需要做哪些其他的检查？

Ophthalmological review has been requested by a physician, who is uncertain if this young adult's optic discs are swollen.

a. What is the investigation shown?

b. What abnormality is demonstrated?

c. What other investigations could be performed?

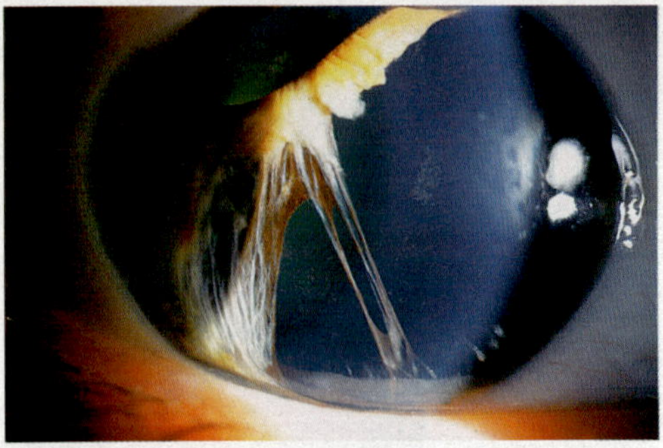

106. 35 岁女性患有青光眼。对侧眼正常。

a. 可能的诊断是什么？

b. 该病其他的形式是什么？

c. 发展为青光眼的比例是多少？

This eye of a 35-year-old woman has glaucoma. The fellow eye is normal.

a. What is the likely diagnosis?

b. What are the other forms of this condition?

c. What proportion of patients develop glaucoma?

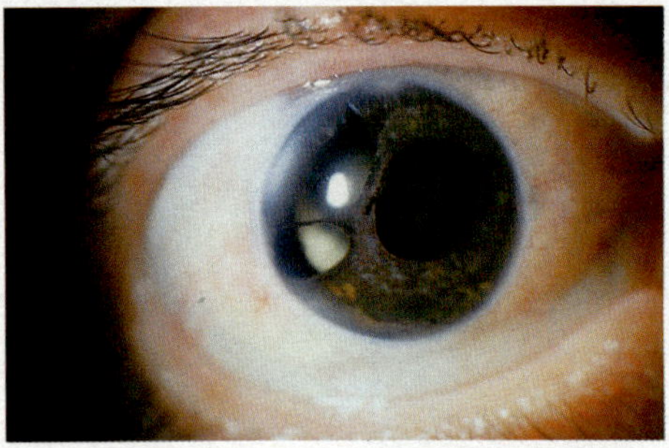

107. 该患者有先天性牙齿和颜面异常，除此之外累及双眼。

a. 描述体征。

b. 诊断是什么？

c. 该病的遗传基础是什么？

d. 该病形成青光眼的比例是多少？在什么年龄？

This patient has congenital dental and facial anomalies as well as this condition, which affects both eyes.

a. Describe the signs.

b. What is the diagnosis?

c. What is the genetic basis of this condition?

d. What proportion of patients develop glaucoma, and at what age?

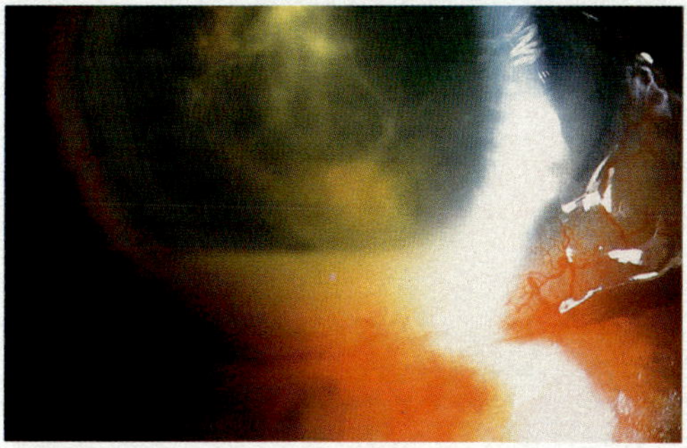

108. 2 天前该眼行白内障手术。

a. 描述体征。

b. 可能的诊断是什么？

c. 怎样治疗？

Cataract surgery was carried out on this eye 2 days earlier.

a. Describe the signs.

b. What is the probable diagnosis?

c. What is the management?

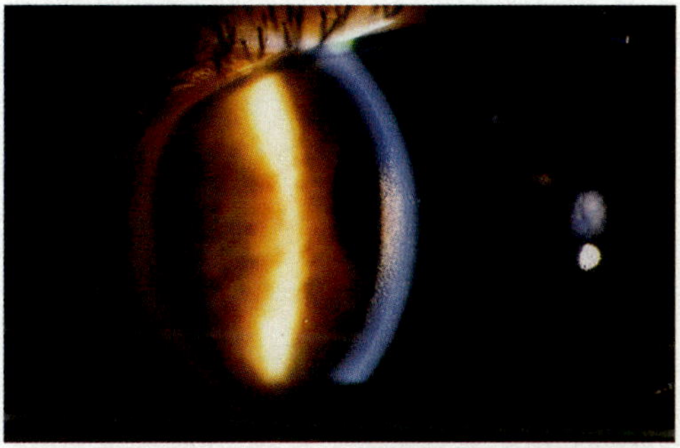

109. 29 岁男性在常规的屈光检查中被发现这种情况。

a. 这种体征是什么？

b. 可能的诊断是什么？

c. 可能的屈光不正是什么？

d. 该病形成青光眼的比例是多少？

A 29-year-old man was found to have this appearance at a routine refraction.

a. What is the sign called?

b. What is the likely diagnosis?

c. What is the probable refractive error?

d. What proportion of patients with this condition are likely to develop glaucoma?

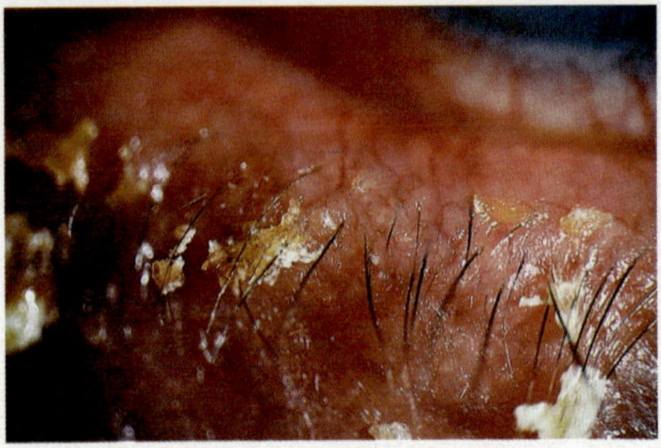

110. 持续的刺激、充血和粘性分泌物，早晨加重。该患者的普通诊所医生让他去看眼科专科医生。

a. 哪些体征明显？

b. 诊断是什么？

c. 怎样治疗？

Persistent irritation, redness and stickiness, worse in the morning, have led this patient's general practitioner to refer him to an ophthalmologist.

a. What signs are evident?

b. What is the diagnosis?

c. What is the treatment?

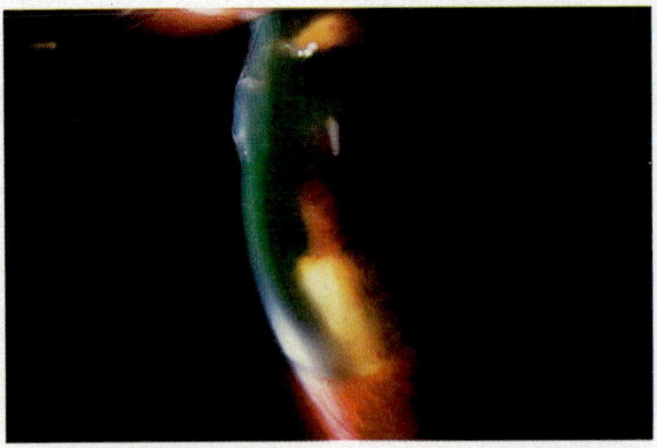

111. 这个青年发生交通事故；没有系安全带。

a. 损伤表现是什么？

b. 怎样处理？

This young man was involved in a car accident; he was not wearing a seatbelt.

a. What injury is shown?

b. How should this be managed?

112. 该患者有青光眼，偶然发生视物模糊伴虹视症；激光治疗后发作结束。

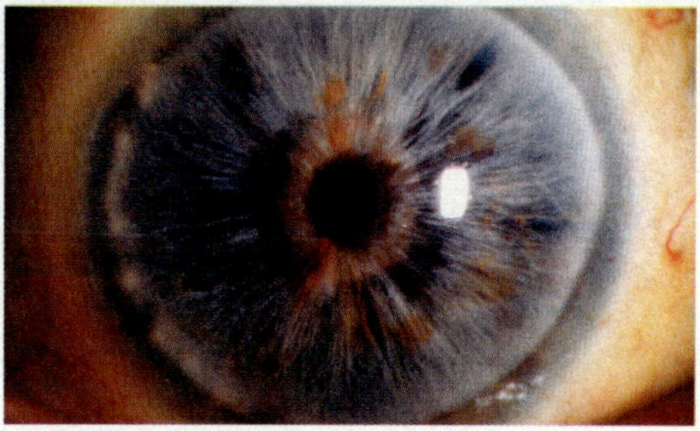

a. 可行什么形式激光治疗？

b. 什么类型的青光眼可出现这些症状？

c. 用于治疗该患者的激光还有什么其他用途。

This patient with glaucoma described episodic blurring of vision associated with rainbows around lights; the episodes ceased following a laser procedure.

a. What form of laser treatment has been carried out?

b. What forms of glaucoma can present with these symptoms?

c. What other uses are there for the type of laser used to treated this patient?

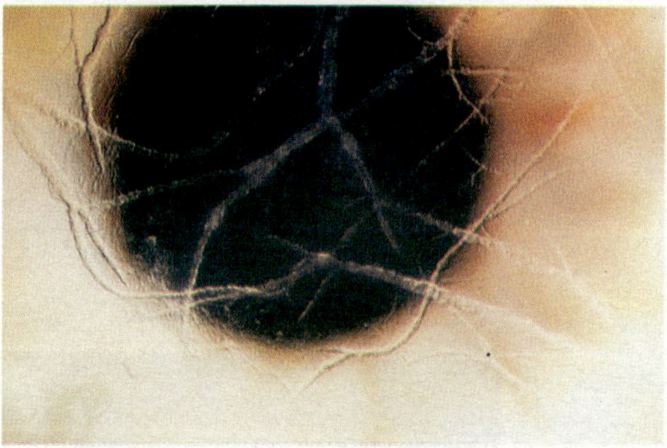

113. 51 岁患者双眼对称性表现，伴视力缓慢下降。

a. 诊断是什么？

b. 该疾病角膜上皮糜烂常复发吗？

c. 该患者需要全层角膜移植吗？

d. 该疾病的其他类型是什么？

This is a symmetrically bilateral appearance in a 51-year-old patient with slowly deteriorating vision.

a. What is the diagnosis?

b. Are recurrent erosions common in this disorder?

c. Will the patient require penetrating keratoplasty?

d. What are the other forms of this disorder?

114. 这是 8 周婴儿的眼底表现。
a. 诊断是什么?
b. 叙述该疾病的不同阶段。
c. 该疾病制定治疗方案的标准是什么?
d. 将采取什么治疗形式?

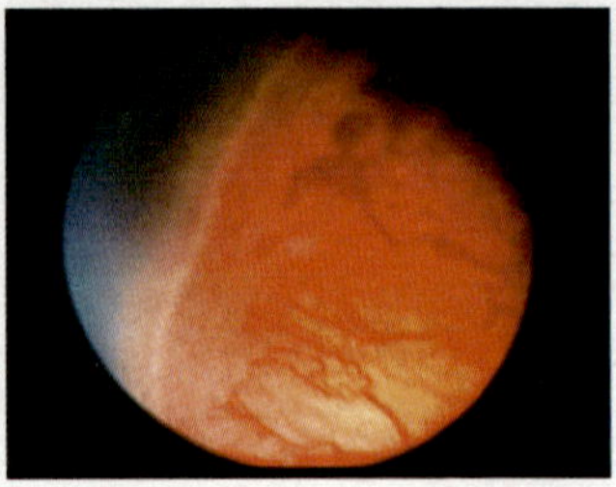

This is the fundus of an 8-week-old baby.
a. What is the diagnosis?
b. Describe the different stages of this disease.
c. What are the criteria for the decision to treat this condition?
d. What form will treatment take?

115. 这是 40 岁男性双眼底表现伴有剧烈头痛。
a. 需做什么临床检查?
b. 为什么黄斑渗出液以这个形状分布?
c. 该疾病还可出现哪些其他的眼底表现?

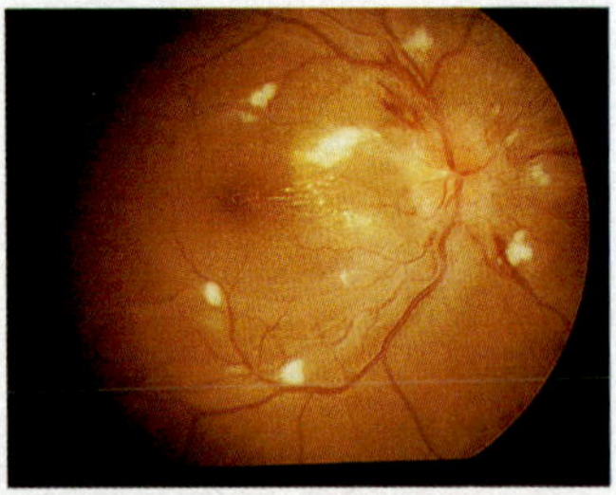

This is the fundus appearance in both eyes of a 40-year-old man with severe headaches.
a. What clinical test is indicated?
b. Why are the macular exudates distributed in the fashion shown?
c. What other fundus signs might be seen in this condition?

116. 34 岁男性的虹膜表现。
a. 体征是什么?
b. 可能的原发全身性疾病是什么?
c. 这种全身性疾病的其他眼部特点是什么?
d. 遗传形式是什么? 基因位点在哪里?

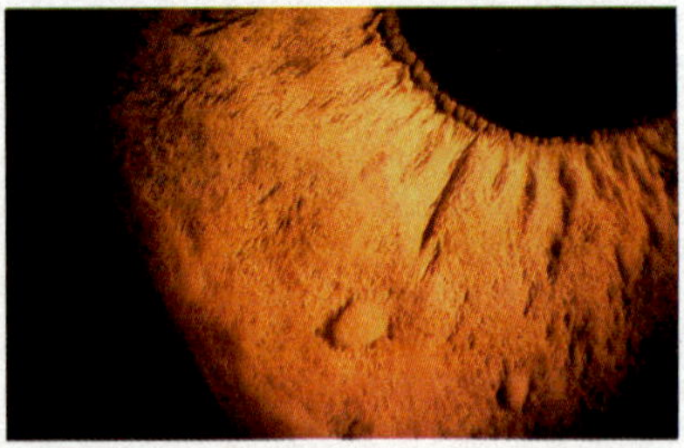

This is the iris appearance in a 34-year-old man.
a. What is the sign?
b. What is the probable underlying systemic disease?
c. What are the other ophthalmic features of the systemic disorder?
d. What is the inheritance pattern, and where is the gene locus?

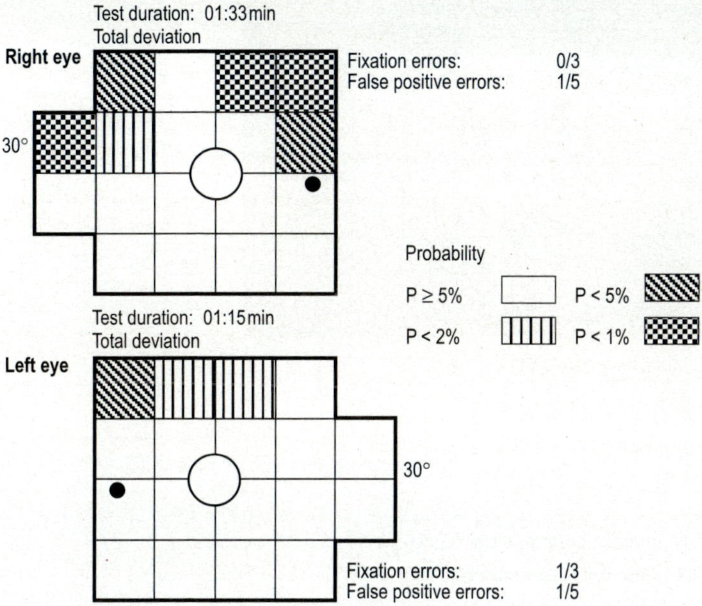

117. 该患者去眼科诊所。

a. 检查所见是什么?

b. 检查原则是什么?

c. 主要的优点是什么?

This patient has been referred to the eye clinic by her optician.

a. What is the investigation shown?

b. What is the principle behind the test?

c. What are its main advantages?

118. 老年印度患者有这些白色的角膜结节已经许多年了。

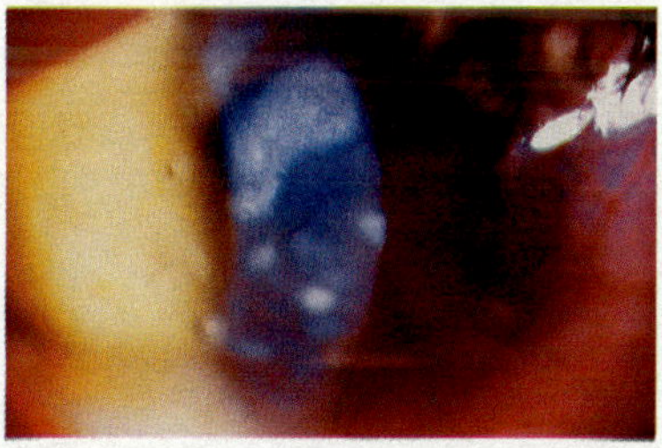

a. 这种病变是什么?

b. 原发眼病可能是什么?

c. 怎样治疗?

This elderly Indian patient has had these whitish corneal nodules for many years.

a. What are the lesions?

b. What is likely to be the underlying eye disease responsible?

c. What is the treatment?

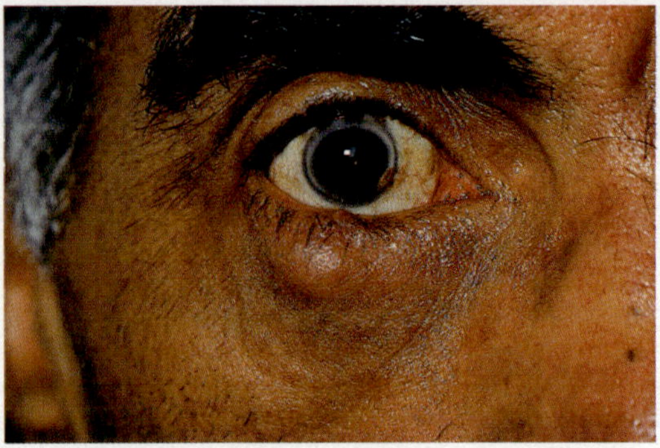

119. 出现无痛肿块几个月。
a. 诊断和发病机理是什么？
b. 相应的结膜病变是什么？
c. 可采用哪种治疗形式？

This painless lump has been present for several months.
a. What is the diagnosis and pathogenesis?
b. What is the corresponding conjunctival lesion?
c. What forms of treatment are available?

120. 该患者的私人医生注意到他眼底的表现。
a. 诊断是什么？
b. 眼部伴随表现是什么？
c. 发病机理是什么？
d. 人群发病率？

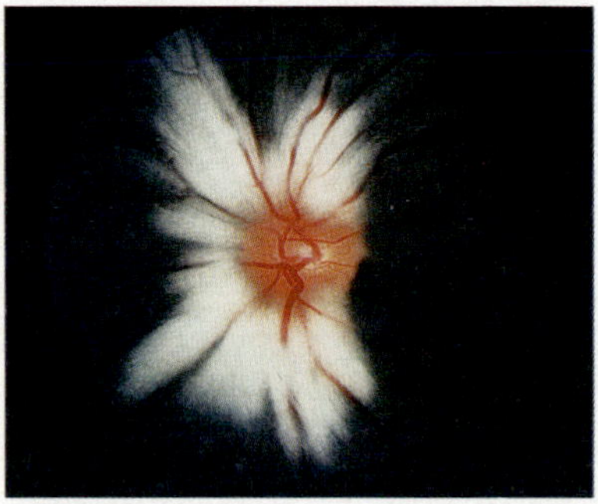

The patient's general practitioner was concerned about this fundal appearance.
a. What is the diagnosis?
b. What are the ocular associations?
c. What is the pathogenesis?
d. What is the population prevalence?

1. a. 虹膜缺损。
   b. 通常在常染色体 11p13 的 *PAX6* 基因。
   c. 发病率大概与一般人一样。虹膜缺损分型：I型虹膜缺损（占患者65%）伴有常染色体显性遗传，没有全身的症状；Ⅱ型虹膜缺损（33%），散发，来自 Wilms 肿瘤（Miller 综合征）的可能性为 30%；Ⅲ型虹膜缺损或Gillespie综合征是常染色体隐性遗传，伴有神经学上的异常。
   d. 眼球震颤、青光眼、白内障、晶状体半脱位、中心凹注视、视神经发育不全和角膜混浊。

   a. Aniridia.
   b. Usually in the *PAX6* gene on chromosome 11p13.
   c. Probably the same as the general population. Aniridia is classified into AN-1 (65% of patients) with autosomal dominant inheritance and no systemic implications, AN-2 (33%), a sporadic form carrying a 30% risk of Wilms' tumour (Miller's syndrome), and AN-3 or Gillespie's syndrome with autosomal recessive inheritance, associated with neurological problems.
   d. Nystagmus, glaucoma, cataract, lens subluxation, foveal and optic nerve hypoplasia and corneal opacity.

2. a. 基底细胞癌（BCC）。
   b. 结节 - 溃疡型（“侵蚀性溃疡”）和硬化型。
   c. 手术切除，包括临床上较宽的（4 mm）正常组织边缘。

   a. Basal cell carcinoma (BCC).
   b. Nodulo-ulcerative ('rodent ulcer') and sclerosing types.
   c. Surgical excision, including a wide (4mm) margin of clinically normal tissue.

3. a. 小梁切除术，滤过手术的一种。
   b. 青光眼。
   c. • 局部应用前列腺素衍生物、β- 受体阻断剂、α- 受体激动剂、碳酸酐酶抑制剂和缩瞳药。
   • 全身应用碳酰酐酶抑制剂。
   • 闭角型青光眼可行激光小梁成形术、睫状体激光光凝术和周边虹膜切开术。

- 非穿透性引流手术（如粘弹剂-小梁切开术）和植入瓣膜（如Molteno）。

d. 5- 氟尿嘧啶和丝裂霉素 C。

a. Trabeculectomy, a form of filtering surgery.

b. Glaucoma.

c. • Topical prostaglandin derivatives, beta-blockers, alpha agonists, carbonic anhydrase inhibitors and miotics.
- Systemic carbonic anhydrase inhibitors.
- Laser trabeculoplasty, cyclodiode and peripheral iridotomy in narrow-angle glaucoma.
- Non-penetrating drainage surgery (e.g. viscocanalostomy) and valve implants (e.g. Molteno).

d. 5-fluorouracil and mitomycin C.

4. a. 多发大量的上睑血管，鹅卵石样结膜乳头。

b. 增生的结膜上皮环绕血管中心和细胞慢性炎症性浸润（淋巴细胞、浆细胞、嗜酸性细胞）。

c. • 隐形眼镜的机械性刺激。
- 对隐形眼镜材料和清洁液的变态反应。
- 对隐形眼镜沉积物的免疫反应。

d. 严重的慢性变应性结膜炎和突出的缝线。

a. There are multiple large, highly vascular, cobblestone-like conjunctival projections.

b. Hyperplastic conjunctival epithelium surrounds a vascular core and a cellular chronic inflammatory infiltrate (lymphocytes, plasma cells, eosinophils).

c. • Mechanical irritation by a poorly fitting lens.
- Allergy to lens material or cleaning solutions.
- Immune reaction to lens deposits.

d. Severe chronic allergic conjunctivitis and a protruding suture.

5. a. Von Hippel-Lindau 综合征（VHL）。

b. 中枢神经系统成血管细胞瘤，肾癌，嗜铬细胞瘤，红细胞增多症，和肾、胰及其他的腹部囊肿。

c. 大约 50%。事实上所有多发的视网膜肿瘤的患者将变成VHL。

d. 常由于视网膜的渗出物，偶尔由于玻璃体出血和视网膜前膜形成。这种病变可行激光光凝、冷冻疗法或点放射治疗（近距离放射疗法）。

a. Von Hippel-Lindau syndrome (VHL).
b. CNS haemangioblastoma, renal carcinoma, phaeochromocytoma, polycythaemia, and renal, pancreatic and other abdominal cysts.
c. Approximately 50%. Virtually all patients with multiple retinal tumours will have VHL.
d. Most commonly by retinal exudation and occasionally by vitreous haemorrhage and epiretinal membrane formation. The lesions can be treated with laser photocoagulation, cryotherapy or plaque radiotherapy (brachytherapy).

6. a. 假性表皮剥脱。
b. 假性表皮剥脱发展为青光眼的危险率5年者大约为5%，10年者为15%，如果对侧眼已经有假性剥脱性青光眼，该眼更易发病。
c. 斯堪的纳维亚半岛。
d. 瞳孔常很难散大，晶状体植入困难。晶状体囊和悬韧带脆性高，导致囊膜破裂和玻璃体脱出的风险增加。手术后，角膜失代偿和囊膜浑浊常发生，晚期植入的人工晶状体可发生脱位。

a. Pseudoexfoliation.
b. The cumulative risk of developing glaucoma in eyes with pseudoexfoliation is about 5% at 5 years and 15% at 10 years, although this is much higher if the fellow eye already has pseudoexfoliative glaucoma.
c. Scandinavia.
d. The pupil frequently dilates poorly, making access to the lens difficult. The lens capsule and zonules are fragile, leading to an increased risk of capsular rupture and vitreous loss. Postoperatively, corneal decompensation and capsular opacification are more common, as is late dislocation of the implant.

7. a. 鼻泪管阻塞。
b. 泪囊按摩。
c. 泪道探通术最好在12个月龄时考虑使用；鼻泪管阻塞的患者需要做泪囊鼻腔造孔术。
d. 先天性青光眼。

a. Failure of canalization of the nasolacrimal duct.
b. Lacrimal sac massage.
c. Probing of the lacrimal system should be considered only at 12 months; dacryocystorhinostomy may be necessary in resistant cases.
d. Congenital glaucoma.

8. a. 脉络膜脱离。
b. 滤过过强伴随低眼压。
c. 被涡静脉的出口限制，脉络膜脱离表现为光滑的褐色球形隆起，不累及后极部。视网膜锯齿缘不限制前面的液体蔓延，因此可见没有裂孔的视网膜脱离。

a. Choroidal detachment.
b. Overfiltration with associated low intraocular pressure.
c. A choroidal detachment appears as a smooth, brown convex elevation that does not involve the posterior pole, being limited by the exit points of the vortex veins. The ora serrata does not limit anterior fluid spread, and thus may be visible without indentation.

9. a. 原发性获得性黑色素沉着症（PAM）。
b. 典型或非典型PAM，后者是基底上皮细胞层内正常黑色素细胞增殖，前者可见大量的黑色素细胞伴突出的核仁和变形性骨炎样的蔓延。
c. 非典型性 PAM 5 年内恶变的可能性约为 50%。
d. 种族性上皮细胞黑色素沉着症和先天性黑色素细胞增生病（与 PAM 相反，深入到结膜且不能被推动）。

a. Primary acquired melanosis (PAM).
b. PAM with and without atypia, the latter a proliferation of normal melanocytes within the basal epithelial layer, the former shows large melanocytes with prominent nucleoli and pagetoid spread.
c. About 50% within 5 years in PAM with atypia.
d. Racial epithelial melanosis and congenital melanocytosis (in contrast to PAM, lies deep to the conjunctiva and cannot be moved over the sclera).

10. a. 室周的脱髓鞘斑点，它们的长轴对齐室缘；该患者有视神经炎伴随多发性硬化症。
b. 视盘可正常（球后视神经炎），通常较少出现水肿或充血（视盘炎）。对侧的视盘可苍白，通常为暂时的。有时出现视网膜的血管鞘。

c. 疼痛，向上看时明显，头痛，眼部触痛，辨色力下降和视野缺损。

d. 眼运动脑神经麻痹,核间的眼肌麻痹，眼球震颤；罕见中间葡萄膜炎和周边视网膜脉管炎。

a. Periventricular demyelinated plaques, their long axes aligned with the ventricular margins; the patient has optic neuritis associated with multiple sclerosis.

b. The optic disc may be normal (retrobulbar neuritis) or, less commonly, swollen and hyperaemic (papillitis). There may be pallor of the contralateral optic disc, usually temporally. Retinal vascular sheathing is sometimes present.

c. Pain, particularly on upgaze, headache, tenderness of the eye, decreased colour vision and visual field loss.

d. Ocular motor cranial nerve palsies, internuclear ophthalmoplegia, nystagmus; rarely, intermediate uveitis and peripheral retinal vasculitis.

11. a. 脑膜炎，脑脓肿和海绵窦血栓形成。

b. 伴随视网膜母细胞瘤和白血病的眶隔前蜂窝织炎，横纹肌肉瘤和眼眶炎症。

c. 结膜和鼻拭子，静脉注射抗生素，监测视神经功能。应该考虑急诊行眼眶 CT 扫描以排除骨膜脓肿。包括耳鼻咽喉的处置，因为窦道冲洗是必须的。

a. Meningitis, brain abscess and cavernous sinus thrombosis.

b. Preseptal cellulitis, rhabdomyosarcoma and orbital inflammation associated with retinoblastoma and leukaemia.

c. Conjunctival and nasal swabs, intravenous antibiotics and monitoring of optic nerve function. Urgent orbital CT scan to exclude periosteal abscess should be considered. Involve otorhinolaryngological colleagues because sinus washout may be required.

12. a. 糖尿病视网膜病变（DR）增殖致视盘新生血管形成。

b. 背景型（单纯型）DR-渗出，圆点和污点状出血；增殖前的DR-深层圆形出血，棉絮状斑和静脉不规则；陈旧性DR -玻璃体出血和牵引性视网膜脱离。

c. 糖尿病的持续时间、血糖控制不良、高血压、肾损害和肥胖，高脂血症和吸烟也应重视。怀孕有时可使病情迅速恶化。

d. 白内障、不稳定的屈光状态、眼球运动神经麻痹、新生血管性青光眼、星形玻璃体变性、视盘病变、虹膜透照缺损和眼眶真菌感染。

a. Proliferative diabetic retinopathy (DR) with disc neovascularization.

b. Background DR-exudates and dot and blot haemorrhages; preproliferative DR-deep round haemorrhages, cotton wool spots and venous irregularity; advanced DR-vitreous haemorrhage and tractional retinal detachment.

c. Duration of diabetes, poor control, hypertension, renal impairment and obesity. Hyperlipidaemia and smoking may also be important. Pregnancy is sometimes associated with rapid deterioration.

d. Cataract, unstable refraction, ocular motor nerve palsies, neovascular glaucoma, asteroid hyalosis, papillopathy, iris transillumination defects and orbital mucormycosis.

13. a. 严重的背景性糖尿病性视网膜病变。

b. • 视网膜的增厚在距黄斑中心 500μm 之内。

• 如果伴有视网膜增厚，渗出物在距黄斑中心 500μm 之内。

• 如果在大小上比一个视盘面积大，视网膜的增厚在距黄斑中心一个视盘直径之内。

c. 局部的氩激光凝固渗漏点（通常是微动脉瘤）或格子激光光凝广泛的渗漏区域。新的方式包括玻璃体内注射类固醇，全身药物治疗和玻璃体切割术。

d. 黄斑中心凹的硬性渗出，明显的局部缺血，弥漫的而非集聚性的水肿，囊样的黄斑水肿和近期视力低下。

a. Severe background diabetic retinopathy.

b. • Retinal thickening within 500μm of the centre of the macula.

• Exudates within 500μm of the centre of the macula if associated with retinal thickening.

• Retinal thickening within one disc diameter of the centre of the macula if greater than one disc area in size.

c. With focal argon laser photocoagulation to points of leakage (usually microaneurysms) or grid laser to diffusely leaking areas. Innovative modalities include intravitreal steroids, systemic pharmaceutical agents and vitrectomy.

d. Hard exudates involving the fovea, significant ischaemia, diffuse rather than focal oedema, cystoid macular oedema and poor visual acuity at presentation.

14. a. 视觉异常，尤其是闪光幻觉。大的病变：直径>5mm，厚度>1 mm，病变表面有橙色色素，有视网膜下积液。青春期后体积增大。

b. 处置则主要根据患者情况（尤其是年龄）、肿瘤体积、位置和患者与医生的选择。对初期的肿瘤有效的方式包括放射性的点状敷贴（近距离放射疗法），外照射放射治疗，局部切除术，整体摘出术，γ 刀立体定向放射治疗和二极管激光器经瞳孔的温热疗法（TTT）。

c. 组织学类型、肿瘤细胞染色体异常、肿瘤体积、患者年龄、巩膜是否有累及和肿瘤的位置（前部的比后部的预后差）。

a. Visual symptoms, especially photopsia. Large lesion size: diameter >5mm, thickness >1mm, orange pigment overlying the lesion, associated subretinal fluid and documented increase in size after puberty.

b. Largely dependent on patient profile (especially age), tumour size and location and preferences of the patient and surgeon. Modalities available for the primary tumour include radioactive plaque application (brachytherapy), external beam radiotherapy, local resection, enucleation, stereotactic radiosurgery using the gamma knife and diode laser transpupillary thermotherapy ('TTT').

c. Histological type, the presence of chromosomal abnormalities in tumour cells, tumour size, patient age, the presence or absence of extrascleral extension and tumour location (anterior worse than posterior).

15. a. 皮脂腺瘤。

b. 结节性硬化症，如 Bourneville 病，是常染色体显性遗传。

c. 大约50%出现视网膜的星形细胞瘤。其他少见的特点包括高颅内压的眼部后遗症（视盘水肿，视神经萎缩和第六脑神经麻痹）和视网膜与虹膜色素减少。

a. Adenoma sebaceum.

b. Tuberous sclerosis, also known as Bourneville's disease, which is inherited in an autosomal dominant pattern.

c. Retinal astrocytomas are present in about 50%. Other rarer features include the ocular sequelae of raised intracranial pressure (papilloedema, optic atrophy and sixth nerve paresis) and hypopigmented retinal and iris spots.

16. a. 视网膜大动脉瘤。
    b. 常见，损伤可致血栓且可自然消退。然而慢性的渗漏可能是视网膜水肿的原因，黄斑可能受累。大动脉瘤破裂可发生出血。
    c. 视力有损害的可用激光，否则可进行观察。

    a. A retinal artery macroaneurysm.
    b. Frequently, these lesions thrombose and undergo spontaneous involution. However, chronic leakage may cause retinal oedema, with the risk of macular involvement. Haemorrhage may occur if the macroaneurysm ruptures.
    c. Laser may be applied to a vision-threatening lesion, otherwise observation is appropriate.

17. a. 小梁切除术成功率低时可以使用人工引流器。包括新生血管性、外伤性和确定的发育性青光眼，严重的结膜瘢痕，虽然做过小梁切除术联合应用抗代谢药但未控制的青光眼。
    b. 长期的大约占 1/3。
    c. 引流过畅（伴浅的/扁平眼前房）、白内障、角膜失代偿、引流器导管缩回或穿透糜烂的结膜、眼内炎和眼外肌不平衡。

    a. Artificial drainage shunts are used when the success rate of trabeculectomy is low. Examples include neovascular, traumatic and certain developmental glaucomas, severe conjunctival scarring and uncontrolled glaucoma despite previous trabeculectomy with adjunctive antimetabolite.
    b. Only about one-third in the longer term.
    c. Overdrainage (with shallow/flat anterior chamber), cataract, corneal decompensation, tube retraction or erosion through the conjunctiva, endophthalmitis and extraocular muscle imbalance.

18. a. 急性后部多发性鳞状色素上皮病（AMPPPE）。
    b. 虹膜炎、玻璃体炎，有时伴有视盘水肿和视网膜静脉周围炎。
    c. 流行性感冒样病和结节性红斑。
    d. 预后好，80% 恢复到 6/12 或更好。

    a. Acute multifocal posterior placoid pigment epitheliopathy (AMPPPE).
    b. Iritis and vitreitis, and sometimes optic disc oedema and retinal periphlebitis.
    c. An influenza-like illness and erythema nodosum.

d. The prognosis is good, 80% of eyes regaining 6/12 or better.

19. a. CT 扫描表明右侧眶底爆裂性骨折。
b. 严重的钝挫伤。
c. 眼周肿胀和擦伤、皮下积气（外伤性气肿）、眼球内陷、眶下神经分布区感觉异常、垂直方向眼球运动受限和眼球损伤。
d. 全身应用抗生素（如果是开放性骨折），避免擤鼻，如果有明显的大面积缺损和软组织嵌顿需手术修复，手术时间选择是有争论的。

a. The scan shows a right orbital floor 'blowout' fracture.
b. Severe blunt trauma.
c. Periocular swelling and bruising, subcutaneous air ('surgical emphysema'), enophthalmos, paraesthesia in the infraorbital nerve distribution, limitation of vertical eye movement and damage to the globe.
d. Systemic antibiotics (as this is a compound fracture), avoidance of blowing the nose, and surgical repair if indicated, usually for larger defects and soft tissue entrapment; timing of surgery is controversial.

20. a. 血管样条纹症；其与弹性纤维假黄瘤相结合就是 Grönblad-Strandberg 综合征。
b. 血管样条纹症包括 Bruch 膜弹力层裂开，是由于视网膜色素上皮细胞与脉络膜毛细管层的渐进性变性和钙沉积等继发性改变所致。
c. “橘皮”（橘样皮肤）指的是黄斑颞侧明显的色素斑纹，可见于血管样条纹症的眼部。
d. Ehlers-Danlos 综合征 6 型，Paget 病和某种血红蛋白可能变异。

a. Angioid streaks; the combination of these and pseudoxanthoma elasticum is known as Grönblad-Strandberg syndrome.
b. Angioid streaks consist of dehiscences in the elastic layer of the Bruch membrane due to progressive degeneration and deposition of calcium with secondary changes in the retinal pigment epithelium and choriocapillaris.
c. *Peau d'orange* ('orange skin'), refers to a pigmented mottling, particularly evident temporal to the macula, seen in eyes with angioid streaks.

d. Ehlers-Danlos syndrome type 6, Paget's disease and possibly certain haemoglobinopathies.

21. a. 瞳孔对光反射 - 近反射分离（Argyll-Robertson 瞳孔），眼睑退缩（Collier阳性），辐辏式回缩性眼震（用视动性眼球震颤滚筒引出），集合和调节局部麻痹（或痉挛）。向下看正常。第一眼位在没有其他运动性异常情况下眼球正位。
    b. 包括中脑和后颅窝动脉瘤的破裂或上述部位的肿瘤。
    c. 中脑导水管狭窄，松果体瘤和脑膜炎。

    a. Light-near dissociation of pupillary reactions, lid retraction (Collier's sign), convergence-retraction nystagmus (elicited with an optokinetic nystagmus drum), paresis (or spasm) of convergence and accommodation. Downgaze is typically normal. The eyes will be straight in the primary position of gaze in the absence of additional motility abnormality.
    b. Stroke or tumour involving the midbrain and posterior fossa aneurysm.
    c. Sylvian aqueduct stenosis, pinealoma and meningitis.

22. a. 白瞳: 白色瞳孔。
    b. 视网膜母细胞瘤，儿童最常见的眼内恶性肿瘤；60%患者出现白瞳，30% 患者双眼受累。
    c. 持续增生性原始玻璃体、Coats病、陈旧性早产儿视网膜病变和弓蛔虫病。

    a. Leukocoria: 'white pupil'.
    b. Retinoblastoma, the most common malignant intraocular tumour in children; 60% of cases present with leukoria and both eyes are affected in 30% of patients.
    c. Persistent hyperplastic primary vitreous, Coats' disease, advanced retinopathy of prematurity and toxocariasis.

23. a. 小囊泡发展为初期的斑丘疹，其后形成溃疡结痂；典型的伴有眼眶周围的水肿。
    b. 是指以鼻尖为中线的一侧皮肤病损，发生眼并发症的风险高。
    c. 急性虹膜炎，角膜炎（上皮细胞的，圆形的，盘状的和神经营养性的），巩膜炎，视神经炎和眼运动神经麻痹。

a. An initial maculopapular rash progresses to form vesicles and subsequently crusting ulcers; associated periorbital oedema is typical.
b. This refers to skin lesions on the side of the tip of the nose and is associated with an increased risk of ocular complications.
c. Acute iritis, keratitis (epithelial, nummular, disciform and neurotrophic), scleritis, optic neuritis and ocular motor nerve palsies.

24. a. 小结节的中心溃疡界限清楚。当其发展为大的中心溃疡时，底部的增生性鳞状上皮细胞含有嗜酸性胞质包涵体，细胞逐渐增大，并随细胞核的丧失而退化。诊断是传染性软疣。
b. 持续性滤泡性结膜炎，是由病毒颗粒从睑缘病变区持续不断的脱落引起。
c. 获得性免疫缺陷综合征（AIDS）。

a. A well-defined nodule with a central crater. The base consists of proliferating squamous cells with eosinophilic cytoplasmic inclusions that enlarge as they progress towards the large central crater, degenerating with loss of their nuclei in the process. The diagnosis is molluscum contagiosum.
b. With a persistent follicular conjunctivitis, caused by continual shedding of viral particles from a lesion on the lid margin.
c. Acquired immune deficiency syndrome (AIDS).

25. a. 正常眼压性青光眼，因为视盘表现为青光眼杯。
b. 已报道的血管现象有：Raynaud 现象，偏头痛，夜间系统性低血压，眼动脉和睫状动脉血流速度减慢，异型球蛋白血症，存在血清抗体。
c. 中心旁暗点，鼻侧阶梯，弓状缺损，环状暗点和末期有小的残留视岛。

a. Normal-tension glaucoma because the disc shows glaucomatous cupping.
b. A range of vascular phenomena have been reported: Raynaud's phenomenon, migraine, nocturnal systemic hypotension, reduced blood flow velocity of the ophthalmic and ciliary arteries, paraproteinaemia and the presence of serum autoantibodies.
c. Paracentral scotoma, nasal step, arcuate defect, ring scotoma and end-stage with a small residual central island.

26. a. 后囊下混浊（PSC）。
 b. 症状与矫正的视力不成比例，例如眩光，在强光或晚上汽车前灯照射时视力下降，阅读困难，是由瞳孔狭窄增强了不透明的程度所致。
 c. 患者可能全身应用类固醇，其促进了 PSC 白内障形成。

 a. Posterior subcapsular (PSC).
 b. Symptoms out of proportion to the corrected visual acuity such as substantial glare, vision worse in bright light or when encountering car headlights at night, and difficulty with reading vision, caused by pupillary constriction enhancing the effect of the opacity.
 c. The patient may have taken systemic steroids, which promote the formation of PSC cataract.

27. a. 视网膜颞上分支静脉闭塞。
 b. Behçet病。在没有其他疾病的情况下，视网膜的静脉闭塞在这个年龄很罕见。Behçet 病对静脉循环的影响较动脉大。
 c. 有效；前葡萄膜炎常伴前房积脓，连同复发性口腔溃疡一起是 Behçet 病的主要诊断指标之一。
 d. HLA-B51。

 a. Superotemporal branch retinal vein occlusion.
 b. Behçet's disease. A retinal venous occlusion is very uncommon in a patient of this age without an underlying predisposing condition. Behçet's affects the venous circulation more than the arterial.
 c. Yes; anterior uveitis, often with a hypopyon, is one of the major diagnostic criteria for Behçet's, along with recurrent aphthous oral ulceration.
 d. HLA-B51.

28. a. 除发病年龄和斜视的变化性之外，应注意家族史、分娩史和全身健康状况。
 b. 视力，立体视觉，确定斜视存在（即排除假性内斜视），测量斜视度，检查眼球运动（特别是排除第六脑神经麻痹），屈光和眼部检查（斜视可以是一些疾病的体征，例如视网膜母细胞瘤和先天性白内障）。
 c. 典型的会出现远视。眼镜矫正通常部分或完全控制斜视，几周后需复查。

a. Besides age of onset and variability of the squint, family history, birth history and general health.
b. Visual acuity, stereopsis, confirm the presence of a deviation (i.e. exclude pseudoesotropia), measurement of the deviation, checking the ocular movements (particularly to exclude a sixth nerve palsy), refraction and ocular examination (a squint can be the presenting sign of pathology such as retinoblastoma and congenital cataract).
c. Typically, a hypermetropic refractive error will be present. Spectacle correction will usually partially or completely control the squint, and the child should be reviewed after several weeks.

29. a. 年龄相关性黄斑裂孔。
b. 视力一般会降至 6/60，虽然假黄斑注视视力可为 6/9。
c. 大多数患者通常伴随裂孔周围的内界膜剥离和眼球内注气，玻璃体切割术可促进裂孔闭合和视力改善。裂孔存在少于一年可得到最好的结果。
d. 5 年上升为 15%。

a. Age-related macular hole.
b. Typically this will be 6/60, though eccentric fixation may permit up to 6/9.
c. Vitrectomy, usually accompanied by peeling of the internal limiting membrane surrounding the hole, and intraocular gas injection, facilitates closure of the hole and visual improvement in most patients. Best results are achieved with holes present for less than a year.
d. Up to 15% at 5 years.

30. a. U 字形的视网膜撕裂。
b. 激光光凝两排。如果撕裂十分靠近周边，可以较早采取冷冻疗法。
c. 近视、格子状变性、无晶状体和人工晶状体（特别当并发玻璃体丢失时）、外伤（陈旧的或新的）和视网膜脱离家族史，尤其是伴随 Stickler 综合征。

a. A U-shaped retinal tear.
b. Laser photocoagulation with two rows of confluent burns. If the tear is very peripheral, cryotherapy may be easier to apply.
c. Myopia, lattice degeneration, aphakia and pseudophakia (particularly when complicated by vitreous loss), trauma (old or recent), and family history of retinal detachment, especially when

associated with Stickler's syndrome.

31. a. 单纯疱疹性角膜炎（HSK）所致树枝状角膜溃疡。
   b. HSK 典型的角膜知觉减退，必须在局麻药滴入之前检查。
   c. 角膜上皮擦伤愈合很可能是诊断困难最常见的原因；树枝状表现的其他原因包括带状疱疹性角膜炎，隐形眼镜所致上皮病，棘阿米巴角膜炎和局部用药所致。
   d. 局部应用阿昔洛韦，更昔洛韦或三氟胸腺嘧啶核苷。一些情况可以清创。必要时长期口服阿昔洛韦可以减少复发率。

   a. Dendritic ulcer due to herpes simplex keratitis (HSK).
   b. Corneal sensation is typically reduced in HSK and must be checked before the instillation of local anaesthetic.
   c. Healing corneal abrasion is probably the most common source of diagnostic difficulty; other causes of a dendritic appearance include herpes zoster keratitis, the epitheliopathy of contact lens wear, acanthamoeba keratitis and topical medication toxicity.
   d. Topical aciclovir, ganciclovir or trifluorothymidine. Debridement is used in some circumstances. Long-term oral aciclovir can be used to reduce the frequency of recurrence if necessary.

32. a. 新生儿结膜炎或“新生儿眼炎”，结膜炎出现在出生第一个月内。
   b. • 化学性结膜炎：出生后的第一周内通常用硝酸银点眼防治淋病双球菌感染。
      • 淋病双球菌：1 ~ 3 周。
      • 单纯疱疹：1 ~ 2 周。
      • 葡萄球菌和其他的细菌：第一周内。
   c. 感染可能包括肺（肺炎）、鼻咽、中耳、阴道和直肠。

   a. Neonatal conjunctivitis or 'ophthalmia neonatorum'-conjunctivitis occurring within the first neonatal month.
   b. • Chemical conjunctivitis: within the first postnatal week is usually due to antiseptic agents although in the past commonly due to silver nitrate gonococcus prophylaxis.
      • Gonococcus: within the first week.
      • Chlamydia: 1-3 weeks.
      • Herpes simplex: 1-2 weeks.
      • Staphylococci and other bacteria: end of first week onwards.
   c. Infection may involve the lungs (pneumonitis), nasopharynx,

middle ear, vagina and rectum.

33. a. 连续画面对确定诊断必须的，这几乎断定是脉络膜新生血管膜。
b. 年龄相关性黄斑退行性病变的湿性形式。
c. 其他较少见的原因包括近视，细孔状的内部脉络膜病，外伤性脉络膜破裂，血管样条纹症，不适当的视网膜激光光凝和视盘玻璃疣。

a. Although a series of frames is ideally required to ascertain the diagnosis, this almost certainly shows a choroidal neovascular membrane.
b. The 'wet' form of age-related macular degeneration.
c. Other, less common, causes include myopia, punctate inner choroidopathy, traumatic choroidal rupture, angioid streaks, inappropriate retinal laser photocoagulation and optic disc drusen.

34. a. 右上斜肌麻痹。
b. 较小的面积是右眼图，表明这是异常眼。右眼图中心的水平比左眼高，显示这是在第一眼位较高的眼。除右上斜肌原发的功能不足之外，还有同侧下斜肌的作用过强（由于随着时间而挛缩），对侧的下直肌（由于 Hering 法则的相等神经支配）作用过强，对侧的上直肌功能不足（由于 Hering 法则，在右下斜肌收缩时需要更少神经支配）。

a. Right superior oblique palsy.
b. The smaller area is enclosed by the chart for the right eye, suggesting that this is the abnormal side. The right chart is centred at a higher level than the left, showing that this is the higher eye in the primary position. In addition to the primary underaction of the right superior oblique, there is overaction (due to contracture with time) of the unopposed ipsilateral inferior oblique, overaction of the contralateral inferior rectus yoke muscle (due to Hering's law of equal innervation), and underaction of the contralateral superior rectus (due to Hering's law, as the contracted right inferior oblique requires less innervation).

35. a. 视网膜出现苍白和水肿，只有黄斑中心凹形成差别明显的“樱桃红斑”。小动脉变细。
b. 视网膜中央动脉阻塞。

c. 用超声，MRI 或常规的血管造影检查颈动脉和心脏影像术，可判定栓子的来源。

d. 玻璃体出血，视网膜分支动脉阻塞，视网膜静脉闭塞，黄斑出血（通常由于黄斑变性），前部缺血性视神经病和视神经炎。

a. The retina appears pale and oedematous, except at the centre of the macula where the contrast gives the appearance of a 'cherry-red spot'. The arterioles are attenuated.

b. Central retinal artery occlusion.

c. Carotid artery assessment by ultrasound (duplex), MRI or conventional angiography, and cardiac imaging, in order to exclude an embolic source.

d. Vitreous haemorrhage, branch retinal artery occlusion, retinal venous occlusion, macular haemorrhage (usually due to macular degeneration), anterior ischaemic optic neuropathy and optic neuritis.

36. a. 这是“典型”视网膜色素上皮细胞的先天性肥大（CHRPE）。

b. 这种病变是孤立的，扁平的，深灰色至黑色，圆形，伴有低色素的镶边和低色素的裂隙。

c. “典型”CHRPE不会导致任何全身性影响，与“非典型”相反（纺锤形或椭圆形，多发，两侧，在一个边缘色素减退）。“非典型”伴有家族性腺瘤性息肉病，Gardner综合征和Turcot综合征。

a. The 'typical' form of congenital hypertrophy of the retinal pigment epithelium (CHRPE).

b. The lesion is solitary, flat, dark-grey to black, round, with a hypopigmented rim and hypopigmented lacunae.

c. The 'typical' form of CHRPE does not carry any systemic implications, in contrast to the 'atypical' form (spindle-shaped or oval, multiple, bilateral, hypopigmentation at one margin), which is associated with familial adenomatous polyposis, Gardner's syndrome and Turcot's syndrome.

37. a. 视网膜赤道部 - 周边骨小体样色素沉着，视盘蜡黄和小动脉变细，是色素性视网膜炎的特征。

b. 一般特性包括视网膜赤道部环状暗点，黄斑病变（囊样水肿，萎缩），后囊膜下白内障，近视和开角型青光眼（3%）。

c. ERG暗适应延缓（和稍后明视），异常EOG，延长的暗适应。

d. 重要的疾病包括 Bassen-Kornzweig 综合征、Refsum 综合征、Usher 综合征、Kearns-Sayre 综合征和 Bardet-Biedl 综合征。

a. Mid-peripheral retinal pigmentary deposits in a bone-spicule pattern, waxy disc pallor and arteriolar attenuation, characteristic of retinitis pigmentosa.
b. Relatively common features include: mid-periphery annular scotomas, maculopathy (cystoid oedema, atrophy), posterior subcapsular cataracts, myopia and open-angle glaucoma (3%).
c. Reduced scotopic (and later photopic) responses in ERG, abnormal EOG, prolonged dark adaptation.
d. Important conditions include Bassen-Kornzweig syndrome, Refsum's syndrome, Usher's syndrome, Kearns-Sayre syndrome and Bardet-Biedl syndrome.

38. a. 轻度右侧上睑下垂和瞳孔缩小。诊断是Horner综合征。患者患侧出汗减少，因为病变使邻近的沿颈外动脉走行的促汗纤维受损。
b. 下眼睑轻度提高，异色症，相对的张力过低，结膜充血和调节过度。
c. 4% 可卡因可阻止去甲肾上腺素重新吸收使瞳孔散大，但不是 Horner 瞳孔表现。1% 羟基苯丙胺可引起从第三交感神经元释放去甲肾上腺素，因此瞳孔散大，在第一神经元病变或第二神经元病变则不起作用。0.1%肾上腺素由于去神经增敏状态，可使第三神经元病变瞳孔散大。

a. Slight right ptosis and miosis. The diagnosis is Horner's syndrome. The patient is actually experiencing reduced sweating on the abnormal side, as the lesion is proximal to the splitting of the sudomotor fibres to travel along the external carotid.
b. Slight elevation of the lower eyelid, heterochromia, relative hypotony, conjunctival hyperaemia and hyperaccommodation.
c. Cocaine 4% dilates a normal pupil due to prevention of noradrenaline (norepinephrine) re-uptake, but not a Horner's pupil. Hydroxyamphetamine 1% causes release of noradrenaline (norepinephrine) from a functioning third-order sympathetic neurone and so will dilate the pupil in first- or second-order lesions as well as the normal pupil. Adrenaline (epinephrine) 0.1% dilates the pupil of a third-order lesion due to denervation hypersensitivity.

39. a. 基质性角膜炎的羽状深基质层的瘢痕和血管虚影。
    b. 如果炎症复发，血管虚影可以再灌注，出血少见。
    c. 骨骼的特征包括马刀状胫骨、鞍鼻、额部隆起、下颌前突、高腭穹、牙齿畸形（Hutchinson 牙与先天梅毒磨牙）和感觉神经性耳聋。

    a. A feathery deep stromal scar and ghost vessels characteristic of interstitial keratitis.
    b. The ghost vessels may refill and, rarely, bleed if the inflammation reactivates.
    c. Bony features include sabre tibiae, saddle-shaped nose, frontal bossing, prognathism, high-arched palate, dental malformations (Hutchinson's teeth and Moon's molars) and sensorineural deafness.

40. a. 晶状体向上半脱位。
    b. Marfan 综合征，15 号染色体原纤维蛋白基因突变。
    c. 身材高，但两臂伸展距离比身高大、肌肉发育不良、疝气、主动脉扩张症和心脏瓣膜疾病、皮肤皱纹和脆性高。
    d. 高胱氨酸尿症、Weill-Marchesani综合征、高赖氨酸血症、亚硫酸氧化酶缺乏、Ehlers-Danlos 综合征和 Stickler 综合征。

    a. The lens is subluxated upwards.
    b. Marfan's syndrome, associated with a mutation of the fibrillin gene on chromosome 15.
    c. Tall, but with arm span greater than height, muscular underdevelopment, hernias, aortic dilatation and dissection, heart valve disease, striae and fragility of the skin.
    d. Homocystinuria, Weill-Marchesani syndrome, hyperlysinaemia, sulphite oxidase deficiency, Ehlers-Danlos syndrome and Stickler's syndrome.

41. a. 90% 或更多患者是 HLA-A29 阳性。
    b. 常见，中度的玻璃体炎是典型特征。
    c. 视网膜电图（ERG），它能提供测量视网膜功能的基础曲线。
    d. 视神经萎缩和慢性黄斑囊样水肿。

    a. 90% or more of patients are positive for HLA-A29.
    b. Yes, moderate vitreitis is typical.
    c. Electroretinography (ERG), which provides a baseline measure of retinal function.

d. Optic atrophy and chronic cystoid macular oedema.

42. a. 关节炎（尤其是膝和踝关节）、足底筋膜炎、Achilles 腱炎、脓性卡他性角化病、口腔溃疡形成、阴茎头炎、附睾炎、睾丸炎和前列腺炎。
b. 急性前葡萄膜炎和偶发浅层点状角膜炎。
c. 70% 病例组织相容抗原分型 HLA-B27 阳性。
d. 主动脉瓣关闭不全。

a. Arthritis (especially knees and ankles), plantar fasciitis, Achilles tendonitis, keratoderma blenorrhagica, mouth ulceration, balanitis, epididymitis, orchitis and prostatitis.
b. Acute anterior uveitis and occasionally punctate epithelial keratitis.
c. HLA-typing will be positive for HLA-B27 in 70% of cases.
d. Aortic incompetence.

43. a. 眼部不适、复视、视力下降和外貌异常。
b. 甲状腺眼病在甲状腺功能亢进（甲亢）的发病率远高于在甲状腺功能减退症（粘液性水肿）的发病率。然而，患者可能在临床上和生物化学检验上甲状腺机能正常。
c. 内转不能。
d. 全身应用类固醇、眼眶放射治疗和手术减压。

a. Ocular discomfort, double vision, reduced vision and cosmetic problems.
b. The incidence is far higher in hyperthyroidism (thyrotoxicosis) than hypothyroidism (myxoedema). However, patients can be clinically and biochemically euthyroid.
c. Failure of adduction.
d. Systemic steroids, orbital radiotherapy and surgical decompression.

44. a. 复发的，无瘢痕化水疱和稀疏的限局性红斑。
b. 睑球粘连（眼球和睑结膜间粘连）、睑缘粘连（上下眼睑外眦间粘连）和严重的干眼。重症者包括继发的严重角膜改变，可能是致盲的原因。
c. 局部适当的应用润滑剂、类固醇和抗生素；结膜下注射丝裂霉素 C；防护性隐形眼镜；全身治疗包括类固醇、氨苯砜、静脉注射免疫球蛋白和细胞毒素。

a. Recurrent, non-scarring blisters and sparse localized erythematous plaques.

b. Symblepharon (adhesions between bulbar and palpebral conjunctiva), ankyloblepharon (adhesions between the lids at the outer canthus) and severe dry eye. Advanced disease can involve severe secondary corneal changes, which may cause blindness.

c. Topical lubricants, steroids and antibiotics where appropriate; subconjunctival mitomycin C; protective contact lenses; systemic options include steroids, dapsone, intravenous immunoglobulins and cytotoxic agents.

45. a. 原发性颅内高压，不过CT或MRI脑扫描是排除占位性病变所必须的。

b. 失明是由于长期的视盘水肿导致的继发性视神经萎缩而引起。

c. 利尿剂、全身应用类固醇、视神经减压术和腰部脊髓腔-腹腔分流术。

a. Idiopathic intracranial hypertension, although CT or MRI brain scan is required to rule out a space-occupying lesion.

b. Blindness may result from secondary optic atrophy due to chronic papilloedema.

c. Diuretics, systemic steroids, optic nerve fenestration and lumboperitoneal shunt.

46. a. 单纯的移植失败是因为内皮失代偿，全眼尚无剧烈反应。而排异反应包括炎症成分（虽然可能较轻）。特殊的上皮体征（不连续的上皮下浸润—Krachmer点）或内皮体征（角膜后沉着物、水肿、明显的炎症）的排异反应明显。失败常常是排斥反应的结果。

b. 主要治疗是局部应用类固醇，然而眼周注射或全身应用免疫抑制剂也是必要的。

c. 眼睑疾病、泪膜异常、前段炎症、角膜的血管化或变薄和难以控制的青光眼。

a. In pure graft failure, which occurs because of endothelial decompensation, the eye is quiet, whereas rejection involves an inflammatory element (although this may be mild). Specific signs of epithelial (discrete subepithelial infiltrates-Krachmer's spots) or endothelial (keratic precipitates, oedema, more marked inflammation) rejection will be evident. Failure is often a consequence of rejection.

b. The mainstay of treatment is topical steroids, although periocular injection or systemic immunosuppression may be necessary.

c. Eyelid disease, tear film dysfunction, anterior segment inflammation, corneal vascularization or thinning and uncontrolled glaucoma.

47. a. 翼状胬肉，变性的血管组织区侵犯角膜多由于热和干燥气候所致。

b. 视力减退（由于散光或视线阻挡），实际上是由于刺激作用和从美容角度考虑。

c. 单纯的切除复发率高。结膜瓣自体移植，放射和抗有丝分裂剂应用是很有效的。

a. A pterygium, an area of degenerative fibrovascular tissue encroaching on the cornea most commonly seen in hot, dry climates.

b. Visual deterioration (due to astigmatism or visual axis obstruction), substantial irritation and cosmesis.

c. Simple removal is associated with a high rate of recurrence. Conjunctival patch autografting, irradiation and antimitotic agent application are more effective.

48. a. 脉络膜褶。

b. 原发性的。因为累及双眼，无症状和存在隐性远视。

c. 眼眶疾病（例如甲状腺眼病、肿瘤）和眼球病变（例如张力减退、脉络膜肿瘤、后巩膜炎、长期的视盘水肿和巩膜折叠术）。

a. Choroidal folds.

b. Idiopathic, because of bilateral involvement, lack of symptoms and the presence of hypermetropia.

c. Orbital disease (e.g. thyroid, tumours) and ocular causes (e.g. hypotony, choroidal tumours, posterior scleritis, chronic papilloedema and scleral buckling).

49. a. 否。双眼颞侧的视野缺损，被确定为两颞侧偏盲。

b. 视交叉被占位性病变压迫，例如脑垂体瘤最需要被排除。“倾斜的” 视盘（在近视者比较常见），可有类似的视野图形，虽然视野缺损典型地横过中线。

c. 脑和眼眶 MRI 检查，包括视交叉在内。

a. No. The defects involve the temporal field of each eye; by definition, a bitemporal hemianopia.
b. Chiasmal compression by a space-occupying lesion such as a pituitary adenoma needs to be excluded urgently. 'Tilted' optic discs, relatively common in myopes, can also give a similar field pattern, although the defects typically cross the midline.
c. MRI of the brain and orbits, to include the optic chiasm.

50. a. 手表现为类风湿性关节炎的典型特点。
b. 基本可以确定她有干眼症：干燥性角结膜炎，即继发的Sjögren 综合征。
c. 裂隙灯检查可见碎屑、泡沫，一个不规则的或边缘为新月形的薄泪膜，泪膜破裂时间短。其他的检查包括角膜和结膜孟加拉玫瑰红染色、荧光素染色和泪液分泌试验。
d. 角膜炎（严重的角膜可融解和穿孔）和巩膜炎。后天性Brown综合征（上斜肌鞘综合征）很少见。

a. The hands show features typical of rheumatoid arthritis.
b. She almost certainly has dry eyes: keratoconjunctivitis sicca, i.e. secondary Sjögren's syndrome.
c. Slit-lamp assessment of the tear film may show debris, froth, an irregular or thin marginal meniscus and a short break-up time. Other tests include staining the cornea and conjunctiva with rose Bengal and fluorescein, and the Schirmer test.
d. Keratitis (which can be severe, with melting and perforation), and scleritis. Acquired Brown's syndrome is very rare.

51. a. 右侧下运动神经元性面神经麻痹。
b. 继发于眼睑闭合不全的角膜暴露，重要的是美容问题。
c. 轻症患者局部用润滑剂足矣。对复发性麻痹，肉毒杆菌毒素诱导的上睑下垂是有用的，但重症必需手术（如上下睑缝合术，眼睑缩短术和神经移植术）。

a. A right lower motor neurone facial nerve palsy.
b. Exposure keratopathy secondary to poor eyelid closure; cosmetic implications may also be substantial.
c. Topical lubricants may suffice in mild cases. Botulinum-induced ptosis is useful in recovering palsies but surgery will be necessary for profound permanent deficit (e.g. tarsorrhaphy, lid shortening and nerve grafting).

52. a. 很可能不是，因为视盘正常。

b. 5 年大约为 10%。

c. 如果视盘非常小，其生理凹陷的实际面积比看到的小很多。

d. 视野，排除青光眼的改变和作为监测病情发展的指标；角膜中心的厚度测量法，对于厚角膜同样可判断眼压高于正常水平；视盘成像，用计算机分析参数更好。

a. Probably not, as the optic discs appear normal.

b. Approximately 10% at 5 years.

c. If the disc is unusually small, the physiological cup size might be considerably smaller than that shown.

d. Visual fields, to exclude glaucomatous changes and act as a baseline for monitoring purposes; pachymetry for central corneal thickness, as the measured intraocular pressure is higher than the true level in eyes with thick corneas; and baseline optic disc imaging, preferably with computed parameter analysis.

53. a. 钙沉积于睑裂部暴露区角膜（带状角膜病）。

b. 一些孩子 JIA 发展为慢性的前葡萄膜炎，它可导致继发性青光眼、带状角膜病和白内障。炎症活动期眼部典型地保持为白色且无不适感，因此诊断会被忽略。

c. 早发小关节病变，存在抗细胞核抗体的免疫血清和HLA-DR5阳性。

a. Corneal calcium deposition in an interpalpebral distribution (band keratopathy).

b. Some children with JIA develop a chronic anterior uveitis, which can lead to secondary glaucoma, band keratopathy and cataract. The eye typically remains white and comfortable despite active inflammation so that the diagnosis may be overlooked.

c. Early-onset pauciarticular disease, the presence of serum anti-nuclear antibodies, and HLA-DR5 positivity.

54. a. 隐形眼镜相关的角膜炎，临床上多由细菌引起。

b. 角膜刮片显微镜检查，细菌培养和药敏试验，然后局部应用广谱抗生素。应该住院治疗。散瞳可以改善和防止虹膜后粘连。口服抗生素往往对接近角膜缘的溃疡是有效的。

c. 棘阿米巴属，真菌，非典型分枝杆菌和单纯性疱疹。

a. Contact lens-related keratitis, which clinically appears to be bacterial.

b. Corneal scraping for microscopy, culture and antibiotic sensitivity testing, followed by intensive topical broad-spectrum antibiotics. Admission to hospital is usually advisable. A mydriatic may improve comfort and prevent posterior synechiae formation. Oral antibiotics are sometimes used for ulcers near the limbus.

c. Acanthamoeba, fungi, atypical mycobacteria and herpes simplex.

55. a. 右侧核间性眼肌麻痹（INO）。

b. 右侧的内侧纵束（MLF）；在MLF损伤侧的眼不能内转（55a中的右眼）。

c. 多发性硬化症。

d. 卒中、肿瘤、外伤、脑炎、药品和脑积水。

a. Right internuclear ophthalmoplegia (INO).

b. The right medial longitudinal fasciculus (MLF); the side of the lesion in the MLF corresponds to the eye that fails to adduct (the right eye in 55a).

c. Multiple sclerosis.

d. Stroke, tumours, trauma, encephalitis, drugs and hydrocephalus.

56. a. 急性视网膜坏死；在这个年龄组水痘是可能的原因。

b. 聚合酶链反应（PCR） 分析房水和玻璃体的病毒 DNA。

c. 无环鸟苷静脉注射10天，然后口服3个月；抗病毒疗法开始后全身应用糖皮质激素 24 小时。

a. Acute retinal necrosis; in this age group, varicella is the likely cause.

b. Polymerase chain reaction (PCR) analysis of aqueous and vitreous for viral DNA.

c. Intravenous aciclovir for 10 days then orally for 3 months; systemic steroids 24 hours after commencement of antiviral therapy.

57. a. 大约50%缺血型CRVO形成虹膜新生血管，然后常常发展成新生血管性青光眼。

b. 糖尿病、视网膜中央动脉阻塞、颈动脉阻塞疾病和慢性眼内炎。

c. 立刻全视网膜光凝，如果未能诱导复原至形成不可逆高压力之前的状态，可进行cyclocliode激光光凝或引流术。视力预后差。

a. Rubeosis iridis, which develops in about 50% of ischaemic CRVOs and often results in neovascular glaucoma.
b. Diabetes, central retinal artery occlusion, carotid obstructive disease and chronic intraocular inflammation.
c. Urgent panretinal photocoagulation. If this fails to induce regression prior to irreversible pressure elevation, cyclodiode laser or drainage surgery can be carried out. The visual prognosis is very poor.

58. a. 角膜混浊，前房浅和瞳孔散大。诊断是急性闭角型青光眼。腹部的症状可能偶然出现这么严重，所以成为主要焦点。眼压测量将确定诊断。
b. 住院治疗，静脉注射乙酰唑胺和局部治疗以降低眼压，然后行双眼激光虹膜切除术。
c. 急性虹膜炎、角膜上皮擦伤、角膜炎和巩膜炎。

a. The cornea is cloudy the anterior chamber shallow and the pupil dilated. The diagnosis is acute angle-closure glaucoma, in which the abdominal symptoms may occasionally be so severe as to constitute the main focus. Intraocular pressure measurement will confirm the diagnosis.
b. Admission to hospital, intravenous acetazolamide and topical agents to lower the intraocular pressure, followed by laser iridotomy to both eyes.
c. Acute iritis, corneal abrasion, keratitis and scleritis.

59. a. 毛细血管瘤或草莓痣。
b. 是的，该损害会导致弱视，因为可合并上睑下垂或斜视。
c. 病变内部注射类固醇。然而，大多数的草莓痣在7岁之前会自发的消退。
d. 极罕见，毛细血管瘤是Maffucci综合征（多发的全身性血管瘤和骨骼损害）或Kasabach-Merritt综合征（血液学的异常情况）的一部分。

a. Capillary haemangioma or 'strawberry naevus'.
b. Yes, because the lesion may induce amblyopia as a result of associated ptosis or strabismus.
c. Intralesional steroid injection. However, most strawberry naevi constitute only a cosmetic problem and can be left alone in anticipation of spontaneous resolution by the age of 7 years.

d. Very rarely, capillary haemangioma is part of a wider syndrome-Maffucci's (multiple systemic haemangiomata and bone lesions)or Kasabach-Merritt (haematological abnormalities).

60. a. 提上睑肌和Müller肌；前者由动眼神经上分支支配，后者由自主神经系统的交感神经支配。

b. • 神经性：第三脑神经、Horner 综合征、Marcus Gunn（颌动瞬目）综合征。
- 腱膜性：退化（年龄相关性）、手术后。
- 机械性：水肿、肿瘤、多余的皮肤、瘢痕。
- 肌性：单纯先天性、睑裂狭小综合征、重症肌无力、进行性眼外肌麻痹、肌强直性营养不良。

c. • 对侧眼突出。
- 眼睑：多余的皮肤悬垂超过睑缘（皮肤松垂）。
- 眼球：小眼、眼球痨。
- 眼肌：垂直运动的肌肉失调。
- 眼眶：眼球内陷。

a. Levator palpebrae superioris and Müller's muscle; the former is supplied by the superior division of the oculomotor nerve and the latter by the sympathetic component of the autonomic nervous system.

b. • *Neurogenic*: third nerve palsy, Horner's syndrome, Marcus Gunn's ('jaw-winking') syndrome.
- *Aponeurotic*: involutional (age-related), postoperative.
- *Mechanical*: oedema, tumours, heavy redundant skin, cicatricial.
- *Myogenic*: simple congenital, blepharophimosis syndrome, myasthenia gravis, ocular myopathy, myotonic dystrophy.

c. • *Proptosis of the contralateral eye.*
- *Eyelid*: redundant skin overhanging lid margin (dermatochalasis).
- *Globe*: microphthalmos, phthisis.
- *Eye muscles*: vertical muscle imbalance.
- *Orbit*: enophthalmos.

61. a. 睑缘皮样囊肿。

b. 迷芽瘤，正常组织在不正常位置的先天性瘤。

c. 对视力有影响、刺激症状或从美容角度考虑。

d. 睑缘皮样囊肿通常是孤立性异常，但可以是Goldenhar综合征、Treacher Collins 综合征或 Jadassohn 痣皮脂综合征的一部分。

a. A limbal dermoid.
b. A choristoma, a congenital growth of normal tissue at an abnormal location.
c. For visual interference, irritation, or cosmesis.
d. Limbal dermoids are usually an isolated abnormality but may on occasion be part of Goldenhar's syndrome, Treacher Collins' syndrome or the naevus sebaceous syndrome of Jadassohn.

62. a. 左眼内转障碍，左侧 Brown 综合征。
b. 弱视所有的眼位检查，屈光间质检查，眼底检查和治疗都很重要。只有在第一眼位有显著偏位，复视或异常头位时才需要手术。
c. 炎症（例如类风湿性关节炎），外伤或上斜肌手术。

a. Failure of elevation of the left eye in adduction, consistent with a left Brown's syndrome.
b. As with all squints, refraction, media and fundus examination and treatment of amblyopia are important. Surgery is needed only if there is significant deviation in the primary position, diplopia or an anomalous head posture.
c. Inflammation (e.g. rheumatoid arthritis), trauma and superior oblique surgery.

63. a. 疑诊巨细胞性动脉炎，要询问关于头痛、头皮触痛、牙关紧闭、肌肉束带状（尤其是颈部）疼痛、不适、体重下降和风湿性多发性肌痛。
b. 红细胞沉降率（ESR）和C反应蛋白（CRP）。可是检验数值低并不能排除这个诊断，也不能因为一次性增高的结果而确诊。
c. 颞动脉活组织检查。必须早期全身（通常静脉注射）应用类固醇，而且在等候活组织检查时不应该延误治疗。

a. Giant cell arteritis should be suspected and enquiry made concerning headache, scalp tenderness, jaw claudication, muscle girdle (particularly neck) aching, malaise, loss of weight and specifically previous diagnosis of polymyalgia rheumatica.
b. Erythrocyte sedimentation rate (ESR) and C-reactive protein (CRP); however, the diagnosis is not excluded by a low result nor categorically confirmed by a high one.
c. Temporal artery biopsy. Systemic (usually intravenous) steroids must be commenced immediately in this situation and should not

be delayed while biopsy is awaited.

64. a. Kearns-Sayre 综合征，其特征是视网膜色素变性和慢性进行性眼肌麻痹。这个孩子可能有共济失调、耳聋、糖尿病和其他的全身性异常情况。
    b. 线粒体 DNA 缺失。
    c. ECG示心脏传导缺陷，CSF不正常，肌肉活组织检查示“溃烂的红色纤维组织”图像。

    a. Kearns-Sayre syndrome, which is characterized by pigmentary retinopathy and chronic progressive external ophthalmoplegia. The child may also have ataxia, deafness, diabetes and other systemic abnormalities.
    b. Mitochondrial DNA deletions.
    c. ECG shows cardiac conduction defects, CSF is abnormal and muscle biopsy shows the 'ragged red fibre' pattern.

65. a. 虹膜分裂，极罕见的虹膜渐进性分裂，进入前后薄层并前层分解。
    b. 眼压高。原理是闭角型青光眼发作伴随极高的眼压导致虹膜变化，而不是虹膜变化导致病变开始。
    c. 激光周边虹膜切除术，随后采取适当的内科治疗。

    a. Iridoschisis, a very rare gradual splitting of the iris into anterior and posterior lamellae with disintegration of the anterior layer.
    b. IOP elevation. It is postulated that episodic angle-closure glaucoma associated with very high IOP leads to the iris changes, rather than the iris changes precipitating the initiating event.
    c. Laser peripheral iridotomy, followed by medical treatment as appropriate.

66. a. 下泪点狭窄。重度内侧睑外翻致泪点离开泪湖。
    b. 进一步评价有两类：①排除眼部刺激的所有原因，特别是由于干眼造成的“反常”流泪；②泪液排泄系统阻塞。泪道冲洗基本可以判定泪小管和鼻泪管阻塞。
    c. 单纯的泪点扩张术或切开（单切或双切），扩大泪小管，如果必要可结合睑外翻矫正术。

    a. Stenosis of the lower eyelid punctum. There is also a degree of medial ectropion resulting in the punctum pointing away from the lacus lacrimalis.

b. Further assessment falls into two categories: exclusion of any cause of ocular irritation, particularly 'paradoxical' lacrimation due to dry eye, and obstruction elsewhere in the lacrimal drainage system. Basic assessment of the lacrimal canaliculi and nasolacrimal duct involves syringing with saline.
c. Simple dilation of the punctum or incisional ('one-' or 'two-snip') enlargement of the canaliculus, combined if necessary with ectropion repair.

67. a. 虽然左侧角膜也出现扩大，右侧还是比左侧大。最可能的诊断是原发性先天性青光眼，然而，其他的大角膜、大眼球和继发的婴儿期青光眼的原因必须排除。
b. 后弹力层断裂（当愈合的时候出现“哈布纹”），异常的前房角和视盘的凹陷杯。
c. 必须在全身麻醉情况下行前房角镜检查、测量眼压和角膜直径。

a. The right cornea is larger than the left, although the left also appears enlarged. The most likely diagnosis is primary congenital glaucoma, although other causes of large corneas, large eyes and secondary infantile glaucoma must be excluded.
b. Breaks in Descemet's membrane ('Haab striae' when healed), an abnormal anterior chamber angle and optic disc cupping.
c. Examination under general anaesthesia will be necessary to facilitate gonioscopy, and measurement of intraocular pressure and corneal diameter.

68. a. 边缘性角膜炎。
b. 不能确定，但应全面考虑所有的临床现象。要点包括：症状平缓，缺乏先期诱因（如戴隐形眼镜）。浸润带平行于角膜缘，被透明区与角膜缘分隔开。特点是浸润的比伴随的上皮缺损大。经常出现慢性的前部睑缘炎。
c. 短期小剂量局部类固醇（例如糖皮质激素）治疗。

a. Marginal keratitis.
b. It is not always possible to be certain but the overall clinical picture should be considered. Important points include: the relatively mild symptoms, the absence of predisposing factors such as contact lens wear, the distribution of the infiltrate in a band parallel to the limbus but separated by a clear zone. Typically the infiltrate is much larger than any associated epithelial defect. Chronic anterior blepharitis is

often present.

c. A short course of weak topical steroid (e.g. fluorometholone).

69. a. 前房积血，是严重钝挫伤的常见并发症；前房积血下沉形成“液平”。

b. 主要的危险是大量出血造成眼压升高，可导致永久性角膜血染。必须考虑到可能损伤眼球前节和后节结构。

c. 严格限制活动，有时需住院治疗。早期每日检查患者。其他的措施包括用阿托品散瞳，口服抗纤溶药物和治疗前葡萄膜炎或高眼压。

a. A hyphaema, a common complication of moderate to severe blunt trauma; blood in the anterior chamber which has settled to form a 'fluid level'.

b. The major risk is of a further bleed with resultant elevation of intraocular pressure, which can potentially lead to permanent corneal bloodstaining. Possible damage to anterior and posterior segment structures must also be assessed.

c. Activity is severely restricted, sometimes with hospital admission. The patient is initially reviewed daily. Other measures may include immobilization of the pupil with atropine, administration of an oral antifibrinolytic agent and treatment of anterior uveitis or raised pressure.

70. a. 角膜上皮擦伤。

b. 典型的严重的擦伤症状：明显的异物感，充血，流泪和畏光。自发的复发性上皮缺损常见（复发性剥脱综合征）。

c. 抗生素油膏，睫状肌麻痹剂可减轻不适，口服止痛药；大的擦伤，眼垫可减轻症状，但不能加速修复。有时用治疗性隐形眼镜。

a. A corneal abrasion.

b. Typically, the symptoms of an abrasion are severe: marked grittiness, redness, lacrimation and photophobia. Spontaneous recurrence of the epithelial defect is common (recurrent erosion syndrome).

c. Antibiotic ointment, cycloplegia to reduce discomfort, and oral analgesia; firm padding of the eye may improve comfort in a large abrasion but probably does not speed resolution. A bandage contact lens is sometimes used.

71. a. 单独左侧第三脑神经（动眼神经）麻痹。
b. 压迫性损害，明显的后交通动脉动脉瘤。
c. 根据临床特征，越来越多的怀疑是压迫性损害，包括累及瞳孔、头痛或眼痛、年轻和缺乏已知的血管危险因素，例如糖尿病。仔细的询问病史和检查另外的神经系统特点是必要的，如果条件适合可做CNS成像。第三脑神经麻痹的病因有许多；25% 是原发性的。

a. Isolated left third (oculomotor) cranial nerve palsy.
b. A compressive lesion, particularly posterior communicating artery aneurysm.
c. Clinical features increasing the level of suspicion of a compressive lesion include pupillary involvement, headache or ocular pain, younger patient age and absence of known vascular risk factors such as diabetes. A careful history and examination for additional neurological features is essential, followed by CNS imaging if appropriate. There is a wide range of causes of third nerve palsy; 25% are idiopathic.

72. a. 增殖性玻璃体视网膜病变（PVR）。
b. 玻璃体混浊和收缩；下半部视网膜可见色素细胞；视网膜裂孔缘卷曲；视网膜表面可见皱纹；视网膜全层皱襞；视网膜下的机化条索。
c. 睫状体平坦部玻璃体切割术，如果需要可用硅油填塞和剥“膜”——视网膜前膜的切除或剥离。

a. Proliferative vitreoretinopathy (PVR).
b. Vitreous haze and condensation; pigment cells on the inferior retina; rolling of the edges of retinal breaks; wrinkling of the inner retinal surface; full-thickness retinal folds; subretinal strands.
c. Pars plana vitrectomy, if necessary using silicone oil tamponade and peeling, segmentation or delamination of epiretinal membranes.

73. a. 玻璃体出血。
b. B 超检查，主要为排除视网膜脱离。
c. 包括增殖性视网膜病变（糖尿病性，视网膜静脉闭塞，Eales 病，早产儿视网膜病变，镰状细胞贫血病），玻璃体后脱离和视网膜撕裂，脉络膜新生血管突破性出血和外伤。

a. Vitreous haemorrhage.

b. B-scan ultrasonography, principally to exclude retinal detachment.
c. Examples include proliferative retinopathies (diabetic, retinal vein occlusion, Eales's disease, retinopathy of prematurity, sickle-cell disease), posterior vitreous detachment and retinal tears, 'break-through' bleeding from choroidal neovascularization, and trauma.

74. a. 黄斑视网膜前膜。厚的前膜为“黄斑皱褶”和薄膜的“透明纸样黄斑病变”。
b. 膜由在玻璃体视网膜交界处增生的视网膜神经胶质细胞组成，经由内界膜破口延伸至视网膜表面。
c. 视网膜手术和激光光凝，外伤性炎症和视网膜血管病变。

a. A macular epiretinal membrane. A dense membrane is usually referred to as 'macular pucker' and a thinner membrane 'cellophane maculopathy'.
b. Membranes consist of retinal glial cells proliferating at the vitreoretinal interface, having reached the retinal surface via breaks in the internal limiting membrane.
c. Retinal surgery and photocoagulation, trauma, inflammation and retinal vascular disease.

75. a. 灌注管（左下），导光纤维和玻璃体切除器。
b. • 孔源性视网膜脱离伴随下列病变：明显的 PVR，屈光间质混浊妨碍看清视网膜（玻璃体出血，晶状体后囊膜混浊），巨大视网膜撕裂和包括黄斑裂孔的后极裂孔。
• 牵引性视网膜脱离，常为糖尿病性或外伤性。
• 长期的玻璃体出血。
• 眼内异物取出。
• 严重的眼内炎。
• 年龄相关性黄斑裂孔。
• 黄斑变性：脉络膜新生血管膜切除，黄斑易位。

a. Infusion cannula (lower left), light pipe and vitreous cutter.
b. • Rhegmatogenous retinal detachment associated with the following: significant PVR, media opacity precluding adequate retinal view (vitreous haemorrhage, posterior lens capsular opacity), giant retinal tears and posterior breaks including macular holes.
• Tractional retinal detachment, usually diabetic or traumatic.
• Persistent vitreous haemorrhage.

- Removal of intraocular foreign body.
- Severe endophthalmitis.
- Age-related macular holes.
- Macular degeneration: excision of choroidal neovascular membranes, macular translocation.

76. a. 十岁复发性角膜上皮糜烂。
    b. 不规则排列的胶原带，Masson三重染色为蓝色，替代Bowman层的缺失。
    c. 常染色体显性遗传，基因位于 10q24。
    d. Reis-Bücklers营养不良（Bowman 层1型），其混浊呈蜂窝形，形成很小的突起。

    a. With recurrent erosions at the end of the first decade.
    b. Irregular bands of collagen, staining blue with Masson trichrome, replace the Bowman layer, which may even be absent.
    c. Autosomal dominant; the gene is located at 10q24.
    d. Reis-Bücklers dystrophy (Bowman layer type 1), in which the honeycomb pattern assumed by the opacities is considerably less prominent.

77. a. 右眼正常外转，但左眼外转受限，伴眼球回缩和睑裂缩小。诊断是左侧 Duane 综合征。
    b. 该患者为 Huber 分类 1 型：
       - Huber1 型：外转受限。
       - Huber2 型：内转受限。
       - Huber3 型：外转和内转均受限。
    c. 屈光参差，眼部组织缺损，小眼球和虹膜异色症。

    a. Normal right abduction but limited left abduction associated with retraction of the globe and narrowing of the palpebral fissure. The diagnosis is left Duane's retraction syndrome.
    b. This patient can be classified as Huber type 1:
       - Huber type 1: limited abduction
       - Huber type 2: limited adduction
       - Huber type 3: limited abduction and adduction.
    c. Anisometropia, coloboma, microphthalmos and heterochromia.

78. a. 视盘扩大，被低色素环环绕。新生血管呈放射状。漏斗形凹陷和含有白色神经胶质组织的中央轴。诊断是牵牛花综合征。

b. 大约 30%。

c. 少见：额鼻的发育异常（包含颜面和正中线神经上的异常情况）和多发性神经纤维瘤 2 型。

a. The disc is enlarged and is surrounded by a hypopigmented ring. The emerging blood vessels manifest a radial pattern. The excavation is funnel-shaped and contains a central core of whitish glial tissue. The diagnosis is morning glory anomaly.

b. Approximately 30%.

c. These are uncommon: frontonasal dysplasia, which includes facial and midline neurological abnormalities, and neurofibromatosis type 2.

79. a. 角膜地形图计算机成像："角膜地形图"或地图。

b. 角膜在不同位置的等高线；红色代表高的角膜部位，平坦的区域表现为蓝色。

c. 角膜外形的表现与圆锥形角膜一致。右眼圆锥体较低，顶端屈光度为 56 D；左侧圆锥体中心屈光度达到 63 D。

a. Computed corneal topographic imaging: 'corneal topography' or mapping.

b. The contour of the cornea at differing locations; colours at the red end of the scale are used to represent steep corneal regions, with the flattest areas shown as blue.

c. The contours demonstrated are consistent with keratoconus. In the right eye the cone is located inferiorly with dioptric values at the apex reaching 56D; in the left the cone is central with values up to 63D.

80. a. 重症肌无力。

b. 疲劳使上睑下垂加重。Cogan 眼睑颤动：重症肌无力患者从静止状态到原位的急促运动。冰试验：冰袋敷 2 分钟，上睑下垂减轻。

c. 乙酰胆碱受体抗体水平测定。

d. 滕喜隆（胆碱酯酶抑制剂）试验：在静脉注射药物后，上睑下垂和 / 或复视明显地暂时性缓解。

a. Myasthenia gravis.

b. Fatigue on sustained upgaze with worsening of ptosis. Cogan's lid twitch-overshoot on moving from depression to primary position in myasthenia. Ice test-reduced ptosis after ice pack applied for 2 minutes.

c. Acetylcholine receptor antibody levels.

d. Edrophonium (an anticholinesterase) testing: significant temporary improvement in ptosis and/or diplopia following intravenous administration.

81. a. 人工角膜或人工角膜移植片。

b. 角膜严重被损坏但是视网膜和视神经保留好的功能，常规的角膜移植术预后不良。

c. 眼内炎，青光眼，人工角膜后膜形成和人工角膜脱落。

a. A keratoprosthesis or artificial corneal implant.

b. When the cornea is severely damaged but the retina and optic nerve retain good function and conventional corneal grafting has an extremely poor prognosis.

c. Endophthalmitis, glaucoma, retroprosthesis membrane formation and extrusion.

82. a. 右侧白内障和虹膜异色症。检查可见星状的角膜后沉着物，可能为 Fuchs 综合征。

b. 青光眼和暂时性严重玻璃体混浊。

c. 局部应用类固醇无益而且促进青光眼和白内障形成。严重的玻璃体混浊眼周注射类固醇有用。

a. Right cataract and heterochromia iridis. These findings, together with the stellate keratic precipitates, suggest Fuchs' uveitis syndrome.

b. Glaucoma, and occasionally severe vitreous opacities.

c. Topical steroids are not beneficial and may promote glaucoma and cataract. Severe vitreous opacities may benefit from periocular steroid injection.

83. a. 明显的后囊膜浑浊。

b. 对比敏感度下降和眩光。

c. Nd：YAG 激光晶状体囊膜切开术。

d. 视网膜脱离，黄斑囊样水肿，晶状体脱位，眼压升高（常是暂时的），人工晶状体损伤和视物不连贯。

a. Significant posterior capsular opacification.

b. Reduced contrast sensitivity and glare.

c. Nd:YAG laser capsulotomy.

d. Retinal detachment, cystoid macular oedema, lens dislocation, intraocular pressure elevation (usually transient) and visually inconsequential pitting of the implant.

84. a. 下睑内翻。
b. 年龄相关性下睑松弛，下眼睑缩肌作用减弱，睑板和眶隔失去牵制眼轮匝肌的收缩作用，伴随眶脂肪脱出。
c. 术式取决于是否存在下睑松弛，包括单纯的外翻缝线术、Wies 法下睑切开术、下睑紧缩肌加固（Jones 术式）和下睑缩短术。

a. A lower lid entropion.
b. Age-related horizontal lid laxity, weakening of the effect of the lower lid retractors and over-riding of the pretarsal by the preseptal orbicularis oculi with associated prolapse of orbital fat.
c. Surgical options depend on the presence or absence of horizontal lid laxity and include simple everting sutures, the horizontal lid-splitting Wies procedure, inferior retractor tightening (Jones procedure) and horizontal lid shortening.

85. a. 大量的玻璃膜疣。
b. 荧光素眼底血管造影能显示CNV，并有助于决定是否需要治疗和采取什么形式的治疗。
c. 给予适当剂量具有特效的抗氧化维生素和矿物补充剂可减低患者 CNV 的风险，包括本病例。

a. Numerous large drusen.
b. Fundus fluorescein angiography would demonstrate CNV and aid in deciding whether treatment is indicated and what form this should take.
c. A specific antioxidant vitamin and mineral supplement regimen reduces the risk of CNV in patients fitting certain criteria, including the situation described.

86. a. 吲哚氰绿血管造影（ICG)；比荧光素眼底血管造影更有效地穿透血液和色素，因此ICG在某些情况下可以更好的显示视网膜的病变。
b. 色素上皮脱离（PED）ICG 晚期。
c. 退化的Bruch膜增厚，阻碍液体从视网膜色素上皮细胞（RPE）向脉络膜运输。
d. PED 无法治疗；激光光凝可造成 RPE 撕裂。有时可自愈。

a. Indocyanine green angiography (ICG); the wavelengths used penetrate blood and pigment more effectively than fluorescein angiography and ICG is therefore superior for investigating retinal pathology in some circumstances.
b. This is a late phase ICG of a pigment epithelial detachment (PED).
c. A thickened degenerate Bruch membrane may impede the transit of fluid from the retinal pigment epithelium (RPE) to the choroid.
d. There is no treatment for PEDs; laser photocoagulation may cause tearing of the RPE. Spontaneous resolution sometimes occurs.

87. a. 几个大的出血，出血中心部白色（Roth 斑），通常被认为是纤维蛋白栓子堵塞血管的裂口。
b. 该患者需要立刻检查。其他的原因包括贫血，细菌性心内膜炎，白细胞过多症和蛋白异常血症。
c. 其他的眼底改变包括棉绒斑，出血，周边视网膜新生血管形成，“豹纹”状眼底和视盘浸润。在该眼的其他部位可发生结膜下出血，眼眶浸润，虹膜炎，假性前房积脓和前房积血。

a. Several large haemorrhages with white centres (Roth spots) which usually represent fibrin emboli occluding ruptured blood vessels.
b. This patient requires urgent investigation. Other causes include anaemia, bacterial endocarditis, leukaemia and dysproteinaemia.
c. Other fundus changes include cotton wool spots, haemorrhages, peripheral retinal neovascularization, a 'leopard spot' fundus and infiltration of the optic nerve head. Elsewhere in the eye, subconjunctival haemorrhage, orbital involvement, iritis, pseudohypopyon and hyphaema may occur.

88. a. 明显的虹膜透光，极白的皮肤和头发，酪氨酸酶阴性。
b. 酪氨酸酶阴性的眼皮肤白化病患者除其他中央视路异常外，在视交叉处交叉的神经纤维数量减少。
c. Chediak-Higashi 综合征（白色 - 细胞 - 相关性免疫缺陷）和 Hermansky-Pudlak 综合征（溶酶体贮存病伴血小板功能缺陷）。
d. 没有，因为只有酪氨酸酶阳性的白化病才与这些综合征有关。

a. Given the marked iris transillumination and the extremely pale skin and hair, tyrosinase-negative.
b. Patients with tyrosinase-negative oculocutaneous albinism have a decreased number of crossing nerve fibres at the optic chiasm, as

well as other central visual pathway anomalies.

c. Chediak-Higashi syndrome (white-cell-related immunodeficiency) and Hermansky-Pudlak syndrome (a lysosomal storage disease with platelet dysfunction).

d. No, because only tyrosinase-positive albinism is associated with these syndromes.

89. a. 脉络膜视网膜萎缩区伴随视网膜色素上皮细胞增生。这种表现最可能的原因是陈旧性先天性弓形体病。

b. 通常青少年发病。然而在免疫缺陷，先天性获得性感染的复发或发生的新感染可在任何年龄发病。

c. 进行弓形体抗体血清学测定，可是滴定度与活性无关。应用玻璃体活检样本的多聚酶链式反应（PCR） DNA测定可以诊断。

a. An area of chorioretinal atrophy associated with retinal pigment epithelial hyperplasia. The most common cause of this appearance is old congenital toxoplasmosis.

b. Usually in the teens to thirties. In the immunocompromised, however, reactivation of congenitally acquired infection or acquisition of new infection commonly occurs at any age.

c. Serology for toxoplasma antibodies but the titre, however, does not correlate with activity. Polymerase chain reaction (PCR) DNA testing of a vitreous biopsy sample may be diagnostic.

90. a. 荧光素眼底血管造影片显示黄斑囊样水肿所特有的花瓣样强荧光图像。

b. 玻璃体从后段生理位置脱出进入眼前段，通常由于不慎使晶状体后囊膜或晶状体悬韧带破裂造成。

c. 增加黄斑囊样水肿、视网膜脱离、眼内炎、葡萄膜炎、青光眼、角膜失代偿和人工晶状体错位的危险。

a. A fluorescein angiogram showing the petalloid hyperfluorescent pattern characteristic of cystoid macular oedema.

b. The prolapse of vitreous gel into the anterior segment from its physiological location in the posterior segment, usually by inadvertent rupture of the posterior capsule or zonules.

c. Increased risk of cystoid macular oedema, retinal detachment, endophthalmitis, uveitis, glaucoma, corneal decompensation and lens implant dislocation.

91. a. 术中放置的硅胶外植块穿透结膜。

b. 在这个阶段可以安全的取出外植块而不会再次脱离。在最初的几个月取出会有 5% ~ 10% 再脱离的风险。

c. 在无菌条件下：如果外植块很松只需从该位置拉出、剪去；如果帖附很牢固，必须切开结膜取出 。

a. A silicone explant, placed during the surgery, has eroded through the conjunctiva.

b. At this stage, it should be safe to remove the explant without precipitating re-detachment. Removal in the first few months, however, carries a 5-10% risk.

c. Under sterile conditions: if very loose, the explant can simply be lifted gently out of its position and any visible sutures trimmed; if firmly attached, conjunctival dissection and suture release is necessary.

92. a. 肉芽肿性葡萄膜炎特有的大的（“羊脂状”）角膜后沉着物。

b. 是的。除外以前存在的确定的全身性疾病，常常考虑肉芽肿性葡萄膜炎。

c. 适当的初期筛查可能包括全血细胞计数、ESR、血清血管紧张素转换酶、梅毒血清学和胸部X线检查（例如肺结核、肉状瘤病）。

a. Large ('mutton fat') keratic precipitates characteristic of granulomatous uveitis.

b. Yes. Granulomatous uveitis should always be investigated, except in the presence of a previously established systemic illness.

c. Where appropriate, initial screening might include a full blood count, ESR, serum angiotensin-converting enzyme, syphilis serology and chest X-ray (e.g. tuberculosis, sarcoidosis).

93. a. 成骨不全。1 型和 2 型伴随蓝巩膜。

b. 蓝色外观是由于胶原异常导致巩膜较薄。

c. 主要包括Ehlers-Danlos综合征（通常是6型，虽然蓝巩膜在其他的类型被报告过），弹性假黄瘤（显性基因2型），Turner综合征。

a. Osteogenesis imperfecta. Types 1 and 2 are associated with blue sclera.

b. The blue appearance is caused by a collagen abnormality leading to relative scleral transparency.

c. The more important include Ehlers-Danlos syndrome (usually type 6, although blue sclera has been reported in other types), pseudoxanthoma elasticum (dominant type 2), and Turner's syndrome.

94. a. 大范围脉络膜视网膜萎缩，近视性黄斑病变。

b. 其他的黄斑改变包括脉络膜新生血管形成（CNV）、没有CNV的出血、漆裂纹样病变（其诱发CNV）、黄斑裂孔和色素增殖（Fuchs斑）。高度近视眼是视网膜脱离、白内障和青光眼的诱因。

c. 接近 30 mm。

a. Extensive chorioretinal atrophy, a form of myopic maculopathy.

b. Other macular changes include choroidal neovascularization (CNV), haemorrhage without CNV, lacquer cracks (which predispose to CNV), macular hole and pigment proliferation (Fuchs spot). Highly myopic eyes have a predisposition to retinal detachment, cataract and glaucoma.

c. Nearer 30 mm.

95. a. 激光原位角膜磨镶术（LASIK），带蒂的角膜瓣是从角膜表面切口，准分子激光消融术是在暴露的基质上完成，角膜瓣被放回原位。

b. 是的，但只有有限的范围：大约 4 D 的远视和 5 D 的散光。

c. 角膜瓣出现孔和角膜穿孔；术后感染，无菌的弥漫板层角膜炎（DLK或“撒哈拉沙漠样改变”），角膜瓣错位或皱褶，永久的上皮缺损和上皮在角膜瓣下生长。

a. Laser in-situ keratomileusis (LASIK), in which a hinged flap as shown is cut from the corneal surface, excimer laser ablation is performed on the exposed stroma and the flap is replaced.

b. Yes, but only to a limited extent: approximately 4D of hypermetropia and 5D of astigmatism.

c. Operative buttonholing of the flap and corneal perforation; postoperative infection, sterile diffuse lamellar keratitis (DLK or 'sands of the Sahara'), flap dislocation or wrinkling, persistent epithelial defects and epithelial ingrowth under the flap.

96. a. 表层巩膜炎（确切地说是单纯的扇形表层巩膜炎，常见类型）。

b. 单纯性或结节性；单纯性可为扇形或弥漫的。

c. 与巩膜炎相反，不需要全身性检查，因为伴随全身性疾病的患病率是极低的。

d. 轻症是自限的，不需要治疗。严重或持续性病例有时需要局部应用类固醇或口服非甾体抗炎药。

a. Episcleritis (strictly simple sectorial episcleritis, the commonest type).
b. Simple or nodular; the former may be sectorial or diffuse.
c. In contrast to scleritis, systemic investigation is not appropriate because the prevalence of an associated systemic disease is extremely low.
d. Mild cases are self-limiting and require no treatment. Topical steroids or oral non-steroidal anti-inflammatory drugs are sometimes needed in severe or persistent cases.

97. a. 自发的结膜下出血（SCH）。
b. 轻度不适。
c. 测血压，因为高血压患者自发的 SCH 是无高血压者的两倍。即使出血在相同位置复发，不需要做更多的检查。如果累及双眼或怀疑其他的出血原因，应该考虑更多的诊断。

a. A spontaneous subconjunctival haemorrhage (SCH).
b. Mild discomfort.
c. Blood pressure should be checked, because spontaneous SCH is twice as common in patients with hypertension as those without. No further investigation is necessary, even if bleeding should recur at the same site. If both eyes are involved or there is other cause for suspicion of a bleeding diathesis, further assessment might be considered.

98. a. 黄斑中心的浆液性视网膜病变，视网膜感觉神经层局限性脱离。
b. 大约 6/12，戴薄的“正”（凸面）透镜会好转。
c. 荧光素眼底血管造影可显示墨渍样渗漏或烟囱样喷出的渐增的强荧光。

a. A localized detachment of the neurosensory retina at the macula-central serous retinopathy.
b. Approximately 6/12, characteristically improved by a weak 'plus' (convex) lens.
c. Fundus fluorescein angiography will usually demonstrate an 'ink-blot' or 'smoke-stack' pattern of increasing hyperfluorescence.

99. a. 间歇性外斜视。

b. 基本型外斜视，看近和看远斜视角相同；集合不足型，看近的斜视角大于看远的；外展过强型，看远的斜视角大于看近的。

c. 与所有的斜视一样，屈光检查是第一步，然后行屈光间质和眼底诊查。眼镜矫正近视可刺激调节以控制斜视。视轴矫正治疗有时有效，但是经常需要手术。

a. Intermittent exotropia.

b. Basic exotropia, in which the angle is the same for near and distance; convergence weakness, where the deviation is greater for near; divergence excess, with a greater deviation for distance.

c. As with all squints, media and fundus examination followed by refraction is the initial step. Spectacle correction of myopia may stimulate accommodation such that the squint is controlled. Orthoptic treatment is sometimes effective but surgery is frequently necessary.

100. a. 在矫正屈光不正后，排除视路病变出现的视力持续不好。

b. 弱视通常发生在斜视，在发育的关键阶段从斜视眼来的图像被大脑抑制。屈光参差（双眼间屈光差异），形觉剥夺（白内障）和屈光不正（双眼高度屈光不正）也可引起弱视。

c. 多重因素决定，根据父母和孩子的诱因和其他的因素，但是通常斜视性弱视为 7 ~ 8 岁，屈光参差可以到 12 岁。

a. Defective visual acuity persisting after correction of refractive error and removal of visual pathway pathology, if present.

b. Amblyopia commonly occurs in association with strabismus, when the image from the deviating eye is suppressed by the brain during the critical developmental period. It can also be caused by anisometropia (difference in refraction between the eyes), stimulus deprivation (cataract) and ametropia (bilateral high refractive error).

c. This varies according to parent and child motivation and other factors, but is probably around 7-8 years in strabismic amblyopia and up to 12 years for anisometropic.

101. a. K-F 环。

b. 铜沉积在后弹力层周边。

c. Wilson病（肝豆状核变性），铜代谢紊乱使得血浆铜蓝蛋白缺乏。

d. 前囊膜葵花状白内障。

e. 肝病和基底核机能障碍。

a. A Kayser-Fleischer ring.

b. Deposition of copper granules in the peripheral region of Descemet's membrane.

c. Wilson's disease, an abnormality of copper metabolism caused by a deficiency of caeruloplasmin.

d. Anterior capsular 'sunflower' cataract.

e. Liver disease and basal ganglia dysfunction.

102. a. 角膜呈现以瞳孔为中心的分枝状、漩涡状图案，由极细的沉着物在上皮内组成：漩涡状角膜病或涡状角膜营养不良。

b. 胺碘酮。

c. 事实上所有服用胺碘酮的患者都会发生角膜的改变。

d. 其他的药包括氯奎和羟氯喹。Fabry病（磷脂沉着综合征），糖脂贮积病也可形成漩涡状角膜病。

a. The cornea shows a branching, whorled pattern with its centre located inferior to the pupil, consisting of very fine deposits within the epithelium: vortex keratopathy or cornea verticillata.

b. Amiodarone.

c. Virtually all patients receiving amiodarone develop corneal changes.

d. Other drugs include chloroquine and hydroxychloroquine. Fabry's disease, a glycolipidosis, is also associated with vortex keratopathy.

103. a. 不对。圆锥角膜极不可能发生在这个年龄。

b. 特定地累及角膜周边而不是中心会使眼科医生考虑该位置好发的疾病。

c. 考虑该患者的病历，没有全身性疾病，没有累及双眼和角膜外观的炎症，可能是 Terrien 边缘性变性。这种病变是罕见的角膜周边原发性无痛变薄：对视力的主要影响是散光。

a. No. Keratoconus is extremely unlikely to present at this age.

b. Involvement specifically of the peripheral rather than central cornea leads the ophthalmologist towards a number of defined conditions having a predilection for this site.

c. Taking account of the patient's gender, absence of known systemic disease, absence of inflammation, involvement of both eyes and the appearance of the cornea, this is likely to be Terrien's marginal degeneration. This condition is an uncommon idiopathic painless thinning of the peripheral cornea; the main visual effect is astigmatism.

104. a. 轴性突眼。
b. 海绵状血管瘤。70% 发生在女性，大多数位于肌圆锥内。
c. 视盘水肿或苍白，脉络膜褶和眼球运动障碍。
d. 手术切除；肿瘤通常有完整的包膜。

a. Axial proptosis.
b. Cavernous haemangioma. 70% of these occur in women and the majority are located within the muscle cone.
c. Optic disc swelling or pallor, choroidal folds and ocular motility disturbance.
d. Surgical excision; the tumour is usually well encapsulated.

105. a. B超检查，组织扫描的二维图像。A超检查为一维扫描，主要用于计算人工晶状体度数。
b. 视盘的高密度信号，符合视盘玻璃疣，这是假性视盘水肿的原因。
c. 荧光素眼底血管造影将证明视盘表面自身荧光，真性视盘水肿没有渗漏。CT 扫描将显示玻璃疣的钙化。

a. B-scan ultrasonography, which produces a two-dimensional section of the tissue scanned. A-scan ultrasonography produces a one-dimensional scan and is principally used in biometric calculation of intraocular lens implant power.
b. A hyperdense signal is evident at the optic nerve head, consistent with optic disc drusen, a cause of pseudopapilloedema.
c. Fluorescein angiography will demonstrate autofluorescence of superficial disc drusen and absence of leakage that would occur in true disc swelling. CT scanning will show any calcification of the drusen.

106. a. 进行性虹膜萎缩，是虹膜角膜内皮（ICE）综合征的变异体，特征的角膜内皮细胞异常增殖越过前房角和虹膜。
b. 虹膜痣（Cogan-Reese）综合征，以弥漫的虹膜痣伴随虹膜萎缩为特征者大约占 50%；Chandler 综合征，主要是角膜病变。

c. 大约50%。

a. Progressive iris atrophy, a variant of iridocorneal endothelial (ICE) syndrome, characterized by a proliferation of abnormal corneal endothelial cells across the anterior chamber angle and iris.
b. Iris naevus (Cogan-Reese) syndrome, characterized by a diffuse iris naevus with associated iris atrophy in about 50% of cases, and Chandler's syndrome, in which corneal changes predominate.
c. Approximately 50%.

107. a. 瞳孔移位（瞳孔异位），虹膜全层缺损（假多瞳症）和白内障。
b. Rieger 综合征，Axenfeld-Rieger 综合征的变异体。
c. 常染色体显性遗传；涉及的基因包括6p25染色体的*FOXC1*基因，4q25 染色体的 *PITX2* 基因。
d. 大约 50%，通常在儿童期或青少年。

a. A displaced pupil (corectopia), full-thickness iris defects (pseudopolycoria) and cataract.
b. Rieger's syndrome, a variant of the Axenfeld-Rieger syndrome.
c. Inheritance is autosomal dominant; genes implicated include *FOXC1* on chromosome 6p25, and *PITX2* on chromosome 4q25.
d. About 50%, usually during childhood or early adulthood.

108. a. 大量前房积脓。
b. 细菌性眼内炎。
c. 最初，玻璃体活检和玻璃体腔内注射抗生素。局部眼周注射和全身应用抗生素的益处不清楚，但经常使用。全身应用类固醇常常用于减轻炎症。只有当视力降至“光感”才采用玻璃体切割术。

a. A large hypopyon.
b. Bacterial endophthalmitis.
c. Initially, vitreous biopsy and intravitreal antibiotics. The benefit of topical, periocular injection and systemic antibiotics is not clear, but are often used. Systemic steroids are often given to reduce inflammation. Vitrectomy is of benefit only if vision is reduced to 'light perception'.

109. a. 克鲁肯贝格梭。
b. 色素播散综合征。

c. 大多数患者是近视。
d. 50% 最后发展为青光眼。

a. A Krukenberg spindle.
b. Pigment dispersion syndrome.
c. Most patients with this condition are myopic.
d. Up to 50% of patients may eventually develop glaucoma.

110. a. 睑缘皮肤变厚、变红和毛细血管扩张，睫毛周围结痂和鳞屑，睫毛根部更明显。
b. 该患者有前睑缘炎，大部分为葡萄球菌型。
c. 治疗：严格的每日保持眼睑卫生，局部应用润滑剂，睑缘涂抹抗生素油膏，间断的全身应用抗生素（例如四环素，强力霉素）和局部应用小剂量类固醇。

a. Thickening, reddening and telangiectasia of the lid margin skin, with crusting and scaling around the lashes, particularly at the bases.
b. This patient has anterior blepharitis, predominantly of the staphylococcal type.
c. An approximate ascending hierarchy of treatment: rigorous daily lid hygiene regimen, topical lubricants, lid margin antibiotic ointment, intermittent systemic antibiotics (e.g. tetracycline, doxycycline) and weak topical steroids.

111. a. 角巩膜的穿通伤伴浅前房。
b. 理想的CT扫描应该可以排除眼球内或眶内的异物。应该在几小时内初期缝合伤口以恢复眼球壁完整和预防感染；应该仔细寻找隐蔽的伤口。适当给予抗生素。记录生命体征的变化，任何危及生命的损伤处理要首先进行。

a. A corneoscleral penetrating injury with a flat anterior chamber.
b. Ideally, CT scanning should be carried out to exclude an intraocular or intraorbital foreign body. Primary wound repair should be undertaken within a few hours with the intention of restoring the integrity of the eye wall and preventing infection; a careful search for occult wounds should be carried out as part of the procedure. Antibiotics are administered as appropriate. It should be remembered that systemic stabilization and management of any life-threatening injuries has priority.

112. a. Nd：YAG（钕：钇-铝-石榴石）虹膜切开术。

b. 突然和严重的眼压升高造成角膜水肿使得间断的原发房角关闭（包括高褶型虹膜综合征）、Posner-Schlossmann 综合征（青光眼-睫状体炎综合征危象）、色素播散综合征、疱疹性角膜色素膜炎和临时地假性剥脱性青光眼。

c. 晶状体囊切开术，前房内玻璃体条索切开和玻璃体后面切开以消除黄斑前血液。

a. Nd:YAG (neodymium: yttrium-aluminium-garnet) iridotomy.

b. A sudden and severe spike in intraocular pressure sufficient to cause corneal oedema can be caused by intermittent subacute primary angle-closure (including plateau iris syndrome), Posner-Schlossmann syndrome, pigment dispersion syndrome, herpetic keratouveitis and occasionally pseudoexfoliative glaucoma.

c. Capsulotomy, disruption of vitreous strands in the anterior chamber and disruption of the posterior hyaloid face to disperse premacular blood.

113. a. 角膜网络状营养不良 3 型或 3a 型；前者很可能是常染色体隐性遗传，后者常染色体显性遗传。

b. 不是。

c. 大多数需改善视力的病例必须全层角膜移植。

d. 1型（Biber-Haab-Dimmer），十岁内发病伴复发性角膜上皮糜烂；2型（Meretoja综合征），全身性淀粉样变性，中年发病伴面瘫并累及角膜。

a. Lattice dystrophy type 3 or 3a; the former is probably of autosomal recessive inheritance and the latter autosomal dominant.

b. No.

c. This is necessary in most cases to improve vision.

d. Type 1 (Biber-Haab-Dimmer), which presents in the first decade with recurrent erosions, and Type 2 (Meretoja's syndrome), a systemic amyloidosis that presents in middle age with facial palsy and corneal involvement.

114. a. 早产儿视网膜病变。

b. 1 期：血管化与非血管化视网膜之间有一条清楚的分界线。

2 期：分界线变成嵴。

3 期：视网膜外的纤维血管增殖（见插图）。

4 期：次全视网膜脱离。

5 期：完全视网膜脱离。

Plus 病：后极血管扩张，玻璃体混浊，瞳孔强直。

c. 疾病阈界定，包括 3 期和 Plus 病累及 5 个连续的时钟位或 8 个非连续的时钟位。4 期与 5 期应行手术。

d. 无（毛细）血管区激光或冷冻疗法。

a. Retinopathy of prematurity.

b. Stage 1: Demarcation line at the border of vascularized and avascular retina

Stage 2: Ridge at the same site

Stage 3: Extraretinal fibrovascular proliferation (shown in the illustration)

Stage 4: Subtotal retinal detachment

Stage 5: Total retinal detachment

Plus disease: Posterior pole vascular engorgement, vitreous haze, poor mydriasis.

c. Threshold disease, consisting of five contiguous or eight non-contiguous clock-hours of stage 3 together with 'plus' disease. Surgery may be carried out for stage 4 or 5.

d. Laser or cryotherapy to the avascular area.

115. a. 测量血压，因为该体征提示严重的高血压性视网膜病变。

b. 因为沉着物位于视网膜的Henle纤维层，沿着纤维的排列分布。

c. 渗出性视网膜脱离（特别是妊高征），Elschnig 斑（局部的脉络膜梗死）和 Siegrist 斑（沿脉络膜血管分布的斑点指示类纤维蛋白坏死）。

a. Measurement of the blood pressure because the signs are highly suggestive of severe hypertensive retinopathy.

b. Because the deposits are located in the retinal layer of Henle and follow the fibre arrangement accordingly.

c. Exudative retinal detachment (particularly in toxaemia of pregnancy), Elschnig spots (focal choroidal infarcts), and Siegrist streaks, (flecks along choroidal vessels indicating fibrinoid necrosis).

116. a. 虹膜结节。

b. 多发性神经纤维瘤 -1 型。

c. 眼睑神经纤维瘤、青光眼、视神经胶质瘤、睑外翻、突出的角膜神经、脉络膜痣与黑色素瘤、视网膜星形细胞瘤和蝶骨眶部的脑膨出。

d. 常染色体显性与不规则的外显率以及表现变异性；基因位点是染色体 17q11。

a. Lisch nodules.

b. Neurofibromatosis-1.

c. Eyelid neurofibroma, glaucoma, optic nerve glioma, ectropion uveae, prominent corneal nerves, choroidal naevi and melanomas, retinal astrocytomas, and spheno-orbital encephalocele.

d. Autosomal dominant with irregular penetrance and variable expressivity; the gene locus is on chromosome 17q11.

117. a. 频率倍增视野检查法的输出纸带（通常指的是频率倍增技术，FDT）。

b. FDT 特异靶器官是大细胞性的神经节细胞，即青光眼早期受损的细胞。其利用低空间频率光栅感受暂时高频逆转引起的频率倍增幻觉。

c. 比常规的自动视野检查法更快，更早。

a. A printout of frequency-doubling perimetry (commonly referred to as frequency-doubling technology, FDT).

b. FDT specifically targets the magnocellular ganglion cells, which are damaged early on in the course of glaucoma. It does this by utilizing the illusion of frequency doubling produced by a low spatial frequency grating undergoing high temporal frequency reversal.

c. It is much quicker and easier to perform than conventional automated perimetry.

118. a. Salzmann 结节性变性。

b. 沙眼是该患者可能的诱因。

c. 常常不需要治疗。如果眼部不适，局部可用润滑剂。重症需角膜表层切除术或板层角膜移植术。

a. Salzmann's nodular degeneration.

b. Trachoma is the likely cause in this patient.

c. Often, no treatment is required. If the eyes are irritable, topical lubricants can be used. Superficial keratectomy or lamellar keratoplasty may be necessary in severe cases.

119. a. 睑板腺囊肿，阻塞的睑板腺对蓄积的分泌物的肉芽肿炎性反应。
b. 结膜肉芽肿。
c. 睑板腺囊肿可自然消退。长期病变通常行切除术，个别的可行局部类固醇注射。急性炎症或感染病灶需局部的或全身的抗生素治疗。

a. A chalazion, which is caused by a granulomatous inflammatory reaction to accumulated secretions in a blocked meibomian gland.
b. A conjunctival granuloma.
c. Chalazia may resolve spontaneously. Persistent lesions are usually treated by curettage and, rarely, by local steroid injection. Topical or systemic antibiotics may be required for an acutely inflamed or infected lesion.

120. a. 有髓神经纤维。
b. 由于视盘周围的病变出现生理暗点扩大，神经末梢损害可出现相应的视野缺损。可伴有近视和弱视，黄斑受累。伴有视网膜血管的异常者罕见。
c. 有髓纤维表示起因于异位的少突神经胶质细胞的迷芽瘤。
d. 大约 1%。

a. Myelinated nerve fibres.
b. An enlarged blind spot may be present with a peripapillary lesion, and peripheral lesions may give corresponding field defects. Myopia and amblyopia may be associated, and symptomatic macular involvement has been reported. Rarely, associated retinal vascular abnormalities can be present.
c. Myelinated fibres may represent a choristoma resulting from ectopic oligodendrocytes.
d. About 1%.

相关词汇英中对照

A

Abducens nerve palsy	展神经麻痹
Abrasion, corneal	角膜剥脱
Acanthamoeba keratitis	棘阿米巴角膜
Acetazolamide	乙酰唑胺
Acquired maculopathies	后天性黄斑病变
Actinic keratosis	光化性角化病
Acute allergic conjunctivitis	急性变态反应性结膜炎
Acute multifocal posterior placoid pigment epitheliopathy (AMPPPE)	急性后部多发鳞状色素上皮病（AMPPPE）
Adenoma sebaceum	皮脂腺瘤
Adenoviral conjunctivitis	腺病毒性结膜炎
Age-related macular degeneration	年龄相关性黄斑退行性改变
AIDS, molluscum contagiosum in	传染性软疣
Albinism	白化病
Amaurosis fugax	一过性黑矇
Amblyopia	弱视
Amiodarone, corneal deposits in	胺碘酮，角膜沉积物
Angioid streaks	血管样条纹症
Angle-recession glaucoma	房角退缩性青光眼
Aniridia	无虹膜
Ankyloblepharon	融合睑
Antioxidants	抗氧化剂
Antiviral agents	抗病毒剂
Artificial corneal implant (keratoprosthesis)	人工角膜移植片（人工角膜）
Astigmatism correction	散光矫正
Astrocytoma, retinal	视网膜星形细胞瘤
Atopic keratoconjunctivitis	特应性的角膜结膜炎
Axenfeld-Rieger syndrome	Axenfeld-Rieger 综合征

B

Bacterial conjunctivitis	细菌性结膜炎
Bacterial endophthalmitis	细菌性眼内炎

Bacterial keratitis	细菌性角膜炎
Band keratopathy	带状角膜病
Basal cell carcinoma	基底细胞癌
Basal cell papilloma	基底细胞乳头状瘤
Behçet's disease	Behçet 病
Best's disease	先天性黄斑变性
Biber-Haab-Dimmer degeneration	Biber-Haab-Dimmer 退化
Bielschowsky test	Bielschowsky 试验
Birdshot retinochoroidopathy	鸟枪弹样视网膜脉络膜病
Blepharitis	睑缘炎
Blepharophimosis syndrome	睑裂狭小综合征
Blow-out fracture	爆裂骨折
Blue sclera	蓝巩膜
Blunt trauma	钝挫伤
Bournville's disease	Bournville 病
Bowman layer dystrophies	Bowman 层角膜营养不良
Brown's syndrome	Brown 综合征（上斜肌鞘综合征）
Bull's eye maculopathy	Bull 黄斑病变
Buphthalmos	牛眼

C

Candidal keratitis	念珠菌属角膜炎
'Candlewax drippings'	白线
Capillary haemangioma	毛细血管瘤
eyelid	眼睑
orbit	眼眶
retina	视网膜
Capsular opacification	后囊膜浑浊
Carotid-cavernous fistula	颈动脉海绵窦瘘
Cataract	白内障
age-related	年龄相关的
infantile	婴儿的
secondary	继发的
Cataract surgery	白内障手术
complications	并发症
methods	方法

Cavernous haemangioma	海绵状血管瘤
Orbit	眼眶
retina	视网膜
Cellulitis, orbital	眶蜂窝织炎
Central serous retinopathy	中心性浆液性视网膜病
Chalazion (meibomian cyst)	霰粒肿（睑板腺囊肿）
Chandler's syndrome	Chandler 综合征
Chediak-Higashi syndrome	Chediak-Higashi 综合征
Cherry-red spot	樱桃红斑
Chlamydial conjunctivitis	衣原体性结膜炎
Choristoma, conjunctival	结膜迷芽瘤
Choroid	脉络膜
detachment	脱离
dystrophies	营养不良
folds	褶
haemangioma	血管瘤
melanoma	黑色素瘤
metastatic carcinoma	转移癌
naevus	痣
neovascularization (CNV)	新生血管形成（CNV）
osteoma	骨瘤
rupture	破裂
Choroideremia	无脉络膜
Choroidopathy, serpiginous	匐行性脉络膜病变
Cicatricial pemphigoid	瘢痕性类天疱疮
Cicatrizing conjunctivitis	结膜瘢痕
Clinically significant macular oedema (CSMO)	临床上明显的黄斑水肿（CSMO）
Cogan microcystic dystrophy	Cogan 微囊肿性角膜营养不良
Cogan-Reese syndrome	Cogan-Reese 综合征（虹膜痣综合征）
Cogan's lid twitch	Cogan 眼睑颤动
Collier's sign	Collier 征
Coloboma	缺损
lens	晶状体
optic disc	视盘
Commotio retinae	视网膜震荡

Computed corneal topographic imaging	角膜地形图
Congenital hypertrophy of the retinal pigment epithelium (CHRPE)	视网膜色素上皮细胞先天性肥大（CHRPE）
Congenital syphilis	先天性梅毒
Conjunctival and corneal intra-epithelial neoplasia (CCIN)	结膜和角膜上皮癌 （CCIN）
Conjunctival tumours	结膜肿瘤
Conjunctivitis	结膜炎
acute	急性
chronic	慢性
cicatrizing	瘢痕
Cornea	角膜
abrasion	上皮缺损
dystrophies	营养不良
epithelial basement membrane dystrophy	上皮基底膜营养不良
foreign body trauma	异物伤
graft	移植
herpes simplex infection	单纯疱疹感染
implant	移植片
pannus	血管翳
size and shape disorders	大小和形状异常
suppurative keratitis	化脓性角膜炎
topographic mapping	地图形
ulceration	溃疡
verticillata	漩涡状
Cotton-wool spots	棉絮状斑
'Cupid's bow' (pseudogerontoxon)	"弓形" 病变（假性老年环）
Cyst of Moll	Moll 腺囊肿
Cystoid macular oedema	黄斑水肿
Cyst of Zeis	Zeis 腺囊肿
Cytomegalovirus retinitis	巨细胞病毒（CMV）性视网膜炎

D

Dacryocystorhinostomy	泪囊鼻腔造孔术
Dellen, corneal	角膜小凹
Dermoid, limbal	角膜缘皮样囊肿

Dermoid cyst	皮样囊肿
Diabetic maculopathy	糖尿病性黄斑病变
Diabetic retinopathy	糖尿病性视网膜病变
Disciform keratitis	盘状角膜炎
Distichiasis	双行睫
Drusen	玻璃疣
macular	黄斑
optic disc	视盘
Dry eye	干眼
Duane's syndrome	Duane 综合征

E

Ectopia lentis	晶状体异位
Ectropion	睑外翻
Eczema of the eyelids	眼睑湿疹
Edrophonium test	滕喜隆试验
Electroretinography	视网膜电图
Elschnig spots	Elschnig 斑
Entropion	睑内翻
Episcleritis	表层巩膜炎
Esotropia	内斜视
Exotropia	外斜视
External hordeolum (stye)	外睑腺炎（麦粒肿）
Exudative retinal detachment	渗出性视网膜脱离
Eyelid	眼睑
benign tumours	良性肿瘤
ectropion	睑外翻
entropion	睑内翻
non-neoplastic lumps	非新生性肿物
premalignant and malignant tumours	癌前病变和恶性肿瘤
see also Blepharitis; Ptosis	见睑缘炎，上睑下垂

F

Fabry's disease	Fabry 病
Foreign body trauma	异物伤
Fourth nerve palsy	第四脑神经麻痹
Frequency-doubling technology (FDT)	倍增频率技术（FDT）

Fuchs' endothelial dystrophy	Fuchs 角膜营养不良
Fuchs' spot	Fuchs 斑
Fuchs' uveitis syndrome	Fuchs 眼葡萄膜炎综合征
Fundal dystrophies	眼底营养不良
Fundus flavimaculatus	黄点状眼底
Fungal keratitis	真菌性角膜炎

G

Giant cell arteritis	巨细胞性动脉炎
Giant papillary conjunctivitis	巨乳头性结膜炎
Gillespie's syndrome	Gillespie 综合征
Glaucoma	青光眼
angle-closure	闭角
primary	原发的
secondary	继发的
congenital	先天性的
developmental	发育的
drainage device	引流物
neovascular	新生血管性
normal-tension	正常眼压性
open-angle	开角
pigmentary	色素的
primary	原发的
pseudoexfoliation	假鳞片样脱皮
secondary	继发的
Glaukomflecken	青光眼性白内障
Granular dystrophy	颗粒状营养不良
Granulomatous uveitis	肉芽肿性葡萄膜炎
Grönblad-Strandberg syndrome	Grönblad-Strandberg 综合征
Gyrate atrophy	脉络膜视网膜回旋形萎缩

H

Haab striae	哈布纹
Haemangioma	血管瘤
choroidal	脉络膜的
retinal	视网膜的
see also Capillary haemangioma; Cavernous haemangioma	见毛细血管瘤；海绵状血管瘤

Haemorrhage	出血
anterior chamber (hyphaema)	前房（前方积血）
in hypertensive retinopathy	在高血压性视网膜病变
retinal, in diabetic retinopathy	在糖尿病性视网膜病变
in retinal vein occlusion	在视网膜静脉闭塞
spontaneous subconjunctival	自发结膜下的
vitreous	玻璃体
Hay fever conjunctivitis	枯草热性结膜炎
Hering's law	Hering 定律
Hermansky-Pudlak syndrome	Hermansky-Pudlak 综合征
Herpes simplex infection	感染单纯疱疹
Herpes zoster ophthalmicus	眼（部）带状疱疹
Hess chart	Hess 屏
Histoplasmosis	组织胞浆菌病
Horner's syndrome	Horner 综合征
Hutchinson's sign	Hutchinson 征
Hypermetropia correction	远视矫正
Hypertensive retinopathy	高血压视网膜病变
Hyphaema	前方积血

I

Ice test	冰试验
Idiopathic intracranial hypertension	原发性颅内高血压
Idiopathic orbital inflammation (pseudotumour)	原发性眼眶炎症（假斑疹伤寒）
Indocyanine green angiography	吲哚氰绿血管造影
Infantile cataract	婴儿白内障
Infective keratitis	感染性角膜炎
Internal hordeolum (acute chalazion)	睑腺炎 （急性霰粒肿）
Internuclear ophthalmoplegia	核间性眼肌麻痹
Intraocular lens implant (IOL)	人工晶状体
Iridocorneal dysgenesis	虹膜角膜的畸形
Iridocorneal endothelial (ICE) syndrome	虹膜角膜内皮（ICE）综合征
Iridodialysis	虹膜根部断离
Iridoschisis	虹膜缺损
Iris	虹膜
atrophy	萎缩

melanoma	黑色素瘤
see also Aniridia	也见无虹膜
Iris naevus syndrome	虹膜痣综合征
Iritis	虹膜炎
Ischaemic central retinal vein occlusion	缺血性视网膜中央静脉阻塞
Ischaemic optic neuropathy	缺血性视神经病变

J

Juvenile idiopathic arthritis	青少年原发性关节炎

K

Kasabach-Merritt syndrome	Kasabach-Merritt 综合征
Kayser-Fleischer ring	K-F 环
Kearns-Sayre syndrome	Kearns-Sayre 综合征
Keratic precipitates	角膜后沉着物
Keratitis	角膜炎
contact lens-related	接触晶状体相关性
fungal	真菌的
herpes simplex	单纯疱疹
herpes zoster	带状疱疹
interstitial	基质性
marginal	边缘性
pseudomonas	假单胞菌
rosacea	红斑痤疮
suppurative	化脓性
Keratoacanthoma	角化棘皮瘤
Keratoconjunctivitis	角（膜）结膜炎
atopic	特异反应性
sicca	干燥的
vernal	春季的
Keratoconus	圆锥角膜
Keratoglobus	大角膜
Keratoprosthesis	人工角膜
Keratosis, actinic	光化性角化病
Krukenberg spindle	克鲁肯贝格梭

L

Lacrimal system probing	泪道探通
Laser in-situ keratomileusis (LASIK)	激光原位角膜磨镶术（LASIK）
Lattice dystrophies	角膜网络状营养不良
Lens disorders	晶状体病
see also Cataracts	也见白内障
Leukaemia	白血病
Leukocoria	白瞳
Limbal dermoid	睑缘皮样囊肿
Lipodermoid	脂质皮样囊肿
Lisch nodules	虹膜结节

M

Macular degeneration *see* Age-related macular degeneration	黄斑变性，见年龄相关性黄斑退行性改变
Macular epiretinal membrane	黄斑前膜
Macular hole	黄斑裂孔
Macular oedema	黄斑水肿
clinically significant	临床上明显的
cystoid	囊样的
Maculopathy	黄斑病变
acquired	后天性
diabetic	糖尿病的
Maffucci's syndrome	Maffucci 综合征
Map-dot-fingerprint dystrophy	地图状－点状－指纹状营养不良
Marcus Gunn syndrome	Marcus Gunn 综合征
Marfan's syndrome	Marfan 综合征
Megalocornea	大角膜
Meibomian gland	睑板腺
cyst (chalazion)	囊肿（霰粒肿）
dysfunction in blepharitis	睑缘炎功能障碍
Melanocytic naevus	黑色素细胞痣
Melanocytoma, optic nerve head	视盘黑色素细胞瘤
Melanoma	黑色素瘤
choroidal	脉络膜的
conjunctival	结膜的

iris	虹膜的
Melanosis, conjunctival	结膜黑色素沉着病
Meretoja's syndrome	Meretoja 综合征
Microcornea	小角膜
Miller's syndrome	Miller 综合征
Molluscum contagiosum	传染性软疣
Mooren's ulcer	角膜侵蚀性溃疡
Morning glory anomaly	牵牛花综合征
Multiple sclerosis	多发性硬化症
Munson sign	Munson 征
'Mutton fat' keratic precipitates	（羊脂状）角膜后沉着物
Myasthenia gravis	重症肌无力
Myelinated nerve fibres	有髓鞘神经纤维
Myopia correction	近视矫正
Myopic maculopathy	近视黄斑病变
Myotonic dystrophy, ptosis	肌强直性营养不良，上睑下垂

N

Naevus	痣
choroidal	脉络膜的
conjunctival	结膜的
melanocytic	黑色素细胞的
Nasolacrimal duct, congenital obstruction	先天性的鼻泪管阻塞
Nd:YAG iridotomy	Nd:YAG 虹膜切开术
Neonatal conjunctivitis	新生儿结膜炎
Neovascular glaucoma	新生血管性青光眼
Nerve palsies	神经麻痹
Neural tumours	神经肿瘤
Neurofibromatosis-1	多发性神经纤维瘤 -1 型
Nuclear sclerosis	核硬化
Nystagmus	眼球震颤症

O

Oculocutaneous albinism	眼皮肤白化病
Oculomotor nerve palsy	眼球运动神经麻痹
Optic atrophy	视神经萎缩
Optic disc	视盘

congenital anomalies	先天异常
normal	正常
Optic nerve glioma	视神经胶质瘤
Optic nerve head	视盘
drusen	玻璃疣
infarction	梗死
melanocytoma	黑色素细胞瘤
Optic nerve sheath meningioma	视神经鞘脑膜瘤
Optic neuritis	视神经炎
Orbital cellulitis	眼眶蜂窝织炎
Orbital floor fracture	眶底骨折
Orbital pseudotumour	眼眶假瘤
Orbital tumours	眼眶肿瘤
Orbital varices	眶静脉曲张
Osteogenesis imperfecta	成骨不全
Osteoma, choroidal	脉络膜骨瘤

P

Papillary conjunctivitis	假性滤泡性结膜炎
Papilloedema	视盘水肿
Parinaud's (dorsal midbrain) syndrome	Parinaud（中脑背侧）综合征
Pars plana vitrectomy	睫状体平坦部玻璃体切割术
Peau d'orange	橘皮状皮肤
Penetrating keratoplasty (corneal graft)	全层角膜移植术（角膜移植片）
Periphlebitis	静脉周围炎
Peters anomaly	Peter 异常
Phacomatoses	斑痣性错构瘤病
Photodynamic therapy	光动力疗法
Phthisis bulbi	眼球痨
Pigmentary glaucoma	色素性青光眼
Pigment dispersion syndrome	色素播散综合征
Pigment epithelial detachment (PED)	色素上皮脱离（PED）
Pilocarpine	匹罗卡品
Pit, optic disc	视盘陷凹
Plexiform neurofibroma	丛状神经纤维瘤
Pneumococcal keratitis	肺炎球菌性角膜炎
Polypoidal choroidal vasculopathy(PCV)	息肉状脉胳膜血管病变

Posterior lens capsular opacification	晶状体后囊膜浑浊
Premature infants, retinopathy	早产儿视网膜病变
Primary acquired melanosis	原发后天性黑色素沉着病
Primary congenital glaucoma	原发先天性青光眼
Proliferative vitreoretinopathy	增殖性玻璃体视网膜病变
Pseudoesotropia	假性内斜视
Pseudoexanthoma elasticum	弹性假黄瘤
Pseudoexfoliative glaucoma	假性剥脱性青光眼
Pseudogerontoxon	假性老年环
Pseudomonas keratitis	假单胞菌属角膜炎
Pseudopapilloedema	假性视盘水肿
Pseudoptosis	假性上睑下垂
Pseudotumour (idiopathic orbital inflammation)	假瘤（自发性眼眶炎症）
Pterygium	翼状胬肉
Ptosis	上睑下垂
Punctum	斑点
stenosis of	狭窄

R

Racial epithelial melanosis	种族性上皮细胞黑色素沉着症
Recurrent erosion syndrome	复发性剥脱综合征
Reis-Bücklers dystrophy	Reis-Bücklers 营养不良
Reiter's syndrome	Reiter 综合征
Retina	视网膜
acute necrosis	急性坏死
astrocytoma	星形细胞瘤
haemangioma	血管瘤
haemorrhages, see Haemorrhages,retina	出血，见视网膜出血
lattice degeneration	格子状变性
retinoblastoma	视网膜母细胞瘤
tear formation	撕裂形成
trauma	外伤
Retinal artery	视网膜动脉
macroaneurysm	大动脉瘤
occlusion	阻塞
Retinal detachment	视网膜脱离

exudative	渗出性的
rhegmatogenous	孔源性的
surgical complications	手术并发症
tractional	牵引性
Retinal vein occlusion	视网膜静脉闭塞
Retinitis	视网膜炎
cytomegalovirus	巨细胞病毒
Retinitis pigmentosa	色素性视网膜炎
Retinoblastoma	视网膜母细胞瘤
Retinopathy	视网膜病
central serous	中心浆液的
Retinopathy(*cont'd*)	视网膜病（伴有全身病）
diabetic	糖尿病的
hypertensive	高血压的
of prematurity	早产儿
sickle-cell	镰状红细胞
Rhabdomyosarcoma	横纹肌肉瘤
Rhegmatogenous retinal detachment	孔源性视网膜脱离
Rheumatoid arthritis	类风湿性关节炎
corneal ulceration	角膜溃疡
keratoconjunctivitis sicca	干燥性角结膜炎
scleromalacia perforans	坏死性巩膜炎
Rieger's syndrome	Rieger 综合征
Rodent ulcer	侵蚀性溃疡
Rosacea keratitis	酒渣鼻性角膜炎
Roth spots	Roth 斑
Rubeosis iridis	虹膜红变

S

Salzmann's nodular degeneration	Salzmann 结节性变性
Sarcoidosis	伯克肉样瘤
Schirmer's test	Schirmer 试验
Sclera, blue	蓝巩膜
Scleritis	巩膜炎
Scleromalacia perforans	坏死性巩膜炎
Seasonal allergic conjunctivitis	季节性变应性结膜炎
Sebaceous gland carcinoma	皮脂腺癌

Seborrhoeic keratosis	脂溢性角化病
Serpiginous choroidopathy	匍行性脉络膜病变
Siegrist streaks	Siegrist 斑
Silicone explant, retinal surgery	视网膜手术硅胶外植块
Sixth nerve palsy	第六脑神经麻痹
Sjögren's syndrome	Sjögren 综合征
Solar (actinic) keratosis	日光性（光化性）角化病
Spring catarrh	春季结膜炎
Squamous cell carcinoma	鳞状细胞癌
Squamous papilloma	鳞状细胞乳头状瘤
Squint see Strabismus, childhood	斜视，见儿童期斜视
Staphylococcal infections	葡萄球菌感染
blepharitis	睑缘炎
keratitis	角膜炎
Stargardt's disease	Stargardt 病
Stevens-Johnson syndrome	Stevens-Johnson 综合征
Strabismus, childhood	儿童期斜视
amblyopia	弱视
Brown's syndrome	Brown 综合征
Duane's syndrome	Duane 综合征
esotropia	内斜视
exotropia	外斜视
Strawberry naevus	草莓痣
Stromal necrotic keratitis	基质坏死性角膜炎
Sturge-Weber syndrome	Sturge-Weber 综合征
Stye	麦粒肿
Subcapsular cataract	囊下白内障
Subconjunctival haemorrhage	结膜下出血
Superior oblique palsy	上斜肌麻痹
Suppurative keratitis	化脓性角膜炎
Symblepharon	睑球粘连
Syphilis, congenital	先天性梅毒

T

Terrien's marginal degeneration	Terrien 边缘变性
Thiel-Behnke dystrophy	Thiel-Behnke 营养不良
Third nerve palsy	第三脑神经麻痹

Thyroid eye disease 甲状腺眼病
Toxocariasis 弓蛔虫病
Toxoplasmosis 弓形体病
Trabeculectomy 小梁切除术
Trachoma 沙眼
Tractional retinal detachment 牵引性视网膜脱离
Trauma 外伤
  blunt 钝性
  corneal abrasion 角膜上皮擦伤
  foreign body 异物
  orbital floor fracture 眶底骨折
  penetrating 穿透的
Trichiasis 倒睫
Tuberous sclerosis 结节性硬化
Tumours 肿瘤
  conjunctiva 结膜
  eyelid 眼睑
  optic nerve head 视盘
  orbit 眼眶
  retina see Retina 视网膜，见视网膜
  uvea 血管膜

U

Ultrasonography 超声波检查法
Uveal effusion 葡萄膜渗出液
Uveal tumours 葡萄膜肿瘤
Uveitis 葡萄膜炎
  anterior 前部的
  intermediate 中间的
  posterior 后部
    infectious 传染性的
    non-infectious 非传染性的

V

Varicella see Herpes zoster ophthalmicus 水痘，见眼（部）带状疱疹
Varices, orbital 眼眶静脉曲张
Vernal keratoconjunctivitis 春季角膜结膜炎

Viral wart, eyelid	眼睑病毒性疣
Vitamin and mineral supplements	维生素和矿物质补充剂
Vitrectomy	玻璃体切割术
Vitritis	玻璃体炎
Vitreous haemorrhage	玻璃体出血
Vitreous 'loss'	玻璃体丢失
Vogt striae	Vogt 纹
Von Hippel-Lindau syndrome	Von Hippel-Lindau 综合征
Vortex keratopathy	漩涡状角膜病

W

White dot syndromes	白色点状综合征
Wilms'tumour	Wilms 肿瘤
Wilson's disease	Wilson 病（肝豆核变性）
Wyburn-Mason syndrome	视网膜动静脉瘤